THE

Hyperthyroid Healing Diet

REVERSE Hyperthyroidism and
Graves' Disease and SAVE Your Thyroid
Through Diet and Lifestyle Changes

Eric M. Osansky, DC, MS, IFMCP

The Hyperthyroid Healing Diet: Reverse Hyperthyroidism and Graves' Disease and Save Your Thyroid Through Diet and Lifestyle Changes

By Eric M. Osansky, DC, MS, IFMCP

Copyright ©2024

Printed in the United States of America

Natural Endocrine Solutions
10020 Monroe Rd. Ste #170-280
Matthews, NC 28105

www.NaturalEndocrineSolutions.com
www.SaveMyThyroid.com

Book design: Adina Cucicov

ISBN: 978-1-66640-712-9

A Word of Caution to the Reader

This book is for educational purposes only and is not intended to diagnose or treat any disease. Please do not apply any of this information without first speaking with your doctor. The content in this book is not intended to be a substitute for professional medical advice, diagnosis, or treatment. Always seek the advice of your physician or another qualified healthcare provider with any questions you may have regarding your health condition. You should also speak with your physician or other healthcare professional before taking any medication or nutritional, herbal, or homeopathic supplements, or adopting any treatment for a health condition.

Dedication

I dedicate this book to people with hyperthyroidism who are looking to do everything possible to preserve the health of their thyroid gland and therefore avoid radioactive iodine and thyroid surgery.

Thyroid-Related Resources

I've included all of the references and many of the resources related to this book on the website listed below. For those wondering why I didn't include the actual resources in this book, over time, some of the resources I use and recommend will change, and it will be a lot easier to make changes to the resources listed on a website than it is to update this book.

To access the references and resources, visit
SaveMyThyroid.com/HHDNotes.

Want to work with my team and I?

If you have hyperthyroidism and want to do everything you can to save your thyroid, then there are a few factors that can prevent someone from restoring their health:

1. Overlooking the fundamentals
2. Lack of full commitment
3. Lack of accountability
4. Not working with a practitioner who has experience with hyperthyroidism

By reading this book you should have a good grasp of the foundations when it comes to using diet and lifestyle to restore your health, although you can also check out my Foundations of Overcoming Hyperthyroidism Online Course at **www.savemythyroid.com/foundations**. Of course only you can make the commitment to do what is necessary to save your thyroid, but if you want more guidance and accountability and would like to learn what it's like to work with my team and I visit **www.workwithdreric.com**.

A SPECIAL INVITATION
The Hyperthyroid Healing COMMUNITY

In 2021 I started my Hyperthyroid Healing Community, which currently consists of over twelve thousand members. I wanted to create an online community where everyone with hyperthyroidism who is looking to save their thyroid can connect with others, ask questions, support one another, discuss the content in my book and podcast, and swap recipes, etc.

You can immediately begin connecting with over twelve thousand like-minded people with hyperthyroidism. Simply visit **SaveMyThyroid.com/community** and request to join the Hyperthyroid Healing Community (Facebook group). It's free to join, and while you'll find many people who are beginning their hyperthyroid healing journey, you'll also find others who were diagnosed with hyperthyroidism months or years ago and will happily share advice, support, and guidance, which in turn can help save your thyroid. In addition to trying to welcome all new members into the group, I try to do live Q&As in the group at least once or twice each month to answer questions.

By the way, I realize not everyone is on Facebook, and for different reasons some people prefer not to be on Facebook, which I completely understand. I can't say that I love Facebook, but I've tried different groups, and the engagement just isn't the same.

Anyway, for those who are interested in joining, I look forward to seeing you in the group!

Best of health,
Dr. Eric

Table of Contents

Introduction

In late 2007 I stepped on the scale and was about seventeen pounds heavier than my ideal weight. I decided to clean up my diet, and while I was already exercising regularly at the time, I started doing so more intensely. It seemed to be working, as I was losing weight at a pretty good pace, and it wasn't too long before I achieved my goal.

I continued to eat well and exercise intensely, and I kept on losing weight. I didn't suspect anything was wrong until one day I visited a Sam's Club and took my blood pressure at one of those automated blood pressure machines. My blood pressure was fine, but my resting heart rate was elevated at 90 BPM. Over the next few days I measured my pulse multiple times per day and saw that it was anywhere from 90 to 110 BPM.

I decided to visit a family physician, and this is when I was diagnosed with hyperthyroidism. This took place in the spring of 2008, and I eventually saw an endocrinologist, which is when I was diagnosed with Graves' disease. Although I started expanding my diet after being diagnosed with hyperthyroidism, I ended up losing a total of forty-two pounds. And while I knew I was going to take a natural treatment approach, there was some concern that I would lose even more weight if I went back on a restrictive diet.

Not Everyone with Hyperthyroidism Loses Weight

Although I definitely plan on addressing weight loss concerns in this book, after I started working with people who had hyperthyroidism, I realized that not everyone with this condition loses weight. Although weight loss is definitely more common, some people do gain weight. Of course this is to be expected if someone takes antithyroid medication such as methimazole or PTU, but I noticed this also happened to some people who weren't taking antithyroid medication.

Without question this book involves more than helping people gain or lose weight, as my ultimate goal is to help people with different types of hyperthyroid conditions (Graves' disease, toxic multinodular goiter, subclinical hyperthyroidism, etc.) save their thyroid and regain their health. In fact, although I have been helping people with hyperthyroidism regain their health since 2009 and created my first thyroid-related website (**www.naturalendocrinesolutions.com**) in 2010, along with my first book *Natural Treatment Solutions for Hyperthyroidism and Graves' Disease* in 2011 (which was revised in 2013 and again in 2023), it wasn't until 2021 until I launched the *Save My Thyroid* podcast (found at **www. savemythyroid.com**), which focuses on helping people with hyperthyroidism avoid radioactive iodine and thyroid surgery and restore their health.

The Role Diet Played in My Recovery

Before discussing the diet I followed when I dealt with Graves' disease, I want to let you know that my diet was quite horrible growing up. I ate plenty of refined foods and sugars, drank a lot of soda and fruit punch (Hawaiian Punch, anyone?), didn't eat any vegetables, etc. It wasn't until after I graduated from chiropractic school back in 1999 that I started cleaning up my diet, and even then I was far from perfect, as while I ate more whole foods and started eating vegetables (although not a lot), I also ate foods such as soy-based chicken nuggets, pizza, and whole wheat bread.

So when I was diagnosed with hyperthyroidism and eventually Graves' disease, while I knew that I would be taking a natural approach, I also knew it wouldn't be easy to change my eating habits. Even though I arguably ate healthier than the average person, I still ate too much pizza and other unhealthy foods. I bring this up because while I realize that some people have no problem eating healthily, for me it was a struggle. So if you hear me talk about how I currently add five to seven servings of vegetables to my daily smoothie, just keep in mind that this wasn't an overnight transition.

As for what I ate when I was dealing with Graves' disease, I was essentially following a Paleo Diet initially. I'll discuss the Paleo Diet (and some other diets) in this book, so I won't go into detail here, but it consists of eating whole, healthy foods while avoiding refined foods and sugars, unhealthy oils, grains, and legumes. This diet was a struggle for me, especially since I wasn't a big fan of eating eggs at the time.

But I did enjoy eating nuts and seeds as a snack, and I continued to do so until I hit a roadblock in my recovery. At the time I wasn't sure if it was related to the nuts and seeds, but I decided to give them up for a few months, and my recovery went more smoothly from that point on. Perhaps it was a coincidence and not related to the nuts and seeds, although I'll say that over the years I've seen similar things from some of my patients who started with a Paleo Diet but then took a break from eating nuts and seeds. This doesn't mean that everyone who continues to eat nuts and seeds won't be able to regain their health, but it's just something to keep in mind.

There Is No Single Diet That Fits Everyone Perfectly

Even though this book is entitled *The Hyperthyroid Healing Diet*, the truth is that there isn't a single diet that is suitable for everyone with hyperthyroidism. So just because I ate a certain way, it doesn't mean that everyone I work with needs to eat the exact same way. The truth is that everyone is different, and while the three diets I discuss in this book serve as starting points, just as was the case in my situation, modifications may need to be made along the way. Due to that, I probably should have named the book *The Hyperthyroid Healing Diets*!

It's also important to mention that I did other things to improve my health. For example, I did adrenal saliva testing, which revealed that I had compromised adrenals. So I also incorporated stress-management techniques as well as took certain supplements to restore my adrenal health. Because improving adrenal health is so important, I have dedicated a separate chapter to stress management in section 4, along with other chapters that will show you how to find and address other potential triggers and underlying imbalances.

Making the Transition from Chiropractor to Functional Medicine Practitioner

Before I was diagnosed with hyperthyroidism, I had already sold my chiropractic practice. There were a few reasons I decided to do this after being in practice for seven and a half years. One was just the stress I was dealing with at the time, which I'm sure was a factor in the development of my Graves' disease condition. Another reason was a chronic wrist injury that affected my ability to perform spinal adjustments at times. Even though I relied heavily on an instrument that is used in chiropractic to adjust patients, it still impacted my wrist injury.

After being diagnosed with Graves' disease and getting into remission by taking a natural treatment approach, I realized that this was my calling. Now, to be honest, I probably didn't realize that it was truly my calling until ten years later, when I was still passionate about what I was doing. Anyway, I mentioned earlier how I created my main website (**www.naturalendocrinesolutions.com**) in 2010, wrote my first book, *Natural Treatment Solutions for Hyperthyroidism and Graves' Disease*, in 2011, released a revised and updated edition of this book in 2013, and updated it again in 2023.

Even though I had plenty of people with hyperthyroidism to work with, for years, I was also trying to help people with hypothyroidism/Hashimoto's, and in 2018 I wrote a book called *Hashimoto's Triggers*. Although I'm still very proud of that book, shortly after the book was released, I finally realized that I should be focusing more on helping people with hyperthyroidism. There were a few reasons for this, but the main reason is that while there are many natural healthcare practitioners who have a lot of experience with people who have Hashimoto's, only a small number have a great deal of experience working with people who have hyperthyroidism.

In fact, when I launched my podcast in 2021, the goal was to have it exclusively focus on hyperthyroidism. You'll notice that the first ten episodes focus on hyperthyroidism. But since people with Hashimoto's thyroiditis also need to save their thyroid (from the damage caused by the immune system), I decided to have episodes that benefited both people with hyperthyroidism and Hashimoto's, but with an emphasis on hyperthyroidism. If you visit the *Save My Thyroid* podcast, you'll notice that while many of the episodes will benefit those with both hyperthyroidism and Hashimoto's, there are also a good number of episodes that focus solely on hyperthyroidism.

Eating Well Is Just a Piece of the Puzzle

While eating healthy is very important, diet alone usually isn't enough to restore one's health. This was the case with me, and it's also true with most of my patients. Most people also need to improve their stress-handling skills, do things to reduce their toxic load, and correct nutrient deficiencies. Some people also have underlying (or overt) infections they need to address, etc. And so while this book will of course focus on diet, sections 3 and 4 will cover other topics necessary to optimize your health.

Will This Book Benefit Those Who Don't Have Graves' Disease?

As you know, I personally dealt with Graves' disease, and most of my hyperthyroid patients also have Graves' disease. However, I've also worked with a lot of patients who have toxic multinodular goiter. While there definitely is overlap with the dietary recommendations, there are some differences as well, which I'll discuss in this book.

Three other hyperthyroid conditions include *subacute thyroiditis, subclinical hyperthyroidism,* and *Hashitoxicosis.* I don't see too many patients with subacute thyroiditis, mainly because this usually self-resolves over time. However, this doesn't mean that you shouldn't take this seriously, as I've seen people with this condition relapse. Viruses are the most common cause of subacute thyroiditis, so just as is the case with Graves' disease, you definitely need to do things to optimize your immune system health.

Hashitoxicosis is essentially Hashimoto's thyroiditis with transient hyperthyroidism. Like Graves' disease, Hashimoto's thyroiditis is an autoimmune condition that affects the thyroid gland. And while the symptom management aspect is different from Graves' disease, there are a lot of similarities with the diet. When I discuss the Level 3 Hyperthyroid Healing Diet in chapter 5, keep in mind that this diet is also suitable for those with Hashimoto's thyroiditis. And I should mention that it's quite common to have the antibodies for both Graves' disease and Hashimoto's.

Subclinical hyperthyroidism can be a little tricky at times. Some people have subclinical Graves' disease, where thyroid-stimulating hormone (TSH) is depressed and the person has elevated thyroid antibodies (i.e., thyroid-stimulating immunoglobulins), but the thyroid hormones are within the lab reference range, and many times within the optimal range. If someone has Graves' disease, then they definitely can benefit from the advice given in this book. If someone has subclinical hyperthyroidism that is non-autoimmune in nature, they can also benefit from reading this book. Just keep in mind that there isn't a specific diet for those with subclinical hyperthyroidism, although they usually respond well to a Level 2 Hyperthyroid Healing Diet (discussed in chapter 6).

Will This Book Benefit Vegans and Vegetarians?

While I can't say that I recommend a vegetarian/vegan diet to most of my patients, this doesn't mean that you can't receive good results if this describes you. Some natural healthcare practitioners try to talk their vegetarian patients into eating meat, and while you don't have to worry about me doing that, after reading this book, you might decide to incorporate meat and/or fish into your diet to ensure you get sufficient protein. On the other hand, you might choose not to do this, and instead might decide to follow a Level 1 Hyperthyroid Healing Diet, which I discuss in chapter 7.

Regardless of whether you eat meat or are a vegan, vegetarian, or pescatarian, you of course want to eat whole, healthy foods while avoiding refined foods and sugars. You also want to avoid unhealthy oils, artificial ingredients, and genetically modified foods. And you want to make sure you address any nutrient deficiencies, which are more common in those who follow a strict vegetarian or vegan diet.

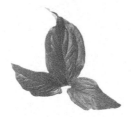

Hyperthyroid Healing
Diet Basics

Where Are You in Your Hyperthyroid Healing Journey?

S ince I started consulting with people who have hyperthyroidism in 2009, I've worked with people at different points in their hyperthyroid healing journey. Some have been just recently diagnosed with hyperthyroidism and haven't made any dietary or lifestyle changes, and others were diagnosed with hyperthyroidism months or years ago and have already made some wonderful changes to their diet. In fact, it's very common for people to tell me that they made these changes by listening to my podcast or reading some of my blog posts, although there are, of course, many other diet-related resources out there.

In fact, there are four common scenarios I encounter in my practice with regard to my hyperthyroid patients:

Scenario #1: They haven't made any changes to their diet. This is common when someone has been recently diagnosed with hyperthyroidism, but many people don't make any changes months or years after being diagnosed. In fact, one can argue that *most* people with hyperthyroidism don't do anything to improve their diet, and this no doubt would have described me if I hadn't become a natural healthcare practitioner. While you have an open mind since you are reading this book, most people simply follow the advice of their endocrinologist, and most of these specialists don't encourage their hyperthyroid patients to make diet and lifestyle changes.

Scenario #2: They have made some changes to their diet. An example of this would be someone who has cut out gluten, but they are still eating some other foods that can cause inflammation and/or have a negative impact on their gut health. Another example involves someone who has started eating more whole foods, including vegetables. Regardless of where you are in your hyperthyroid healing journey, even small changes to your diet deserve celebration. In the introduction I mentioned how I didn't eat any vegetables while growing up, and I ate plenty of gluten, so I understand it's not easy for everyone to make these changes.

Scenario #3: They have made some extreme changes to their diet for one to two months. A lot of people I've worked with have followed a strict diet for one or two months. For example, someone with Graves' disease might have read about the autoimmune Paleo (AIP) diet and decided to follow it for a month or two, but then stopped, either because they found it to be too restrictive, didn't notice enough positive changes in their health, and/or didn't know how long they should follow the diet.

Scenario #4: They have made some extreme changes to their diet for three months or longer. This is similar to scenario #4, with the main difference being that the person has followed a strict diet (i.e., AIP) for a longer period of time. I've had patients follow such a diet for six months or longer before they started working with me. Some were still following the strict diet at the start of their health journey with me, while others had followed a strict diet in the past but eventually stopped because they weren't seeing the desired results.

Do You Need to Follow a Restrictive Diet?

I think it's safe to say that nobody enjoys following a restrictive diet. I certainly didn't like to eliminate certain foods when I was dealing with Graves' disease . . . especially pizza! Okay, I realize that pizza is an extreme example, as everyone knows that pizza isn't a healthy food (yes, even when it's organic and gluten-free). But what's the deal with diets that eliminate foods that have some good health benefits, such as eggs, nuts, seeds, and legumes?

As I mentioned in the introduction, there is no single diet that fits everyone perfectly . . . including those with hyperthyroidism. So while I think the AIP Diet can be beneficial in many cases, it's crazy to think that this is the perfect diet for everyone with Graves' disease and other autoimmune conditions. Similarly, it would be foolish to conclude that there is a specific diet that everyone with toxic multinodular goiter should follow, or those with subclinical hyperthyroidism.

That being said, you need to start somewhere, and if you are to be successful in regaining your health, at the very least you need to eat an anti-inflammatory diet consisting of whole, healthy foods. As you know, there are hundreds, if not thousands, of diet books out there, and many of them recommend whole, healthy foods. The problem is that there is a difference in opinion as to what is considered to be healthy and which foods may cause inflammation.

For example, many sources recommend eating eggs since they are nutrient dense, while others recommend avoiding eggs since they are a common allergen and there are compounds in the egg whites that can be problematic for some people. Similarly, it's common for certain "health experts" to recommend avoiding grains and/or legumes, yet these are staples of a Mediterranean Diet, which is one of the most well-known diets. In this book I will not only discuss the different foods so you can better understand which ones you should eat and which ones you should avoid while trying to heal, but I will also give multiple Hyperthyroid Healing Diet options to choose from, while at the same time trying to guide you toward the one that's the best fit for you.

Have You Made Any Changes to Your Diet?

Although many people with hyperthyroidism ate horribly prior to their diagnosis, this isn't the case with everyone. In fact, some people are shocked upon being diagnosed with hyperthyroidism, as they feel they have been eating a healthy diet and living a healthy lifestyle overall. Sometimes this is true, but many times one's diet isn't as healthy as they think it is. And while there is no question that some foods are more problematic than others, the truth is that it's possible for our bodies to react to foods one wouldn't suspect to cause problems. I talk more about this in chapter 11.

If you ate poorly like I did for many years, then it might not be a surprise that you developed hyperthyroidism. Of course, I was still surprised when I was diagnosed since I was eating much better than I was when I was a teenager and young adult, although I'm sure taking antibiotics many times throughout the years when I was younger didn't help. While you can't turn back time, the good news is that you can make changes now that not only will help you to reverse your hyperthyroidism, but also can prevent you from developing other health issues in the future.

If you were eating healthily throughout the years, then your hyperthyroidism diagnosis probably was a bigger shock to you. Once again, perhaps there were foods you thought were healthy but actually weren't, or perhaps they were healthy but for some reason they just weren't a good fit for your body. Another thing to keep in mind is that eating well is just a piece of the puzzle, which I mentioned in the introduction. While it's essential to eat a healthy, anti-inflammatory diet to regain your health, many times there are other factors, which I'll discuss in sections 3 and 4. So while you still might need to make some small changes to your diet, you also might need to do other things to regain your health.

What Type of Hyperthyroidism Do You Have?

Although most people with hyperthyroidism have Graves' disease, there are also non-autoimmune hyperthyroid conditions. And while everyone needs to eat a healthy diet regardless of what type of hyperthyroid condition they have, there are some differences depending on the type of hyperthyroidism. I will talk more about this when discussing the different types of Hyperthyroid Healing Diets.

Here are the main different types of hyperthyroidism:

- Graves' disease
- Toxic multinodular goiter
- Subacute thyroiditis
- Hashitoxicosis
- Subclinical hyperthyroidism
- Iodine-induced hyperthyroidism

Just about all of these hyperthyroid conditions can benefit from the information given in this book. However, sometimes iodine-induced hyperthyroidism can be tricky. If this leads to Graves' disease, then usually there are other factors responsible for the autoimmune component that need to be addressed. On the other hand, if someone's hyperthyroidism was caused by excess iodine and their condition isn't autoimmune in nature, sometimes simply following a low-iodine diet for awhile may be the answer. It really does depend on the situation.

Wait . . . Is Iodine Bad in Those with Hyperthyroidism?

I'm sure some reading this have questions about iodine, and I will discuss iodine more in section 2. I'll say here that I'm not anti-iodine, and I actually have had a good experience with iodine in the past. However, iodine can be a big problem for some people. I mentioned iodine-induced hyperthyroidism before, and admittedly this is more of a problem when taking medications high in iodine (i.e., Amiodarone), iodine supplements, and even iodine contrast agents. But in some people, foods very high in iodine, such as sea vegetables, can also be a problem, which I will discuss in section 2.

Can Diet Be Used to Manage Your Hyperthyroid Symptoms?

Many people with hyperthyroidism consult with an endocrinologist, and the three treatment options given are almost always the following: (1) antithyroid medication, (2) radioactive iodine, and (3) thyroid surgery. I think it's safe to say that most people reading this book are looking to avoid options 2 and 3. And while many are open to taking antithyroid medication such as methimazole, some people want to do everything they can to avoid taking medication. If this describes you, then you might be wondering if cleaning up your diet will help to manage the symptoms.

Before I go any further, you might wonder why I'm talking about symptom management, as the goal of this book is to help you regain your health, not just manage your symptoms. While this is true, you want to be safe while trying to restore your health. And while eating an anti-inflammatory diet is necessary to help you regain your health, the truth is that eating well alone usually isn't enough to manage your symptoms. Of course there are exceptions, as someone might make some dietary changes and see a quick and dramatic decrease in their thyroid hormones. But this isn't too common.

The goal of this book isn't to discuss symptom management, as I do this in my book *Natural Treatment Solutions for Hyperthyroidism and Graves' Disease.* I will say that when my hyperthyroid patients choose not to take antithyroid medication (or are unable to due to side effects), then I will recommend natural agents to help with this *in addition* to following a hyperthyroid healing diet. I never tell anyone to stop taking their medication, and keep in mind that everything comes down to risks versus benefits. Some people do need to take antithyroid medication, preferably while addressing the underlying cause. But either way, eating well is an essential piece of the hyperthyroid healing puzzle.

5 Steps to Set You Up for Success from This Point On

My goal isn't to have you read this book only to make a few dietary changes and then quit. I want you to do everything you can to get the most out of this information. If you follow these five steps, it will increase your chances of being successful:

Step #1: Choose a single diet to follow. I'll discuss the different Hyperthyroid Healing Diet options in section 2, and while I don't want you to think that you need to follow a Hyperthyroid Healing Diet permanently, I do think it's important to choose one and then stick with it for awhile. This might sound like common sense, but some people struggle with this, as a person might want to follow the most restrictive diet, but they know they will be more compliant with a different diet. In this situation I'd say it's probably best not to choose the most restrictive diet, although you can transition to a different diet in the future.

Step #2: Make changes at your own pace. After choosing a single diet to follow, don't feel like you need to make all of the necessary changes immediately. Some people might go cold turkey and give up all the foods they love right away, while for others it will be a more gradual process. I'd rather you make small changes (i.e., add a new vegetable each week) if it means not getting stressed out and overwhelmed trying to incorporate all of the changes at once. Don't get me wrong, as I don't want you to take too long to make the transition to a healthier diet, and I'm sure you want to regain your health sooner rather than later. But just remember that everyone is different, so you never want to compare yourself to someone else who might have made changes to their diet quicker than you.

Step #3: Have specific goals in mind. Everyone reading this book has the goal of reversing their hyperthyroidism and regaining their health. But to accomplish this, it's wise to break it down into smaller goals. For example, goal #1 might be to choose a single diet and follow it for at least three months. You can even break down each goal into further goals. Here's an example:

1. Write down your goal. For example, if you choose the Level 2 Hyperthyroid Healing Diet (discussed in chapter 6), then write down, "I will follow the Level 2 Hyperthyroid Healing Diet."
2. Decide when you will start. I recommend choosing a specific date. For example, write down, "I am going to start my Level 2 Hyperthyroid Healing Diet on Monday, January 27th."
3. Decide when you will achieve the goal. For example, if your goal is to follow the diet for three months, the achievement date would be April 27th, and you also should write this down: "I am going to start my Level 2 Hyperthyroid Healing Diet on Monday, January 27th, and follow it until at least April 27th."
4. Identify any potential obstacles. Examples of obstacles that might cause you to stray from the diet and prevent you from reaching your goals would be birthdays, anniversaries, parties, etc. Being aware of and preparing for these potential obstacles is perhaps the best way to prevent them from becoming obstacles in the first place.

Step #4: Join a support group. I wouldn't say that this step is essential to succeed, but it's nice to not have to go through this alone. I'd love for you to join my free hyperthyroid healing community at savemythyroid.com/community, which is a group specifically for those with hyperthyroidism, but even if you choose to join another group, that's perfectly fine. You might even find an accountability partner, although this definitely is optional.

Step #5: Read this entire book. The truth is that many people who invest in this book will only read a few chapters and won't take action. This actually is true with most books, and I've been guilty of doing this many times as well. But I don't want *you* to do that. In fact, I want you to think of this book as a $5,000 investment. This might sound crazy to you, but the information in this book can truly be life-changing.

I'd like to end this first chapter by thanking you for investing in this book and taking responsibility for your health. Although I mentioned in the introduction how diet alone usually isn't enough to restore one's health, there is no question that it is an important part of your hyperthyroid healing journey. I do go beyond food in this book, so in the upcoming chapters you will learn other things that are essential to helping you save your thyroid and regain your health.

To access the book references and resources, visit
SaveMyThyroid.com/HHDNotes.

How Is Diet Related to Hyperthyroidism?

If you are working with an endocrinologist and ask them about diet and hyperthyroidism, there is an excellent chance they will tell you that improving your diet won't have any positive effects on this condition. This is true whether someone has Graves' disease, toxic multinodular goiter, or a different hyperthyroid condition. Obviously this isn't true, or else I wouldn't have taken the time to write this book.

And this isn't just my opinion, which is why just about all natural healthcare practitioners recommend dietary changes for those with virtually any chronic health condition. Regarding autoimmune conditions such as Graves' disease, there is plenty of research showing that food can positively affect the immune system. As for other hyperthyroid conditions such as toxic multinodular goiter, there isn't any research I'm aware of showing that eating a healthy diet can be beneficial, but this doesn't mean that diet doesn't play a role, and I'll explain how. In the next few sections, I will discuss how diet can help with the different types of hyperthyroidism, starting with Graves' disease.

How Eating Well Can Help With Graves' Disease

As you probably know, Graves' disease is an autoimmune condition that affects the thyroid gland. And with all autoimmune conditions there is something called the *triad of autoimmunity*, which is also known as the three-legged stool of autoimmunity. Here are the three components of this triad:

- Component #1: a genetic predisposition
- Component #2: exposure to one or more environmental triggers
- Component #3: an increase in intestinal permeability (leaky gut)

I'd like to go ahead and take a deeper look at each of these components:

Component #1: Genetic Predisposition

Obviously you can't do anything to change your genetics, although it is possible to change the expression of genes through diet and lifestyle. The good news is that addressing components #2 and #3 can help to put a person with Graves' disease into a state of remission . . . hopefully permanently. I've been in remission since 2009, and while I feel like I've been cured, there is always a risk of relapsing, especially if one doesn't do a good job of maintaining their health thereafter. But even if I were to relapse today, I would have no regrets, as I would do whatever it takes to save my thyroid.

Component #2: Exposure to One or More Environmental Triggers

There are four main categories of triggers I commonly discuss:

1. **Food.** Common allergens such as gluten, dairy, corn, and even too much refined salt can be triggers. I'll discuss this in greater detail in future chapters, but this is one way the food you eat can be a factor in the development of Graves' disease.

2. **Stress.** Everyone deals with stress, but chronic stress is a concern. I'll discuss this more in chapter 20.

3. **Environmental toxicants.** Heavy metals, xenoestrogens, and even myco-toxins from mold can be factors in the development of Graves' disease. In chapter 24 I'll show you what you can do to reduce your toxic load.

4. **Infections.** Viruses such as Epstein-Barr, bacteria such as *H. pylori* and *Yersinia enterocolitica*, and even parasites can all be triggers. One also needs to consider Lyme disease and some of its co-infections. In 2018 (ten years after my Graves' disease diagnosis) I was diagnosed with chronic Lyme disease and bartonella, and while I definitely experienced symptoms at the time (mostly neurological), thankfully I have been able to keep it under control since then.

Component #3: An Increase in Intestinal Permeability

An increase in intestinal permeability is the medical term for a "leaky gut," which is when someone has a compromised intestinal barrier, which in turn allows larger food proteins, microbes, and toxicants to enter the bloodstream, resulting in an immune response. Certain foods can play a role in this increase in intestinal permeability, especially those containing gluten, and potentially certain foods higher in lectins and other compounds. I'll discuss this in greater detail throughout this book, but this is yet another example of how food can play a role in the development of Graves' disease (and other autoimmune conditions). It's also worth mentioning that other factors can cause a leaky gut, including certain gut infections, as well as candida overgrowth or SIBO (small intestinal bacterial overgrowth).

Other Factors

In addition to these three components, there can be other contributing factors. For example, while I don't look at nutrient deficiencies as a trigger, they definitely can make someone more susceptible to developing an autoimmune condition such as Graves' disease. While all of the nutrients are, of course, very important, some of the more important ones relating to Graves' disease include selenium, zinc, vitamin D, and omega-3 fatty acids. And of course all of these can be obtained through the diet, although the main source of vitamin D (which is actually more of a prohormone) is the sun.

Although the goal of this book isn't to get into great detail when it comes to all of the different triggers of Graves' disease, I definitely will discuss food triggers in greater detail in chapter 11. I probably should mention that all of this also applies to other autoimmune conditions, including Hashimoto's thyroiditis. If someone has hyperthyroidism caused by Hashitoxicosis or has the antibodies for both Graves' disease and Hashimoto's, then they would also want to do things to find and remove triggers as well as heal the gut.

How Eating Well Can Help with Toxic Multinodular Goiter

Up until this point I've focused on Graves' disease, but two of the main causes of having toxic multinodular goiter include insulin resistance and problems with estrogen metabolism.[1,2] Food is a factor in both of these conditions. Regarding insulin resistance, I'm sure many people reading this know that eating an unhealthy diet consisting of refined sugars and large amounts of carbohydrates can cause blood sugar imbalances, leading to an insulin-resistant state. While eating well is essential to reverse insulin resistance, sometimes nutritional supplements can be helpful (i.e., chromium, berberine), and oftentimes there is an inflammatory component that needs to be addressed. I discuss blood sugar imbalances, including insulin resistance, in chapter 14.

As for estrogen metabolism, this can also be positively influenced by certain foods, including cruciferous vegetables (broccoli, broccoli sprouts, cauliflower, Brussels sprouts, etc.). In addition, eating an unhealthy diet can have a negative effect on the gut microbiome, and this in turn can have a negative effect on estrogen metabolism. In fact, some comprehensive stool panels test for an enzyme called *beta glucuronidase*, an enzyme that deconjugates estrogens into their active forms.[3] When this process is impaired through dysbiosis of the gut microbiota, the decrease in deconjugation results in a reduction of circulating estrogens.[3]

In other words, imbalances of the gut microbiota can negatively affect the excretion of estrogen from the body, resulting in an estrogen-dominant state. This in turn can cause a lot of health issues, but it also can play a role in the formation of thyroid nodules.[4] In chapter 6 I'll give some specific dietary recommendations for toxic multinodular goiter.

How Eating Well Can Help with Subacute Thyroiditis

Most cases of subacute thyroiditis are viral induced, and while it usually self-resolves, there is always a chance one can relapse in the future. One way to prevent this from happening, and perhaps to speed up your recovery if you're currently dealing with subacute thyroiditis, is to do things to optimize the health of your immune system. One way of doing this is by eating a healthy diet consisting of whole, healthy foods. Of course other factors are important as well, including incorporating stress management, getting sufficient sleep, and doing things to reduce your toxic load.

How Eating Well Can Help with Subclinical Hyperthyroidism

In the literature there is no evidence I'm aware of that shows that eating a healthy diet can help with subclinical hyperthyroidism. But you probably realize by now that eating a healthy diet is important for just about any chronic health condition. If someone has subclinical Graves' disease (depressed TSH [thyroid-stimulating hormone], elevated TSI [thyroid-stimulating immunoglobulin], normal thyroid hormones) then remember that this is an autoimmune condition, and as I explained earlier, eating well definitely is important for any autoimmune condition.

If you have a non-autoimmune case of subclinical hyperthyroidism, I can't say that there is a specific diet that will reverse your condition. What I can say is that I've had success with patients who had subclinical hyperthyroidism by having them follow one of the Hyperthyroid Healing Diets I recommend in this book (usually a Level 2 Hyperthyroid Healing Diet). This doesn't mean that diet will help 100 percent of people with this condition, but this is true of all health conditions, and I'll actually talk more about this shortly.

How Diet Impacts the Mitochondria

You might already know that the mitochondria are the energy powerhouses of the cells. Most of the cells in your body include mitochondria, and healthy mitochondria are necessary for optimal health. It's important to understand that mitochondria are nutrient dependent. In addition, hyperthyroidism involves a lot of oxidative stress, which can have negative effects on the mitochondria, and eating a healthy, anti-inflammatory diet can help reduce this oxidative stress.

Some of the nutrients that can protect against oxidative stress include omega-3 fatty acids, antioxidants (vitamin C and zinc), members of the vitamin B family (vitamin B_{12} and folate), and magnesium.[5] In addition to vitamin C and zinc, other antioxidants include vitamin E, beta-carotene, lutein, alpha-lipoic acid, coenzyme Q10, lycopene, zeaxanthin, and selenium. You, of course, want to do as much as you can through food (which is what this book is all about), although there is also a time and place for supplementation.

Can Diet Alone Reverse Hyperthyroidism?

You should know the answer to this now, as there are people who have reversed their hyperthyroidism with diet alone. That being said, diet is usually just a piece of the puzzle, although it is an important piece of the puzzle, and it's a great place to start. And the good news is that most people can do things to improve their diet, although I realize it's not always easy to do this.

As you know, everyone is different, and I've seen people give up gluten alone and receive amazing results in both the way they feel and their tests. I've also had patients follow a strict elimination diet for a few months and not feel any better and/or see improvements in their follow-up tests. This doesn't mean that the diet isn't helping. Eating a whole food, anti-inflammatory diet is essential for anyone with hyperthyroidism, but there very well may be other triggers and/or underlying imbalances that also need to be addressed.

So I want you to think of food as part of your hyperthyroid healing journey, and not the complete cure for your hyperthyroid condition. I think you'll agree that it won't cause you any harm to eat well, and no matter how you feel, improving your diet will have a dramatic effect on your health, both in the short term and long term. On the other hand, if you consistently eat inflammatory foods, including refined foods and sugars, fast food, etc., then there is an excellent chance that you won't regain your health.

Don't Listen to Your Endocrinologist

In the opening paragraph of this chapter, I mentioned how most endocrinologists will tell you that improving your diet won't have any positive effects on your hyperthyroidism. Hopefully after reading this chapter you understand that not only can eating well be beneficial, but it is an essential component if you want to heal. And I think you'd agree that nobody with hyperthyroidism has a deficiency of methimazole or PTU, and most don't have an absolute need to get their thyroid gland removed or ablated.

On the other hand, most people are deficient in nutrients and have inflammation, compromised adrenals, a leaky gut, and too high of a toxic load. There is no way that you can address these imbalances and not improve your health. And while diet alone might not accomplish this (which is why this book goes beyond diet), it's crazy for endocrinologists to say, "Improving one's diet won't help, so let's go ahead and remove your thyroid."

Now when I say don't listen to your endocrinologist, I'm not saying to refuse to take medication. Although I took the herbs bugleweed and motherwort to manage my symptoms, there is a time and place for antithyroid medication. There is even a time and place for thyroid surgery. But I'm confident that if you follow the advice given in this book, you will be on the path to regaining your health. When you do regain your health, I want you to visit your endocrinologist and let him or her know how much of an impact diet and lifestyle had on your health.

Hopefully you now understand how diet can play a role in the development of your hyperthyroid condition. This is the case whether you have Graves' disease, toxic multinodular goiter, subacute thyroiditis, or even subclinical hyperthyroidism. And if your endocrinologist tells you that diet isn't a factor, just remember that medical school doesn't train them to address the actual cause of thyroid and autoimmune thyroid conditions.

Chapter 2 Highlights

- With all autoimmune conditions, including Graves' disease, there is a triad of autoimmunity.
- The three components of the triad of autoimmunity include (1) a genetic predisposition, (2) exposure to one or more environmental triggers, and (3) an increase in intestinal permeability.
- The four main categories of triggers include (1) food, (2) stress, (3) environmental toxicants, and (4) infections.
- Certain foods can cause a leaky gut, including gluten and certain foods higher in lectins and other compounds.
- Eating well can help with Graves' disease, toxic multinodular goiter, subacute thyroiditis, and subclinical hyperthyroidism.
- Hyperthyroidism involves a lot of oxidative stress, and eating a healthy, anti-inflammatory diet can help reduce oxidative stress.
- When it comes to restoring your health, diet is usually just a piece of the puzzle.
- Most endocrinologists will tell you that improving your diet won't have any positive effects on your hyperthyroidism.

To access the book references and resources, visit
SaveMyThyroid.com/HHDNotes.

CHAPTER

3

4 Main Food Allergens to Avoid

While I recommend choosing one of the Hyperthyroid Healing Diets I'll be discussing in section 2, at the very least I suggest avoiding the main allergens mentioned in this chapter. In fact, even after restoring your health, I think it's a good idea to minimize your exposure to them . . . especially the first three allergens I'll be focusing on. Just keep in mind that there is a reason why I also recommend avoiding other foods during the healing process, but I'll be discussing these others in different chapters.

The four allergens I'll be focusing on in this chapter include gluten, dairy, corn, and soy. These days, many people are aware of the concerns with gluten, so assuming you're not already gluten-free it might not be too difficult to convince you to take a break from it. Dairy can be more challenging for some to give up, especially with people being concerned about where they'll get their calcium, which will be covered in this chapter.

Corn is another allergen people might find challenging to give up, especially if they're not primarily eating whole, healthy foods. The reason for this is that corn is found in a lot of products, especially those that are gluten-free. Soy is one of the more controversial allergens, and the reason for this is that there are actually some good health benefits from eating organic fermented soy. But unfortunately this isn't the type of soy most people eat, and there definitely are some concerns with soy in general while trying to restore your health.

Allergen 1: Gluten

Before discussing why it's wise to avoid gluten, I'd like to explain what gluten is. Gluten is a mixture of prolamin proteins present mostly in wheat, but also in barley and rye. Gliadin is the most problematic protein found in gluten, specifically wheat, with glutenin being another protein found in wheat that is responsible for the elastic properties of dough. There are other proteins as well, including hordeins (found in barley), secalins (found in rye), and avenins (found in oats). Speaking of oats, even though they are technically gluten-free, oats are commonly cross-contaminated with gluten.

Five Reasons to Avoid Gluten While Trying to Reverse Your Hyperthyroidism

Now that you have a basic understanding of what gluten is, let's discuss some of the main reasons why people with hyperthyroidism should completely avoid gluten while trying to restore their health.

Reason #1: Many people are sensitive to gluten. When I say *sensitive*, I don't just mean having celiac disease, which is an autoimmune condition involving gluten. Many people have a non-celiac gluten sensitivity, also known as non-autoimmune gluten sensitivity, which is defined as a condition in which symptoms are triggered by gluten ingestion in the absence of celiac-specific antibodies and classical celiac villous atrophy.[1] As for why many people have food sensitivities to begin with, certain sequences of amino acids are more likely to cause the production of antibody formation, which is one reason why certain foods such as gluten and dairy are more likely to result in food allergies and sensitivities. Another reason is that an increase in intestinal permeability (leaky gut) can lead to the development of food sensitivities, and a lot of people have a leaky gut.

Reason #2: Gluten cannot be completely digested. If you don't have an allergy or sensitivity to gluten and don't experience an improvement in your symptoms and/or a decrease in thyroid antibodies when avoiding gluten, is it okay to eat foods with gluten? Well, even if you don't have a gluten sensitivity and you don't experience any symptoms when consuming it, the gluten proteins of wheat, rye, and barley can't be completely broken down by human digestive enzymes. This has to do with the high proline content of gluten molecules.[2] One of the consequences of not being able to fully degrade these prolines is that there are large proline-rich gluten fragments, which can cause an increase in proinflammatory cytokines.[2]

Reason #3: Gluten causes a leaky gut in *everyone*. Some studies show that eating gluten causes an increase in intestinal permeability in every single person,[3] even those who don't have a sensitivity to gluten. Since having a leaky gut is a component of the triad of autoimmunity I discussed in chapter 2, eating gluten can be a major roadblock for someone who has Graves' disease and is trying to get into remission. But having a healthy gut is also important if you have a non-autoimmune hyperthyroid condition.

Reason #4: Gluten is a potential trigger of thyroid autoimmunity. As I just mentioned, gluten causes an increase in intestinal permeability, which is a factor in autoimmunity. In addition, gluten also can lead to a loss of oral tolerance, which is characterized by a decrease in regulatory T cells.[4, 5] I discuss oral tolerance in greater detail in Chapter 11. As for regulatory T cells (Tregs), they help to keep autoimmunity in check, and so you want to have an abundance of these cells.

Some also believe that gliadin has an amino acid sequence that resembles that of the thyroid gland. Although I was unable to come across any research demonstrating this, some experts feel strongly about this similarity in amino acid sequence resulting in a molecular mimicry mechanism between the immune response to gluten and some of the proteins that are involved in thyroid function.

Assuming this molecular mimicry theory is correct, if your body develops antibodies to gliadin, the immune system can also mistakenly attack the cells of the thyroid gland. This might explain why so many people with Graves' disease (and Hashimoto's) feel significantly better upon avoiding gluten, and it would also explain why many people experience a decrease in their thyroid antibodies when going on a gluten-free diet.

Now, you might be wondering why everyone who eats gluten doesn't develop an autoimmune condition. First, you need to remember the two other components of the triad of autoimmunity. In addition to having a leaky gut, you also need to have a genetic predisposition for Graves' disease and be exposed to an environmental trigger. I also discussed how you need to have a loss of oral tolerance, which can take years to develop. This is why someone can consume gluten for many years without a problem but develop autoimmunity later in life. Also, we need to keep in mind that gluten isn't always a factor in the development of thyroid autoimmunity, but it is a big factor for many people.

Reason #5: You should focus on eating whole foods. When trying to restore your health, you want to focus on eating whole, healthy foods. No good reason exists to eat bread, pasta, pastries, etc. This is true even if you eat gluten-free versions of these foods, as just because a food is gluten-free doesn't mean it's healthy for you. I'm not suggesting that you need to eat 100 percent whole foods permanently, as I can't say that I never indulge in unhealthy foods now that I am in remission, but you should strive to do this while trying to restore your health.

Even after reading this, some people might think that eating a small amount of gluten every now and then isn't a big deal. Truth be told, for some people, it might not be, but if someone has Graves' disease or any other autoimmune condition, eating even a small amount of gluten might prevent them from getting into remission. This is true even if you don't experience any symptoms when eating gluten.

Gluten can potentially cause a leaky gut in everyone, and in order to have a healthy immune system, you need to have a healthy gut. Thus, for this reason alone, I would try to avoid eating gluten while restoring your health. This is not just the case with those who have Graves' disease, but non-autoimmune hyperthyroid conditions as well.

But what if you have been tested for a gluten sensitivity and it came back negative? First of all, most people who test for gluten antibodies don't obtain comprehensive testing. For example, many people only get the alpha gliadin antibodies tested, and I have had other patients who only tested tissue transglutaminase IgA and nothing else. These are individual components of a celiac panel.

In addition, if someone gets a complete celiac panel and it comes back negative, this doesn't rule out a non-celiac gluten sensitivity. Even if the person obtained more comprehensive testing for gluten that came back negative (i.e., the Array #3 from Cyrex Labs or the Wheat Zoomer by Vibrant Wellness), eating gluten can still increase the permeability of the gut, regardless of whether or not someone is sensitive to it. Thus, it's important to understand that even if you don't have a gluten allergy or sensitivity, avoiding it is still important in order to heal the gut.

Is It Safe to Eat Gluten after Getting into Remission?

If someone has celiac disease, then they should strictly avoid gluten permanently. Eating even a tiny amount of gluten can cause inflammation and an increase in autoantibodies. If someone has a non-celiac gluten

Hyperthyroid Healing Diet Basics

sensitivity, then in my opinion, it is also wise to avoid gluten permanently. I realize it's not easy to completely avoid gluten, and what makes it even more challenging is that there are many hidden sources of gluten, many of which I discuss in chapter 12. Even if you purchase a packaged food that is gluten-free, it still might have traces of gluten in it, especially if it's not certified gluten-free.

According to the US Food and Drug Administration, one of the criteria proposed is that foods bearing the claim "gluten-free" cannot contain 20 parts per million (ppm) or more gluten.[6] The problem is that some people with celiac disease or a non-celiac gluten sensitivity problem might react to trace amounts of gluten. Also, if you are trying to avoid gluten and plan on purchasing packaged gluten-free foods, you ideally want to make sure that the food is "certified gluten-free," which means that there is a third party confirming that the food, drink, nutritional supplement, or herb meets the standards for being labeled as gluten-free.

So far, we have established that you should avoid gluten if you have celiac disease or a non-celiac gluten sensitivity. I'll also add that many healthcare professionals recommend that everyone with any autoimmune condition should avoid gluten permanently, whether or not they have celiac disease or a non-celiac gluten sensitivity problem. While I can't say I have been 100 percent gluten-free since I've been in remission, when you do the research, it makes sense, as gluten can be an autoimmune trigger in many people, and it causes a leaky gut. Thus, if you want to be on the safe side, then after you get into remission, you should ideally avoid gluten permanently.

Gluten vs. Glyphosate

In chapter 26 I discuss how glyphosate can be a factor in why so many people have problems with gluten. In other words, there is the possibility that some people don't have a problem with gluten but instead have a problem with the

26

glyphosate that's sprayed on wheat and other grains. Others suggest that the hybridization of wheat is the main culprit.

In his book *Eat Wheat: A Scientific and Clinically-Proven Approach to Safely Bringing Wheat and Dairy Back into Your Diet,* Dr. John Douillard discusses how the problem with gluten and dairy relates to congested lymphatic vessels in the brain and central nervous system. According to Dr. Douillard, this congestion can lead to food sensitivities, including those related to gluten and dairy. While he isn't necessarily encouraging everyone to eat gluten, he does say that improving upper digestion and having a healthy intestinal tract can help decongest the lymphatic system, which, in turn, will allow many people to tolerate gluten.

He adds that if you have weak digestion or a congested lymphatic system, then eliminating wheat and dairy won't do anything to address the root cause of the issue. Not surprisingly, the quality of the food you eat can make a big difference though. For example, concerning grains, he discusses sourdough bread and ancient wheat such as einkorn.

My goal isn't to confuse you by presenting different sides to the story, and I'm not encouraging you or anyone else with hyperthyroidism and Graves' disease to eat gluten, but I want to encourage you to keep an open mind. Avoiding gluten even after restoring their health is probably the best option for everyone who has Graves' disease. However, I realize that some will choose to reintroduce gluten in the future, regardless of what the research shows.

You might wonder what my opinion is on this subject. As I already mentioned, I think that those with celiac disease or a non-celiac gluten sensitivity should completely avoid gluten permanently. Every now and then I'll be asked if it's okay for someone who has celiac disease to eat sourdough bread. This question is based on a few small studies that showed sourdough wheat baked goods degrading the gluten and thus being supposedly safe for those with celiac disease.[7, 8] However, a more recent study shows that this is not considered to be safe for those with celiac disease.[9]

As for whether someone with Graves' disease who doesn't have celiac disease or a non-celiac gluten sensitivity can safely reintroduce healthier forms of wheat or other forms of gluten (i.e., rye, barley) upon improving their digestion and lymphatic system, this remains controversial. Some people who get into remission might be able to occasionally tolerate small amounts of gluten without relapsing, but the problem is that there is no way to know for certain if you are one of these people, which is why many healthcare professionals recommend avoiding gluten permanently. In fact, many healthcare professionals recommend avoiding *all* grains, even after achieving a state of remission.

Although I do my best to avoid gluten, I can't say that I've been 100 percent gluten-free since being in remission. Once again, I usually avoid gluten, especially in my home, and even when going out to eat. But I can't say that I never get exposed to gluten, and while I'm grateful that this hasn't resulted in a relapse, this isn't the case with everyone. After restoring their health, some people are able to eat gluten on an occasional basis without a problem, while others will need to avoid it on a permanent basis. And assuming you don't have celiac disease or a non-celiac gluten sensitivity, the only way to know how you'll respond to gluten is to reintroduce it, which is a decision that only you can make.

Allergen 2: Dairy

Many people don't do well when consuming dairy. During my childhood and teenage years, I drank plenty of cow's milk, which many people still perceive as being healthy. Although drinking cow's milk is very healthy for baby cows, it's not necessarily healthy for humans.

That being said, dairy has some potential health benefits. In addition, some people do well when consuming raw dairy, while others do fine consuming dairy from a goat or a sheep. However, I recommend that my patients with hyperthyroidism avoid all types of dairy while trying to get into remission. While some people do fine with raw dairy or other forms of dairy, everyone is different, and some people do react to these healthier forms of dairy products. I'm not asking you to give up dairy forever (although some people will need to do this), but try to avoid it while restoring your health.

Why Is It Important to Avoid Drinking "Conventional" Cow's Milk?

Many people still think of cow's milk as being healthy and drink it regularly. Why is commercial cow's milk bad for you? Here are four reasons:

1. **The hormones.** In addition to the growth hormone that is commonly added, cow's milk also contains estrogens, which, in some people, could stimulate the growth of hormone-sensitive tumors.[10] While drinking organic cow's milk would be a healthier choice, it's important to understand that organic milk might not have growth hormones added but may have estrogens because it's common for the milk to be collected from cows while they are lactating. Due to these and other factors I'm about to discuss, avoiding cow's milk altogether is probably best, regardless of whether it's organic or non-organic.

2. **The pasteurization process.** The pasteurization process, developed by Louis Pasteur in 1864, involves heating the milk to a specific temperature in order to kill harmful bacteria. When you think about pasteurization, this might sound like a great idea. However, heating the milk decreases many of the nutrients, such as vitamins B_1, B_2, B_{12}, C, and E, as well as folate.[11]

   In addition, the pasteurization process modifies the proteins of dairy and can potentially lead to a greater increase in food allergies, although some argue that the opposite occurs, as denaturing the proteins might make someone less susceptible to a dairy allergy. You might wonder if the pasteurization process will inactivate estrogens, but the research shows that pasteurized organic and conventional dairy products do not have substantially different concentrations of estrogens.[12]

3. **The homogenization process.** Why is commercial milk homogenized? The process of homogenization helps to give milk its white color and smooth texture and might help with the digestibility of milk.[13] Homogenization changes the physical structure of milk fat and, because of this, might alter the health properties of milk. A review of studies shows an increased risk of cardiovascular disease and type 2 diabetes in those who drink homogenized milk.[14] To be fair, most of these were observational studies, and it's difficult to use these to prove a direct correlation between milk consumption and these diseases.

4. **The mTORC1 pathway.** There is something called the *mammalian TOR complex 1* (mTORC1), and this signaling pathway plays a big role in the development and progression of several different health conditions, including conditions such as acne[15,16] as well as chronic conditions such as obesity,[17,18] type 2 diabetes,[19] and cancer.[20,21,22]

Does this mean that drinking commercial milk will always lead to a condition such as obesity, type 2 diabetes, or cancer? While some people do fine drinking milk, others don't. As with gluten, it's unnecessary to drink cow's milk, although I admit that unlike gluten, dairy has certain health benefits, and it is also very tasty.

Many people are aware of the glycemic index, and milk has a low glycemic index. However, cow's milk, along with other types of dairy, has a high insulin index,[23] which means that it causes a high insulin response. This doesn't mean that you will develop insulin resistance if you regularly consume dairy from a cow, but the persistent consumption of foods categorized by either a high glycemic index or a high insulin index causes beta cells to release more insulin to initiate glucose uptake into body cells, leading to insulin insensitivity.[23] You might wonder if it's healthier to drink other types of milk, such as from a goat or sheep. There hasn't been as much research on these types of milk, although it appears their insulin index is similar to cow's milk.

Another Problem with Cow's Milk: Beta Casein A1

Cow's milk consists of both casein and whey protein, with approximately 80 percent of it consisting of casein. Although many people are lactose intolerant, it's also common to be sensitive to casein. Other dairy products include casein, such as yogurt and cheese. There are different types of casein in dairy cows. The most common forms of beta-casein in dairy cattle breeds are A1 and A2.

It is thought that beta-casein variant A1 yields the bioactive peptide beta-casomorphin-7 (BCM-7). This may play a role in the development of certain human diseases, such as diabetes mellitus and ischemic heart disease. There also might be a relationship between BCM-7 and sudden infant death syndrome.[24]

Some people react to beta-casein A1 but do perfectly fine when consuming beta-casein A2. The challenge is finding out where the dairy you purchase is coming from. Unfortunately, most of the milk in the United States comes from A1 cows. Raw milk is a better option than conventional milk. However, from what I understand, not all raw milk is made from A2 cows, which might explain why some people don't do well when drinking raw milk.

What's the best way to get milk that has beta-casein A2? You might need to go directly to the source, which means contacting local farmers to find out whether they have A1 cows or A2 cows. I have seen A2 milk sold at my local Whole Foods store, although it is pasteurized. Goat and sheep milk don't have BCM-7, which is probably why many people do better when drinking these types of milk.

What about Other Types of Dairy?

Most of this information focuses on the risks associated with drinking cow's milk, but is it okay for people with hyperthyroidism to consume other types of dairy? I recommend that my patients avoid all forms of dairy while trying to restore their health. This includes not only milk but also yogurt, cheese, kefir, and whey because some people are sensitive to these other forms as well.

Since butter is low in casein, you might feel that it is fine to consume. This might be true in some cases, but if someone has a known or suspected casein allergy or sensitivity, then I would still recommend they avoid it. They also need to consider the type of casein they're consuming. It admittedly can be challenging at times to know exactly what a person should and shouldn't eat, but I would rather play it safe and have them avoid all types of dairy while they are restoring their health.

How about ghee? This is clarified butter, and it has even fewer dairy proteins than regular butter. Although for years I've recommended that people avoid ghee if they are strictly avoiding dairy, the truth is that many people who don't tolerate most forms of dairy are able to tolerate ghee. As a result, some health-care practitioners allow ghee in moderation as part of their autoimmune-friendly diets, and I allow it in all three Hyperthyroid Healing Diets.

Although some healthcare professionals think that everyone with Graves' disease should avoid both gluten and dairy permanently, some people can eventually reintroduce dairy into their diet once they get into a state of remission. After all, not everyone has problems with dairy, and consuming certain types of dairy has some health benefits.

However, it does depend on the person, as some people might need to avoid dairy permanently. There admittedly are risks of reintroducing dairy, especially if someone has a sensitivity to dairy proteins such as casein or whey.

Thus, some people choose to avoid dairy permanently, while others choose to reintroduce healthier forms of dairy (i.e., raw dairy) in the future.

Yet Another Problem with Dairy: Cross-Reactivity

While someone can have a direct sensitivity to dairy, it is also possible for one or more of the dairy proteins to cross-react with gluten. This is one of the main reasons why many natural healthcare professionals recommend that their patients with autoimmune conditions such as Graves' disease avoid dairy permanently.

If you insist on eating dairy, then, in this situation, you might want to consider ordering a test such as the Gluten-Associated Cross-Reactive Foods & Foods Sensitivity by Cyrex Labs (Array #4). This tests for sensitivity to cow's milk, along with the following individual proteins of dairy: alpha-casein and beta-casein, casomorphin, milk butyrophilin, whey protein, and milk chocolate. If you test positive for any of these, then Cyrex Labs recommends avoiding dairy permanently. However, some other foods on this panel can be reintroduced once the gut has been healed.

Where Will You Get Your Calcium?

Many people are concerned about getting enough calcium if they are avoiding dairy. Although dairy is the primary source of calcium for many people, there are other foods high in calcium. Kale is high in calcium, so you can eat steamed kale and/or add kale to a smoothie.

Chinese cabbage is also an excellent source of calcium.[25] Collard greens, broccoli, and blackstrap molasses can also provide a sufficient amount of calcium. Sardines and other fish with the bones in them are also good sources of calcium. Thus, there are plenty of non-dairy sources of calcium to choose from.

Allergen 3: Corn

This is yet another common allergen, and one that cross-reacts with gluten. Research has shown that the proteins from corn can cause a celiac-like immune response due to similar or alternative pathogenic mechanisms to the proteins found in wheat.[26] In other words, eating corn can cause a similar response as eating gluten.

Zein is a class of prolamine protein found in corn. And the research shows that zein can cause persistent mucosal damage in some people with celiac disease.[26] Another smaller study revealed a higher incidence of serum antibodies against corn in those with celiac disease,[27] along with barley and oats.

You might be thinking to yourself, "These studies relate to those with celiac disease," which is true. But there are other studies conducted in those who don't have celiac which show that corn is a common food allergen.[28,29,30]

The Challenges with Avoiding Corn

Anyone who eats processed foods regularly is most likely exposed to corn. This is especially true if you are eating gluten-free processed foods such as gluten-free cookies, crackers, cereals, etc. If you are trying to avoid corn, then obviously you will want to avoid ingredients such as corn starch and corn syrup. However, there are many other ingredients that contain corn, including the following: ascorbic acid, caramel, confectioners' sugar, hydrolyzed vegetable protein, corn-based maltodextrin, modified food starch, and xanthan gum. Keep in mind that this is just a small sample of ingredients that may include corn.

In addition to corn being a common allergen, most corn in the United States is genetically modified. If you do choose to eat corn or a product that includes corn, make sure that it is either certified organic or labeled as being non-GMO. Just keep in mind that many people are sensitive to corn, even when it's non-GMO. This is why I recommend avoiding corn while following any of the Hyperthyroid Healing Diets.

Allergen 4: Soy

I want to begin by mentioning that there are numerous health benefits associated with organic fermented soy, including miso, natto, and tempeh. One study showed how fermented soybean products have beneficial effects on neurodegenerative diseases.[31] Another study showed that the consumption of fermented soy was inversely associated with the risk of cardiovascular disease in women.[32] Yet another study showed that a higher intake of fermented soy was associated with a lower risk of mortality.[33]

So why in the world should you avoid soy? As I mentioned earlier, most soy that people consume isn't fermented soy. But while organic fermented soy has many health benefits, soy is a common allergen, and this is true even with fermented soy. Let's go ahead and take a look at some of the main concerns with soy:

Soy is a common allergen. The Food and Agriculture Organization of the United Nations includes soy in its list of the eight most significant food allergens, and at least sixteen potential soy protein allergens have been identified.[34] And I'm not just talking about an IgE-mediated soy allergy, as many people have a sensitivity to soy. So, for example, if you go to an allergy doctor and test negative for soy, this usually doesn't rule out a soy sensitivity.

Most soy is genetically modified. Unfortunately, most soy is genetically modified. There are a few studies that suggest that genetically modified soy might be less allergenic than non-GMO soy.[35,36] But the problems with GMOs don't just relate to allergies. One of the main concerns is that genetically modified soybeans contain high residues of glyphosate, which I discuss in chapter 26. Obviously, you can avoid GMO-soy simply by eating organic.

Soy is very high in lectins. Soybean agglutinin (SBA) is a non-fiber carbohydrate-related protein and the main anti-nutritional factor that exists in soybean or soybean products.[37] Although heating can reduce the lectin content of SBA, even after heating, a considerable quantity is still found. SBA can have a negative effect on the intestinal structure,[38] barrier function,[39,40] and the mucosal immune system.[41]

However, while heat alone won't significantly decrease the lectin content of soy, the fermentation process can have a dramatic effect. Most fermented soy products have been analyzed to contain very small amounts of lectins and other antinutrients (i.e., phytates, trypsin inhibitors) when compared with raw soybean.[42,43] Almost all lectins in soybeans are destroyed during fermentation processes over seventy-two hours.[44]

As a result of this, one can make a good argument that if a soy allergy and sensitivity are ruled out, then eating organic fermented soy might be acceptable. And if someone is a vegan, then soy very well might be one of their main sources of protein. That being said, organic fermented soy is excluded from all three Hyperthyroid Healing Diets discussed in section 2, but if someone is certain they don't have a soy allergy or sensitivity, then I'd say they can eat some as part of a Level 1 Hyperthyroid Healing Diet.

A Note to Those with Non-Autoimmune Thyroid Conditions

I realize a lot of the focus has been on the impact of these common allergens (especially gluten) in those with Graves' disease, and the reason for this is that an increase in intestinal permeability is part of the triad of autoimmunity. However, if you don't have an autoimmune hyperthyroid condition, this doesn't mean that you can't develop one in the future. And so regardless of whether you have Graves' disease, toxic multinodular goiter, or a different hyperthyroid condition, you really do want to take a break from these four allergens during the healing process.

Chapter 3 Highlights

- Gliadin is the most problematic protein found in gluten, specifically wheat.
- Even though oats are technically gluten-free, they are commonly cross-contaminated with gluten.
- People with hyperthyroidism should avoid gluten for five reasons: (1) many people are sensitive to gluten, (2) gluten can't be completely digested, (3) gluten can potentially cause a leaky gut in everyone, (4) gluten is a potential trigger of thyroid autoimmunity, (5) you should focus on eating whole foods.
- I recommend that my patients with hyperthyroidism avoid all types of dairy while trying to get into remission.
- Cow's milk is bad for you for the following four reasons: (1) the hormones, (2) the pasteurization process, (3) the homogenization process, (4) the mTORC1 pathway.
- Although dairy is the primary source of calcium for many people, there are other foods high in calcium, including kale, collard greens, broccoli, and sardines.
- Corn is another common allergen and cross-reacts with gluten.
- A few reasons to avoid soy is because soy is a common allergen, most soy is genetically modified, soy is very high in lectins.

To access the book references and resources, visit
SaveMyThyroid.com/HHDNotes.

CHAPTER

4

Carbohydrates, Proteins, and Fats

A common question I am asked is, "How many grams of protein, carbo-hydrates, and fats should I eat?" This can get confusing, as different sources provide different recommendations. I'll also add that most people aren't going to keep track of the number of macronutrients (protein, fats, and carbohydrates) they eat on a daily basis. For years I didn't think it was important to keep track of your macronutrient intake, but upon doing the research for this book, I learned that it's important for us to at least know how much protein we're consuming each day.

As for carbohydrates, while you can keep track of this, if you eat an abundance of vegetables and some fruit on a daily basis and try your best to avoid refined foods and sugars, then you should be consuming an adequate number of carbohydrates. With fats, make sure to have at least one or two servings of healthy fats per day in the form of avocados, olives, and healthy oils (i.e., coconut oil, olive oil, avocado oil). Depending on the type of Hyperthyroid Healing Diet you're following, you might also be able to eat certain nuts, which are a good source of fat. If you eat meat, this also will provide some fat along with protein.

As for how to track your intake of protein, as well as carbohydrates and fats, you can use a program such as Cronometer. With this you enter everything you eat in a day, and it will tell you approximately how many grams of protein, carbohydrates, and fats you have eaten, along with the vitamins and minerals.

Why Is Protein So Important?

I'm going to start out by discussing the importance of protein, and then I'll talk about healthy fats, followed by carbohydrates. These days a lot of people follow a ketogenic diet, so they're aware of the importance of healthy fats. But many don't get enough protein, which is the building block of all body tissues.

Adequate intake of protein is one of the key nutritional factors to prevent loss of muscle mass and strength, frailty, and associated comorbidities in later life.[1,2,3] A gradual decline in muscle mass is observed from the third decade of life,[4] with a 30–50 percent decrease reported between the ages of 40 and 80.[5] This age-related loss of muscle mass, strength, and quality is known as *sarcopenia*. Eating sufficient protein can at least help to minimize this loss of muscle mass.

The Role of Protein in Immune System Health

It's also important to mention that eating sufficient protein is important for optimal immune health. This, of course, is relevant to those who have Graves' disease, but it also can impact those with other hyperthyroid conditions. Research shows that a deficiency of dietary protein or amino acids has long been known to impair immune function and increase the susceptibility of animals and humans to infectious diseases.[6] Findings from recent studies indicate the important role of amino acids in immune responses by regulating the following: (1) the activation of T lymphocytes, B lymphocytes, natural killer cells, and macrophages; (2) cellular redox state, gene expression, and lymphocyte proliferation; and (3) the production of antibodies, cytokines, and other cytotoxic substances.[6]

If you're deficient in protein, this can potentially make you more susceptible to infections. Infections are a potential trigger of Graves' disease, and for those who have subacute thyroiditis, this is usually caused by a virus. This doesn't mean that if you eat sufficient protein you'll never get an infection, but if you do eat enough protein, your immune system will be in a much healthier state. In January 2022 I got hit hard by SARS-CoV-2, and thinking back, I wonder if not eating enough protein was at least one factor as to why it affected me the way it did. Up until that point I'd never even gotten the flu, and when I dealt with chronic Lyme disease in 2018, my symptoms weren't too extreme when compared to those of many others with tick-borne infections.

Essential vs. Nonessential Amino Acids

There are twenty known amino acids in total, with nine of them being essential, and the other eleven nonessential. *Essential* means that we need to get them in the food we eat. The nine essential amino acids include phenylalanine, valine, tryptophan, threonine, isoleucine, methionine, histidine, leucine, and lysine. As for the nonessential amino acids, our body can synthesize these using only the essential amino acids.

Three of the essential amino acids are known as *branched-chain amino acids* (BCAAs); these are valine, leucine, and isoleucine. It's common to see amino acid supplements that only include these three amino acids. Some claim that the BCAAs alone will help to stimulate muscle protein synthesis, but the research doesn't support this,[7] as all of the essential amino acids are important.[7]

Animal vs. Plant Sources

In general, animal-based foods are considered to be a superior source of protein because they have a complete composition of essential amino acids, with high digestibility and bioavailability.[8] Proteins found in milk, whey, egg, casein, and beef have the highest *protein digestibility corrected amino acid*

(PDCAA) score (1.0), while scores for plant-based proteins are as follows: soy (0.91), pea (0.67), oat (0.57), and whole wheat (0.45).[9] In addition, animal-based foods provide heme-iron, cholecalciferol, vitamin B_{12}, creatine, taurine, carnosine, and conjugated linoleic acid (CLA), which are compounds not present in plant-based foods.[10]

Although protein content and amino acid composition vary between plant species, in general, the protein found in legumes is limited in methionine and cysteine; cereals are limited in lysine and tryptophan; vegetables, nuts and seeds are limited in methionine, cysteine, lysine, and threonine; and seaweed is limited in histidine and lysine.[11] In addition, the digestibility and bioavailability of plant proteins are lower than those from animal sources, and the reason for this is that plants have a high amount of trypsin inhibitors, phytates, saponins, and tannins.[12] This doesn't mean that you can't get protein from plant sources, but it's another argument for why it might be a good idea to include some animal protein in your diet.

How Much Protein Do You Need to Consume?

The Dietary Reference Intake is 0.8 grams of protein per kilogram of body weight, or 0.36 grams per pound. For example, according to the DRI, someone who weighs 150 pounds should eat approximately 54 grams of protein per day. However, there is strong evidence that for optimal muscle protein synthesis and to prevent muscle loss, an aging adult would benefit from an increase (>1.2 g/kg/bw) in protein intake.[13,14] One kilogram equals approximately 2.2 pounds, so based on this number, if someone weighs 150 pounds (68 kilograms), then they should eat a minimum of 82 grams of protein per day.

Some sources suggest that it's not just the total daily protein intake that you want to pay attention to, but ideally you should consume protein three times a day, eating at least 25 to 30 grams of high-quality protein during each meal.[15,16,17,18] If this is true, then in the past I definitely wasn't getting enough protein most days, and this is probably true with a lot of others as well. Some suggest even higher amounts, as I've interviewed practitioners on my podcast (*Save My Thyroid*) who recommend eating 1 gram of protein for every pound you weigh, which means that if you weigh 150 pounds, you should eat 150 grams of protein!

After doing research for this book, I think that a good daily protein intake goal is at least 75 percent of your ideal body weight in pounds. For example, if your ideal body weight is 120 pounds, you should aim for at least 90 grams of protein per day. Divide this up into two or three meals, which is reasonable since most people won't be able to eat 90 grams of protein in a single serving. So, for example, when I dealt with Graves' disease, I lost 42 pounds, and at one point my actual weight was 140 pounds, but my ideal weight was around 165–170 pounds. If I followed these recommendations back then, I would have wanted to eat at least 75 percent of my ideal weight (165–170 lbs.), and not my actual weight (140 lbs.).

Is More Protein Necessary for Those with Hyperthyroidism?

Not surprisingly, it's common for people with hyperthyroidism to experience a decrease in muscle mass. In fact, many will have decreased creatinine on a comprehensive metabolic panel, which is common with lower skeletal muscle mass.[19] There isn't a lot of research on this, although I did come across one study that showed that hyperthyroidism caused a 25 percent to 29 percent increase in protein breakdown, and this increased muscle protein degradation may be a major factor in the development of skeletal muscle wasting and weakness in hyperthyroidism.[20]

I think a good argument can be made that those with hyperthyroidism can benefit from eating more protein, although some studies show that over time, muscle mass and muscle strength can be restored just by normalizing the thyroid hormones.[21,22] Even though I have a separate chapter on exercise and hyperthyroidism (chapter 23), I want to mention here a study that showed that resistance training accelerates the recovery of skeletal muscle function and promotes weight gain based on muscle mass improvement.[23] So while I think it's reasonable to increase your protein intake, you need to do things to lower the thyroid hormones, and some resistance training can also help.

"How in the World Will I Get Enough Protein?"

You might wonder how you can eat enough protein, and it's a fair question. If you're not a vegan or vegetarian, then the easiest way to increase your protein intake is by eating more meat, poultry, and fish. Of course you would want to make sure it's of good quality (i.e., grass-fed, pasture raised). Depending on the type of Hyperthyroid Healing Diet you choose to follow, eggs can also be a good source of protein.

You can also consider supplementing with protein powders. Hydrolyzed beef protein or bone broth powder are good options. Many people add collagen to their smoothies, and while this is an incomplete protein, it's still a good option. You just wouldn't want to rely on collagen alone as your protein source. If you're a vegan or vegetarian, then a good-quality organic pea protein is an option to consider. Although peas aren't allowed on the Level 2 and 3 Hyperthyroid Healing Diets (to be discussed in chapters 5 and 6), for most people, adding a good quality pea protein (in the form of pea protein isolate) to a smoothie doesn't seem to negatively affect their progress.

In the past I would only have animal protein once per day and would supplement with protein powders a couple of times per day (hydrolyzed beef or organic pea protein). Although I still add protein powder to my smoothies, I now eat animal protein two or three times per day. So it's not uncommon for me to eat two or three eggs for my first meal along with half of my smoothie, and then have animal protein for lunch with the other half of my smoothie.

And then when I eat dinner, I will also have animal protein. In addition to loading my smoothie with vegetables, when I eat lunch and dinner, I also have a couple of servings of vegetables.

Will a High-Protein Diet Damage the Kidneys?

Some people are concerned that diets high in protein can damage their kidneys. According to the research, if someone already has kidney disease, then it can be harmful to eat a high-protein diet. However, while higher-protein diets do increase renal workload, if someone has healthy kidneys, then they should be able to handle protein intakes above the RDA.[24]

Since hyperthyroidism can have a negative effect on bone density, I think it's also worth mentioning that dietary protein can benefit bone health and help prevent osteoporosis.[25] This doesn't necessarily mean that a high-protein diet can further increase bone density, but that not eating enough protein can have a negative effect on bone density. I also wanted to bring this up because there are some concerns that eating too much protein can actually have a detrimental effect on bone health, but this has proven not to be the case.[26]

How to Keep Track of Your Protein Intake

Keeping track of your protein intake isn't too difficult with the help of certain apps, such as Cronometer. With Cronometer you simply add the foods you eat on a daily basis, and it will tell you approximately how much protein you're getting. It will also let you know approximately how many fats and carbohydrates you're consuming. Another app you can check out is called Protein Pal, where you can set your protein target for a specific day, as well as review your history of protein intake. However, this isn't a free app, as there is a seven-day free trial before being billed monthly or annually.

Getting Enough Protein

You can actually use Cronometer to determine how much protein is in a specific food. For example, if you click on "Add Food" and add "Chicken Breast, Skinless," you'll see that an ounce is equal to 8.8 grams of protein. Three to four ounces is what most people will eat for lunch and dinner, so this would equal 26 to 35 grams of protein. If you do a search for cooked eggs, you'll see that one large egg has approximately 6.3 grams of protein.

The Best Sources of Protein

I'm not going to get into too much detail here, as I simply want to list some of the food sources highest in protein (data obtained from Cronometer):

- Chicken breast, skin removed before cooking: 8.8 grams per ounce
- Eggs, cooked: 6.3 grams per large egg
- Hamburger or ground beef, 80 percent lean: 7.2 grams per ounce
- Beef steak, sirloin: 8.5 grams per ounce
- Turkey breast, skin removed before cooking: 40.7 grams per cup
- Wild salmon: 7.2 grams per ounce
- Large white beans: 17.4 grams per cup
- Kidney beans: 15.3 grams per cup
- Jelly beans: 0 grams per cup
- Lentil sprouts, cooked: 10.9 grams per cup
- Walnuts: 0.2 grams per 1 gram of walnuts
- Brazil nuts: 0.4 grams per 3 grams of whole pieces

The Scoop on Healthy Fats

Fats are an essential macronutrient of the human diet. Fats are essential in providing the body with energy. Every single cell in your body has a membrane that protects it from damage. These membranes are made of proteins, fat, and cholesterol. Fat keeps us warm and protects the organs in our body. Fats are crucial for proper absorption of the fat-soluble vitamins A, D, E, and K.

The Different Types of Fat

- **Saturated fats.** These fats are found in animal products (beef, pork, chicken, dairy, etc.) and tropical oils (coconut oil, palm oil). They are called *saturated* because each saturated fat molecule's carbon has two hydrogens attached, making saturated fats solid at room temperature. While some claim that eating a lot of saturated fat causes oxidative stress, some studies show that a diet high in saturated fat doesn't cause an increase in inflammation and oxidative stress.[27]

- **Monounsaturated fats.** These fats are found in nuts and fruits (olives, avocados, peanuts, ground nuts, tree nuts, etc.) and contain one double bond. Not all carbons in the molecule have hydrogens stuck to them. This breaks the chain and makes these types of fats liquid at room temperature. Most foods that are high in monounsaturated fats are considered to be healthy forms of fats, although there are exceptions (i.e., peanuts).

- **Polyunsaturated fats.** These fats are found in foods such as fish, nuts, seeds, and vegetable oils. They contain more than one double bond, and not all carbons in the molecule have hydrogens stuck to them, so they are also liquid at room temperature. There are four types of polyunsaturated fats:

  - **Omega-3s.** These fats are found in fish as EPA (eicosapentaenoic acid) and DHA (docosahexaenoic acid) and are found in smaller amounts in walnuts, flaxseeds, and soybeans. Many people don't get enough EPA and DHA, which is why I commonly recommend a fish oil supplement to my patients. However, you can also do an omega-3 index test to determine if you need to eat more food sources and/or take an omega-3 supplement.

- **Omega-6s**—These fats are found in nuts and seeds, whole grain cereals and breads, meats, and vegetable oils (soybean oil, corn, and safflower oils). You need omega-6 fatty acids, but the problem is that many people eat too many omega-6 fatty acids and don't get sufficient omega-3 fatty acids. Many people consume a ratio of 15 to 1 omega-6 to omega-3, when you ideally don't want it to exceed 3/1 or 4/1. You can test for the omega-3 index through the blood, which ideally should be above 8 percent.

I also want to briefly mention arachidonic acid. Arachidonic acid (ARA) is a long-chain omega-6 fat derived from linoleic acid that can be pro-inflammatory in high amounts. However, it also provides some important health benefits. ARA is an integral constituent of biological cell membranes, conferring it with fluidity and flexibility, so it's necessary for the function of all cells, especially in the nervous system, skeletal muscle, and immune system.[28] Metabolites derived from ARA oxidation do not initiate but contribute to inflammation and most importantly lead to the generation of mediators responsible for resolving inflammation and wound healing.[28]

- **Conjugated linoleic acids (CLA)**—CLA is mainly consumed by humans in the form of meat and dairy products. CLA appears to modify body composition favorably and has beneficial actions on blood sugar, atherosclerosis, and cancer.[29] If you're a vegan, then you very well might be deficient in CLA.

- **Trans fats**—These types of fats naturally occur in meat and dairy products in small amounts but are also made when unsaturated fats are altered during processing to extend shelf life. Anything that has the word "hydrogenated" on the label is considered a trans fat. Trans fats are used for many different reasons, as they are less likely to go rancid and can be used for deep frying, but the main reason is because they are cheap to use.

Foods That Contain High-Quality Fats:

- **Avocados.** I can't say I love eating avocados, although I do like adding them to smoothies. According to the research, avocado consumption is associated with improved overall diet quality, nutrient intake, and reduced risk of metabolic syndrome.[30]

- **Coconuts.** Coconuts can be eaten raw, dried, or flaked, and coconut flour can be used in baking and other recipes. Coconut oil can be used for cooking and oil pulling, and topically as well. One study researched all components of the coconut plant and found it to have antiviral, antiparasitic, antibacterial, and antifungal properties.[31] The same study showed that it has antioxidant, renal protective, cardioprotective, hepatoprotective, and antidiabetic properties, and it increases bone volume.[31]

- **Meat.** Eating meat is a good way to get high-quality saturated fats along with B vitamins, minerals, and quality protein. I recommend that my patients eat organic, free-range, and pasture-raised meat whenever possible, as these types of quality meats are higher in nutrients. For example, numerous studies show that grass-fed beef has a significantly higher level of total omega-3 fatty acids compared to grain-fed beef.[32,33] Poultry has significant amounts of monounsaturated fatty acids, and one study showed that eating poultry reduces the risk of obesity, cardiovascular disease, and type 2 diabetes.[34]

- **Olives.** The possible health benefits associated with the consumption of olives are thought to be primarily related to the effects of monounsaturated fatty acids on cardiovascular health, the antioxidant capacity of vitamin E and its role in protecting the body from oxidative damage, and the anti-inflammatory and antioxidant activities of hydroxytyrosol.[35]

- **Fish.** Fish and shellfish are the richest sources of the omega-3 fatty acids DHA and EPA, which decrease inflammation in the body. Seafood effectively prevents cardiovascular disease, regulates body weight, decreases the risk of type 2 diabetes, reduces inflammation, and protects against Alzheimer's.[36]

While there is no question that seafood has many health benefits, there are also risks associated with seafood consumption. One of the main concerns is the mercury found in fish, although there are other environmental toxins as well, including polychlorinated biphenyls (PCBs) and microplastics. As a result, while some healthcare professionals recommend eating fish on a daily basis, I would limit your consumption of seafood to two to three times per week. I will discuss this in greater detail in chapter 5, including any concerns you may have when it comes to the iodine content in seafood.

- **Nuts and Seeds.** Nuts are off-limits for those following a Level 3 Hyperthyroid Healing Diet (discussed in chapter 5), but for those who choose to eat nuts or have reintroduced them after eliminating them for a few months, they are a wonderful source of healthy fats. Nuts are nutrient-rich foods with wide-ranging cardiovascular and metabolic benefits that can be readily incorporated into healthy diets.[37]

However, while eating a small amount of raw nuts on a daily basis provides some health benefits, keep in mind that they are still higher in omega-6 fatty acids, and they are also high in oxalates (I discuss oxalates in chapter 16), so I wouldn't consume too many nuts while healing. However, as I'll discuss later in this book, some nuts are lower in oxalates than others. You probably know that you should avoid eating nuts that contain unhealthy oils (i.e. vegetable oil, peanut oil), but I want to briefly mention it here just to play it safe.

The Concern with Nut-Based Products

I just want to add that on a wellness basis, I eat nuts regularly. And while nuts have some great health benefits, eating too many can be problematic for the reasons I just discussed. Some people don't eat a lot of nuts in their whole form but instead consume a lot of nut milks, nut butters, almond yogurt, almond ice cream, almond flour, etc. While I can't deny that I love eating an almond-based chocolate chip cookie every now and then, you want to be careful about consuming too many nuts in these other forms, which I discuss further in chapter 6.

How Much Fat Should You Eat Daily?

The USDA recommends that healthy adults over the age of nineteen consume between 20 and 30 percent of their daily calories from fat.[38] While you don't necessarily want to rely on the guidelines from the USDA, in this case I would agree. Because fat is so important, you definitely don't want your fat intake to be too low, but I also don't recommend it to be too high. Yes, I realize that a high-fat, low-carbohydrate diet is still followed by many people, and I'm definitely an advocate of eating plenty of healthy fats. But you also want to make sure you're getting sufficient protein.

Healthy Fats and Oils to Consider

Not all of the fats and oils I'm about to mention are permitted on each of the Hyperthyroid Healing Diets, but overall these are considered to be healthier oils. For more specifics about which oils you can and can't eat with each diet, please refer to section 2, where I discuss each of the Hyperthyroid Healing Diets in detail.

- Avocado oil
- Butter

- Tallow
- Coconut oil
- Duck fat
- Flax oil
- Hazelnut oil
- Lard
- Macadamia oil
- Olive oil
- Walnut oil

The Carbohydrate Controversy

A few decades ago many people tried doing everything they could to avoid eating fat, and while I can't say the same is true with carbohydrates these days, a lot of people realize that minimizing carbohydrates can be an effective weight loss strategy in some cases. This is one of the big reasons why a ketogenic diet is so popular, and without question it has helped many people lose weight.

That being said, while I don't recommend going crazy with the carbohydrates, I also don't recommend following an extremely low-carbohydrate diet. Even though we can survive without carbohydrates, they do have some positive health benefits, as they act as an energy source, help control blood glucose and insulin metabolism, participate in cholesterol and triglyceride metabolism, and help with fermentation.[39] The problem is that many people eat too many carbohydrates, and most of the carbohydrates people eat are unhealthy, consisting of bread, pasta, pastries, and other unhealthy carbs.

One of the challenges with hyperthyroidism is that many people lose weight. This isn't true for everyone, and I discuss weight loss and weight gain in greater detail in chapter 13. But what I will say here is that it's common for people who are losing weight to consume larger amounts of carbohydrates in order to counteract the weight loss. And I do think it's fine to eat good-quality carbohydrates, consisting of some fruit and mostly vegetables.

So while I'm not suggesting that people with hyperthyroidism should follow a low-carbohydrate diet, I do recommend avoiding refined carbohydrates while restoring your health. I also advise that you focus more on getting quality proteins and fats. Once again, I understand if you feel the need to eat more carbohydrates than usual, especially if you have lost a lot of weight, and if you absolutely feel the need to do this, then I would stick with the healthier carbohydrates and then perhaps cut back as your health improves.

Glucose vs. Fructose

Glucose is a simple sugar that is mainly found in plant-based foods, including fruits and vegetables. One of the main roles of glucose is that it serves as a source of energy for cells. While small amounts of glucose are usually well tolerated, larger amounts can cause problems, such as insulin resistance.

Like glucose, fructose is another simple sugar that is mainly found in fruits and vegetables. However, it is processed differently than glucose, as fructose gets shunted to the liver for conversion into glucose or fat. While small amounts of fructose are fine to consume (i.e., from fruits and vegetables), too much from sources such as high-fructose corn syrup can lead to health issues.

Even though it's fine to get fructose from fruits and vegetables, you might wonder if you can overdo it. In other words, is it problematic to eat a lot of fruit? I do think it depends on the person. For example, if someone has a candida overgrowth, then they might want to limit fruit to a couple of servings per day, although some natural healthcare practitioners would recommend avoiding fruit altogether in this situation. If someone has insulin resistance, you can also minimize the amount of fruit you eat, although it's important to keep in mind that eating a lot of fruit usually won't cause insulin resistance.

What You Need To Know About Fiber

In an attempt to make it easier to understand, let's look at the different types of fiber and discuss their characteristics:

Soluble fiber. Soluble fiber attracts water and turns into a gel during digestion.[40] In other words, it gets dissolved during the digestive process, which is why it's referred to as being soluble. This type of fiber is found in foods such as oat bran, barley, nuts, seeds, beans, lentils, peas, some fruits and vegetables.[40] Psyllium is also a form of soluble fiber.

Pectin, gums, and fructans are soluble types of fiber. With regard to fructans, short-chain fructans are referred to as *fructooligosaccharides*, whereas longer chain fructans are called *inulins*. Food sources of fructan include chicory, Jerusalem artichokes, and onions. Beta-glucans are prominent in mushrooms, but they are also found in certain grains, some types of seaweed, and they are mostly soluble. In general, soluble fiber provides better support for blood sugar balance and cardiovascular health when compared to insoluble fiber.

Soluble fibers are also more completely fermented and have a higher viscosity than insoluble fibers. However, not all soluble fibers are viscous (e.g., partially hydrolyzed guar gum and acacia gum), and some insoluble fibers may be well fermented.[41] But what is the difference between viscous soluble and non-viscous soluble fiber? Well, soluble fibers that are viscous are gel-forming and have greater cardiovascular benefits than non-viscous soluble fibers. In fact, viscous soluble fiber can bind with cholesterol and help with its excretion in the stool.

Insoluble fiber. While soluble fiber seems to play a greater role in cardiovascular health, as well as helping to regulate blood sugar levels, insoluble fiber adds bulk to the stool and thus seems to provide a greater benefit in the prevention of constipation. Food sources of insoluble fiber include vegetables, legumes, nuts, and whole grains.

While some foods can be classified as being strictly soluble or insoluble, many foods will have a combination of different types of fiber. For example, although beans and other types of legumes are excluded from both a Level 2 and Level 3 Hyperthyroid Healing Diet, it's worth mentioning that they are good sources of fiber. And most beans will include both soluble and insoluble fiber. This also describes most vegetables, as most have both soluble and insoluble fiber, although starchy vegetables are typically higher in soluble fiber.

Resistant starch. This is insoluble and isn't broken down by digestive enzymes, and thus reaches the large intestine and is fermented by bacteria, which classifies it as a type of fermentable fiber. There are four categories of resistant starch, known as RS1, RS2, RS3, and RS4.[42] RS1 is found in whole grains and legumes. RS2 consists of foods such as raw potatoes and high-amylose corn starch. An example of RS3 foods include potatoes cooled after cooking. RS4 is found in breads and cakes. Food sources of resistant starch include plantains, potatoes, and legumes.

Short-chain fatty acids (SCFAs). The main SCFAs include acetate, proprionate, and butyrate. When you eat resistant starch, the good bacteria will feed on this and will produce SCFAs through fermentation. Bacteria in the colon use these short-chain fatty acids as their energy source, with butyrate being the main SCFA. The production of SCFAs can also help to reduce inflammation, and they can inhibit the growth of pathogenic organisms by reducing luminal and fecal pH.[43] SCFAs also help regulate sodium and water absorption and can increase the absorption of certain minerals, such as calcium, magnesium, copper, zinc, and iron.[43]

How Much Fiber Should You Consume Each Day?

The recommended fiber intake for children and adults is 14 grams of fiber per 1,000 calories.[44] According to this, if you consume an average of 2,000 calories per day, then you should be eating 28 grams of fiber per day. If you average

2,500 calories per day, then you should aim for 35 grams of fiber per day. If you aren't sure how many calories you consume on a daily basis, you can use a free program such as **www.myfitnesspal.com**, where you can enter your food diary and it will tell you approximately how many calories you consume on a daily basis. In fact, you can also use MyFitnessPal to keep track of how much fiber you are consuming, although you will have to change the default settings.

However, some sources suggest that we need to consume more fiber than this. There is some evidence that our ancestors ate up to 100 grams of fiber each day![45] I don't expect anyone to eat this much fiber, but there is justification to aim for at least 50 grams of fiber consumption per day.

Good vs. Bad Carbohydrates

One of the main characteristics of fiber is that digestive enzymes are unable to break it down into monosaccharides, and as a result the fiber passes through the digestive tract mostly intact. Two of the main functions of fiber are to feed the good bacteria in the gut and to add bulk to the stool. With regard to feeding the good bacteria, you probably have heard about prebiotics, and all prebiotics are considered to be a type of fiber. Resistant starch is considered to be a type of prebiotic. And since all prebiotics are fiber and resistant starch falls under the category of prebiotics, then this means that resistant starch is a type of fiber.

Which Healthy Carbohydrates Can You Eat?

With all three of the Hyperthyroid Healing Diets, and especially with the Level 2 and Level 3 Diets, you will get most of your carbohydrates from fruits and vegetables. Many people wonder how much fruit they should eat, and while this may vary depending on the person, I'd say that most people can have two to three servings of fruit per day. If someone has moderate to severe candida overgrowth, then they might want to stick with a single serving of fruit per day in the form of berries.

Some people are afraid of eating fruit, and while I can't say I eat a lot of fruit each day, it's not out of fear of causing blood sugar imbalances or feeding candida. Sure, if someone already has one or both of these issues, then they probably will want to exercise caution. But we need to remember that fruit can be a good source of vitamins, minerals, phytochemicals, and fiber.

That being said, you definitely want to eat more vegetables than fruits. Before my Graves' disease diagnosis, I definitely was eating more fruits than vegetables, so I realize that for some people, this won't be an easy transition. But like fruit, vegetables also are a wonderful source of vitamins, minerals, phytochemicals, and fiber. I'll discuss some of the different fruits and vegetables you can and should consume in section 2.

In summary, you want to make sure you consume sufficient protein, getting at least 75 percent of your ideal body weight in grams of protein on a daily basis. And don't be afraid of eating fats, especially healthy fats such as avocados and coconut oil. As for carbohydrates, you mostly want to get them from the vegetables and fruits you eat, and you definitely want to avoid refined sources of carbohydrates. You also want to make sure you consume enough fiber.

Chapter 4 Highlights

- Adequate intake of protein is one of the key nutritional factors in preventing the loss of muscle mass and strength, frailty, and associated comorbidities in later life.
- Research shows that a deficiency of dietary protein or amino acids has long been known to impair immune function and increase the susceptibility of animals and humans to infectious diseases.
- In general, animal-based foods are considered to be a superior source of protein because they have a complete composition of essential amino acids, with high digestibility and bioavailability.
- I think that a good goal is to aim for a protein intake that's at least 75 percent of your ideal body weight in pounds.
- For example, if your ideal body weight is 120 pounds, you should aim for at least 90 grams of protein per day.
- Because it's common for those with hyperthyroidism to experience a decrease in muscle mass, I think a good argument can be made that those with hyperthyroidism can benefit from eating more protein.
- Since hyperthyroidism can have a negative effect on bone density, I think it's also worth mentioning that dietary protein can benefit bone health and help prevent osteoporosis.
- Many people eat too many omega-6 fatty acids and not enough omega-3 fatty acids.
- You should get between 20 and 30 percent of your daily calories from fat, but just make sure they're healthy fats.
- Some of the healthier oils include avocado oil, coconut oil, olive oil, and macadamia oil.
- While I don't recommend going crazy with carbohydrates, I also don't recommend following an extremely low-carbohydrate diet.
- With all three of the Hyperthyroid Healing Diets, you will get most of your carbohydrates from fruits and vegetables.

To access the book references and resources, visit
SaveMyThyroid.com/HHDNotes.

The Different Hyperthyroid Healing Diets

Hyperthyroid Healing Diet Level 3

I n this chapter I will discuss the "Level 3 Hyperthyroid Healing Diet." This is the most restrictive diet, and it's similar to an Autoimmune Paleo (AIP) Diet, also known as the Autoimmune Protocol. However, there are a few important differences, which I'll discuss shortly.

You might wonder why I'm starting with the Level 3 Diet, and the reason for this is that most people with hyperthyroidism have Graves' disease, and ideally, those with Graves' disease would start with this diet (although there are exceptions, which I'll discuss toward the end of this chapter). This doesn't mean that those with a different type of hyperthyroidism can't benefit from this diet, as it really depends on their situation. For example, since this diet can greatly benefit the health of the gut, someone with a non-autoimmune hyperthyroid condition who has a known or suspected gut issue can follow this diet.

The problem is that you can't always go by symptoms. For example, it's very possible for someone to have a leaky gut, yet not experience any symptoms. Based on this, I can make the argument that everyone should follow a Level

3 Diet, but since it is restrictive, I would say that the main people who should follow this diet are those with Graves' disease, or perhaps someone with a non-autoimmune hyperthyroid condition who has a known gut issue. Otherwise you can begin with one of the other two Hyperthyroid Healing Diet options that I'll discuss in the next two chapters.

Which Foods Can You Eat On an AIP Diet?

If you're familiar with an AIP Diet, then you know it is similar to a "standard" Paleo Diet, although it excludes eggs, nuts, seeds, and nightshades. Here is a bulleted list of foods that are allowed on an AIP Diet:

- Lean meats and poultry (beef, pork, lamb, chicken, turkey)
- Organ meats (liver, heart, kidney, etc.)
- Fish and other types of seafood (salmon, trout, sardines)
- Fresh fruits
- Vegetables (excluding the nightshades)
- Mushrooms
- Healthy oils (olive oil, coconut oil, avocado oil)
- Spices (excluding seed-based and nightshade-based spices such as cayenne, celery seed, chili powder, fenugreek, and paprika)
- Honey and pure maple syrup (in moderation)
- Certain flours (coconut flour, tapioca flour, cassava flour)
- Green tea in moderation (due to the caffeine), herbal teas

What's the Purpose of This Diet?

One purpose of the Level 3 Diet is to focus on eating nutrient-dense foods while at the same time avoiding inflammatory foods, including common allergens such as gluten, dairy, and corn. These foods can cause inflammation and/or exacerbate an existing inflammatory condition.

Another goal of the diet is to exclude foods higher in certain compounds that can have a negative effect on the gut. Some examples of these compounds include lectins, alkaloids, and glycoalkaloids. While many people understand that gluten can cause or contribute to a leaky gut, even gluten-free grains can be harsh on the gut, which is why they are not only excluded from this diet but from a Level 2 Diet as well, and are allowed minimally on a Level 1 Diet. Legumes are treated similarly.

This is especially important in autoimmune conditions such as Graves' disease, as you need a healthy gut in order to have a healthy immune system, and most of the immune system cells are located in the gut. So while trying to restore the health of the immune system, it makes sense to avoid foods that can have a negative effect on the gut.

Are There Concerns with a Restrictive Diet and Hyperthyroidism?

Although not everyone with hyperthyroidism loses weight, many people do, and this included me when I dealt with Graves' disease. In fact, I lost forty-two pounds, and while this was a concern, I understood that the reason why I lost so much weight was related to the elevation in thyroid hormones. Don't get me wrong, as a restrictive diet can also cause someone to lose additional weight.

That being said, while following any of the three Hyperthyroid Healing Diets, you shouldn't be restricting calories. While you might not be eating as many carbohydrates as you normally do, you definitely want to make sure you're eating sufficient protein and healthy fats, which I discussed in chapter 4. If you do this and also do what is necessary to lower your thyroid hormones, then your weight loss concerns should be minimal.

If, for any reason, you continue losing weight once your thyroid hormones have normalized and you're not restricting calories, then this usually indicates a problem with the gut. It could be related to small intestinal bacterial overgrowth

(SIBO), inflammatory bowel disease, or another gastrointestinal condition. Please refer to chapter 21, where I discuss healing the gut in great detail.

Why Are Eggs Excluded?

Eggs are a nutrient-dense, whole, healthy food. As a result, in general, if someone enjoys eating eggs and can eat eggs without experiencing symptoms, then it makes sense for them to eat them. However, for those with an autoimmune condition such as Graves' disease, there are a few reasons to consider taking a break from eggs for awhile.

First of all, eggs are a common allergen. This is why they are excluded from many elimination diets. In addition to someone having a possible egg allergy or egg sensitivity, there are compounds in egg whites that can have a negative effect on gut health, specifically a protease called *lysozyme*. Lysozyme is a proteolytic enzyme with 129 amino acid residues, and it's also produced in mucosal secretions such as saliva and tears.[1]

Dr. Sarah Ballantyne, author of the books *The Paleo Approach* and *Nutrivore*, along with the websites **www.thepaleomom.com** and **www.nutrivore.com**, has an article on eggs that discusses the problems with lysozyme. In her article, Dr. Sarah explains how "lysozyme has the ability to form strong complexes with other proteins" and how it is "resistant to digestion by our digestive enzymes." She also explains how when lysozyme passes through the intestinal barrier, other proteins can bind to it and pass through into the bloodstream, where they shouldn't be, and therefore can trigger an immune system response. So essentially the problem isn't with lysozyme itself, but the protein complexes it forms, which in turn pass through the cells of the small intestine.

I'll add that while eggs are excluded from a Level 3 Hyperthyroid Healing Diet, egg yolks are one of the first foods you can try to reintroduce. So while

I understand that you might miss eating eggs for breakfast each morning, you'll probably be able to reintroduce them again before you know it. That being said, it's common for people to ask what they should eat for breakfast, and while you can refer to the recipes in the bonus chapter (available in the resources), it's common for people who follow this diet to have leftovers from dinner for breakfast. At the very least it's an option to consider.

The Problem with Nightshades

The nightshades are members of a family of plants called Solanaceae. Some of the common foods in this family include tomatoes, white potatoes, and eggplant, as well as most types of peppers (black pepper is excluded). First of all, I should mention that these foods have some positive health benefits, so I'm not suggesting that you should avoid these permanently.

The reason why people with autoimmune conditions such as Graves' disease should initially avoid nightshade foods is because they have compounds that can cause inflammation and/or affect the health of the gut. These include lectins, as well as alkaloids and glycoalkaloids, which I briefly mentioned earlier.

While there are actually some health benefits of lectins, in susceptible individuals, eating foods high in lectins can potentially cause damage to the intestinal lining, which in turn can cause an increase in intestinal permeability (a leaky gut). And since a leaky gut is common in autoimmune conditions, it would make sense to avoid foods that have higher amounts of lectins while trying to restore your health.

As for alkaloids and glycoalkaloids found in nightshades, capsaicin is an alkaloid found in spicy peppers. Capsaicin is also the active ingredient in pepper spray and is highly responsible for the acute inflammation and burning feeling when sprayed and might even cause bronchoconstriction.[2] In fact, there have been numerous reports of pepper spray-related injuries,[3,4] and this very well might be because some people are highly sensitive to capsaicin.

This doesn't mean that everyone will have a negative reaction when consuming hot peppers, but it's something to keep in mind, and like tomatoes, these probably should be initially avoided while trying to restore your health. But it's not just hot peppers that should be avoided. If you are trying to avoid the nightshades, then you will want to avoid other types of peppers as well.

Solanine is a glycoalkaloid found in nightshade foods, especially eggplant and potatoes, although it's also found in tomatoes and peppers. Solanine has fungicidal and pesticidal properties, due to compounds inside the plant that are used as a form of protection. Solanine affects insects who feed on these plants by the inhibition of acetylcholinesterase,[5] which breaks down acetylcholine.

Acetylcholine inhibitors can lead to problems with the nervous system and can cause other health issues such as hypotension, bronchoconstriction, and hypermotility of the GI tract. This doesn't mean that everyone who eats these foods will have problems breaking down acetylcholine, but many people do react to the solanines and experience significant relief in some of their symptoms upon avoiding these foods.

I just want to reinforce that many of the foods I just mentioned have some positive health benefits, but they can potentially cause health issues in those with autoimmune conditions such as Graves' disease. Just to play it safe, I would recommend avoiding these foods at least for the first few months during the healing process.

Do You Need to Eat a Lot of Meat?

Before discussing how much meat you should eat, I need to mention that if you are a strict vegan or vegetarian, then you probably should follow a Level

2 or Level 1 Hyperthyroid Healing Diet. The reason for this is that if you're a vegan or vegetarian, you probably won't be able to get enough protein if you're following a Level 3 Diet. Like I discussed previously, eating sufficient protein is very important, especially since it's common for those with hyperthyroidism to experience a decrease in muscle mass.

In chapter 4 I discuss how you want to consume at least 75 percent of your ideal body weight in pounds of protein, which means that if your ideal weight is 120 pounds, you would want to eat 90 grams of protein per day. And while you certainly can add a good-quality protein powder to a smoothie while following any of the Hyperthyroid Healing Diets, with the Level 3 Diet, you will need other sources of protein, and animal protein in the form of meat, poultry, and fish is the main thing I would focus on.

And it's not just about protein, as meat, poultry, and fish are also excellent sources of micronutrients. You can get many of these micronutrients by eating vegetables and fruits, but not all of them. As a result, I recommend eating a combination of meat, poultry, fish, vegetables, and fruits in order to optimize your micronutrient intake.

If you're a vegan or vegetarian, I don't want you to feel like I'm pressuring you to eat animal sources of protein, as over the years I've had vegan and vegetarian patients restore their health. It just can be more challenging to get sufficient protein as a vegetarian, and especially as a vegan. In addition, proteins from animal food sources are referred to as *high-quality proteins* due to the presence of all nine essential amino acids (EAA) in high quantities as well as the greater bioavailability of these EAA.[6,7]

It goes without saying that you want to only eat good-quality animal sources of protein. Ideally, all meat and poultry should be organic, with beef being 100 percent grass-fed. If possible poultry should be pasture-raised, but if not, just eating organic poultry is fine. Avoid processed meats as much as you can, as while these will provide a good amount of protein, they also commonly include nitrates and/or nitrites, sometimes other ingredients that should be avoided, although you can find healthier versions of these in many grocery stores.

What's the Deal with Organ Meats?

There is no question that organ meats are very nutrient dense, which is why many advocates of a Paleo or AIP Diet recommend that people eat them. While this is true, I must admit that I didn't eat any organ meats while I was dealing with Graves' disease. And these days I also don't eat organ meats, although I recently started supplementing with organ meat capsules.

But just because I don't eat organ meats doesn't mean that you shouldn't eat them. Supplementing with organ meat capsules isn't as beneficial as eating organ meat, however, and there definitely are ways you can sneak organ meat into your diet. For example, if you're eating a beef burger (with no bun, of course!), you can grind up liver (or a different organ meat) and mix it with the beef.

Dr. Sarah Ballantyne recommends a 1:1 to a 1:2 ratio of liver to ground meat if you have a mild-flavored liver (i.e., bison, lamb, or chicken). So, for example, if you have two pounds of ground meat, you would add one or two pounds of liver. On the other hand, for stronger-flavored livers (i.e., beef and pork), she recommends using a 1:3 to a 1:5 ratio.

How much organ meat should you ideally eat per week? Dr. Terry Wahls, author of the Wahls Protocol, recommends eating a total of twelve ounces of organ meats per week. She recommends having six ounces of liver per week and six ounces of other organ meats. By the way, Dr. Wahls reversed her autoimmune condition (multiple sclerosis) in part by eating a nutrient-dense diet.

Level 3 Hyperthyroid Healing Diet Variations

As I mentioned earlier, this diet is similar to an AIP Diet, but with the following variations:

- **Follow a low- to moderate- iodine diet.** I don't have anything against iodine, as I realize it's an important mineral, and in the past I actually had a positive experience when supplementing with iodine. The truth is that everyone is different, as some people do perfectly fine with eating foods higher in iodine, such as sea vegetables. On the other hand, in some people with hyperthyroidism, a higher iodine diet might exacerbate their condition and prevent them from restoring their health. So whether you have Graves' disease, toxic multinodular goiter, or a different hyperthyroid condition, you might want to at least consider eating a low- to moderate-iodine diet while trying to restore your health.

But what do I mean by a low- to moderate-iodine diet? Well, some practitioners recommend not exceeding 200 mcg of iodine per day. I don't think most people need to stay this low if they're getting iodine mostly from food sources. That being said, if you're someone who enjoys eating sea vegetables on a daily basis, then I'd be cautious, especially when eating kelp.

I find that many people with hyperthyroidism, including those with Graves' disease, can tolerate at least 500 mcg/day of iodine. So, for example, if someone takes a multivitamin that has 150 mcg of iodine, they most likely can still eat some other foods that have some iodine, including seafood that isn't too high in iodine. (I'll include additional information about iodine in food in the resources.)

It's worth mentioning that while wild fish is preferred, on average, wild fish tends to exhibit higher iodine concentrations than farmed fish.[8] However,

69

one study showed that no significant differences were observed between wild and farmed Atlantic salmon, rainbow trout, and turbot.[8]

That being said, a number of different factors can influence the iodine content of seafood. It's also worth mentioning that on average, shellfish are higher in iodine than marine and freshwater fish.[8] And marine fish are typically higher in iodine than freshwater fish.[8] Shellfish is divided into crustaceans (shrimp, crab, lobster) and mollusks/bivalves (clams, mussels, oysters, scallops, octopus, squid, snail). Not all of these are extremely high in iodine, as while oysters and lobsters tend to be higher in iodine, squid isn't as high.

Some people tend to run into trouble when taking higher-dose iodine supplements, and while some people have successfully used high-dose iodine as a way of managing hyperthyroidism, because iodine is involved in the production of thyroid hormone, too much iodine can cause more harm than good in some people. Since everyone is different, I would try to limit foods that contain very high amounts of iodine, especially sea vegetables.

- **Eat fish and other types of seafood no more than three times per week.** I have already expressed some concern about iodine and seafood, but there are other reasons you should be concerned about eating too much fish. While in a perfect world I'd love for people to get most of their omega-3 fatty acids from fish, I'm definitely concerned about the environmental pollutants. And it's not just heavy metals in fish (and other types of seafood), but other potentially harmful chemicals, including organochlorine pesticides and polychlorinated biphenyls (PCBs). Some healthcare practitioners and researchers feel that it's still fine to eat seafood daily, while others recommend completely avoiding fish because of the toxicants, but everything comes down to risks versus benefits, and the truth is that these days almost every food has some level of contamination.

Microplastics are a big concern, as once in the environment, plastic objects degrade and give rise to smaller fragments, which can directly enter the food chain or indirectly contaminate it due to the leaching of their potentially harmful chemicals.[9] The ingestion of food and water contaminated with microplastics is the main route of human exposure.[10] Once ingested, microplastics reach the gastrointestinal tract and can be absorbed, causing oxidative stress, cytotoxicity, and translocation to other tissues.[10]

If you choose to eat fish, I would focus on eating oily coldwater, wild-caught fish, such as wild salmon. Feel free to also eat freshwater whitefish. If you like sardines, these are also a good option. If you're not allergic to shellfish, this can also be an option, although remember that you want to be cautious about eating shellfish that's higher in iodine, such as lobster and oysters.

- **Eat plenty of plant-based foods.** For those following a Paleo or AIP Diet, it's common to eat a lot meat. And while it might be a good idea to increase your meat consumption in order to get sufficient protein, for all three Hyperthyroid Healing Diets I would try to eat at least five servings of vegetables per day. For those who already eat a lot of vegetables, this probably won't be too big of a deal, but for others it will be a challenge.

I personally didn't eat a lot of vegetables when I was a child, teenager, and young adult. In fact, I really didn't eat any vegetables as a child and teenager, and while I finally started eating some vegetables in adulthood, it wasn't until after my Graves' disease diagnosis that I began eating them regularly. Even at that point I can't say that I immediately started eating five servings of vegetables per day, as it was admittedly a gradual process.

And I need to mention that it's not just the quantity of vegetables that's important, but also the variety. In fact, this might be even more important than the quantity. But either way, I would try to eat at least ten to fifteen different vegetables per week.

71

The Different Hyperthyroid Healing Diets

If you're currently only eating two or three different vegetables in total, then I realize this probably will be a gradual process. Try to add one new vegetable per week until you're eating at least ten different ones on a weekly basis. Of course on a daily basis I don't expect you to eat ten different vegetables (although you could if you wanted to!), as once you build up to ten veggies per week I'd say to try to eat at least three to five different vegetables each day. I'm personally at the point where I have five to seven different vegetables per day, but it took me awhile to get to this point.

Should you eat your vegetables raw or cooked? I recommend a combination of both, as while I'd say that approximately 75 percent of the vegetables I eat are raw, it's perfectly fine to eat 50 percent raw and 50 percent cooked. But you also need to listen to your body. If you are unable to tolerate raw vegetables at this time, then feel free to stick with cooked vegetables, and hopefully as your health improves you'll be able to introduce some raw ones.

- **Limit very-high-oxalate foods.** Chapter 16 is dedicated to oxalates, and if you're not familiar with oxalates, then I definitely would read that chapter. But I'll say here that eating a lot of high-oxalate foods can cause health issues, and some of the foods high in oxalates include spinach, Swiss chard, sweet potatoes, beets, blackberries, and raspberries. This doesn't mean that you need to eliminate all of these, but at the very least I would greatly minimize spinach, Swiss chard, blackberries, and raspberries. The reason for this is that you can easily substitute other green leafy vegetables (i.e., arugula, green leaf lettuce) and berries (i.e., blueberries).

I know some reading this might be shocked that I mentioned sweet potatoes, and I discuss this in greater deal in chapter 16. All I'll say here is that if you do enough searching on the internet, you can find a reason to avoid most healthy foods, and you can definitely overdo it when following a restrictive diet. As a result, I still have my patients with hyperthyroidism eat sweet potatoes.

- **Eat some healthy fats.** Whereas a ketogenic diet focuses on eating a high amount of fat, both an AIP and standard Paleo Diet focus more on eating a higher amount of protein. And while I agree that you want to get a good amount of protein, I also would make sure you are eating a good amount of healthy fats on a daily basis. I spoke about fats in chapter 4 and mentioned how you want to get between 20 and 30 percent of your daily calories from fat.

To Ghee or Not to Ghee?

Speaking of healthy fats, ghee is a form of dairy, and an AIP Diet excludes dairy, so it would make sense that ghee should also be excluded, right? This was the approach I took for many years, but then I realized that some advocates of the AIP Diet, including Julie Michelson, who I interviewed on the *Save My Thyroid* podcast, allow their autoimmune patients to consume ghee. They probably wouldn't do this if it wasn't well tolerated, so having some ghee is probably okay for many people with Graves' disease.

My Thoughts on the Carnivore Diet

I'm sure some reading this are familiar with the carnivore diet, which is a diet that involves eating only animal-based foods (red meat, poultry, organ meat, fish, eggs) while avoiding all plant-based foods (vegetables, fruit, nuts, seeds, grains, legumes). The main reason why these foods are excluded is to avoid certain toxins that are present in plant-based foods, which include lectins, phytates, glycoalkaloids, and oxalates.

While there isn't much in the research when it comes to the carnivore diet and autoimmune conditions such as Graves' disease, if you visit online forums and groups related to the carnivore diet, you no doubt will find people with different autoimmune conditions who greatly benefited from following this type of a diet. Based on this you may wonder if you should eat any plant-based foods, let alone eat as many as I suggested earlier in this chapter.

As you know by now, there is no diet that fits everyone perfectly. And even though there are three different Hyperthyroid Healing Diet versions mentioned in this book, this doesn't mean that you can't modify them further. While over the years I've found that most people do fine eating a combination of animal-based and plant-based foods, including myself when I dealt with Graves' disease, some people might find they do better sticking solely with animal-based foods on a short-term basis.

I'm just concerned about the long-term impact of the carnivore diet on the gut microbiome. I realize that the proponents of the carnivore diet claim that fiber isn't necessary for the health of the gut microbiome. But this isn't supported by the research, as there are many studies showing the health benefits of fiber.

I should mention that a 2021 journal article looked at the changes in the gut microbiota after a four-week intervention with a vegan versus a meat-rich diet, and it showed that alpha diversity and beta diversity did not differ significantly between these two diets.[11] However, this involved a small number of people over a short period of time, so it will be interesting to see what future studies show involving following such a diet for many months, and even years.

How Long Should You Follow a Level 3 Diet?

The Level 3 Diet isn't meant to be a long-term diet, although how long someone needs to follow this for depends on the person. For example, the Level 3 Diet also serves as an elimination diet, and many healthcare professionals recommend for their patients to follow an elimination diet strictly for thirty days. This is the approach I take in my practice, although ninety days would be even better.

Ultimately it's up to you, as after thirty days some people choose to slowly reintroduce some foods, while others will continue to follow the diet for a couple of additional months. If after thirty days someone is thriving while following the diet, then it makes sense for them to continue to follow it for at least a few additional months. If someone feels worse after thirty days of following the diet, then it might be best for them to reintroduce foods.

It's worth mentioning that some people aren't necessarily thriving after thirty days, but they are feeling somewhat better, yet they find following this diet to be a major struggle. In this situation it probably is best to have the person continue with the diet and re-evaluate after two to four weeks. While some people will experience physical symptoms, there is a mental aspect as well.

For example, if someone started following the Level 3 Diet with the mindset that they would need to be strict for three months, this would be more mentally challenging than planning on being strict with the diet for thirty days and then taking it on a month-to-month basis after that. Of course, everyone is different, as some people don't find following such a restrictive diet to be a struggle at all (at least that's what some patients tell me!), while others are thinking about reintroducing foods after one or two weeks.

More on Reintroductions and a Level 3 Diet

Two questions you might have are, "When can I reintroduce foods?" and, "In what order?" As I just mentioned, ideally you would want to follow a Level 3 Diet for at least three months. At this point, if you want to go longer, it's fine, but if you're ready to reintroduce foods, that's also perfectly fine. And if you're stressed out and struggling after thirty or sixty days then it's okay to reintroduce foods earlier. As for how to reintroduce foods and in what order, I would refer to chapter 11 for more information.

Should Everyone with Graves' Disease Follow a Level 3 Diet?

Ideally, a Level 3 Diet should be the starting point for those with Graves' disease. However, I realize that there isn't a single diet that fits everyone perfectly, which of course is why there are other diet options in this book. If you have Graves' disease and feel stressed out about following a Level 3 Diet, then feel free to begin with a Level 2 or Level 1 Diet instead. Those are still very healthy diets.

I have already mentioned a couple of times in this chapter that you should listen to your body. If you start with a Level 3 Diet but after a few days or weeks don't feel like it's a good fit for you, then of course feel free to switch to a different one. But how do you know if it's a good fit for you? In other words, if you start with the Level 3 Diet (or any other diet), how do you know if it truly is the best diet for you to follow?

The truth is that there is no surefire way to know that any diet is the best one for you initially after starting it. Obviously, if someone is completely miserable, then they probably can conclude that it's not a good fit. On the contrary, if someone feels truly amazing upon following it, then they probably can conclude it's a good fit. But how about if someone doesn't feel any better or worse?

This actually describes a lot of people who follow diets in general, as while it's common for people to notice an improvement in their symptoms upon eating whole, healthy foods, this isn't the case with everyone. This doesn't necessarily mean that the diet isn't benefiting you, but it likely means that there are other triggers and/or underlying imbalances that need to be addressed. So I wouldn't be discouraged if you don't notice any symptomatic improvements within a few weeks of changing your diet, as everyone is different.

What Diet Did I Follow When I Dealt with Graves' Disease?

Just as a reminder, I was diagnosed with Graves' disease in 2008, and I didn't have the knowledge that I have now. So I initially followed a standard Paleo Diet, although at the time I wasn't a big egg eater, and I also didn't eat many nightshades, other than some tomato sauce and white potatoes. I did give these up while I was trying to regain my health, but I didn't give up nuts and seeds, mainly because I didn't know any better.

To make a long story short, before achieving a state of remission, I hit a roadblock in my recovery. Overall, my health was improving, but on the saliva panel I did, there's a marker called *secretory IgA* that was depressed initially, and upon retesting a few months later, it remained depressed, even though my adrenal markers (cortisol and DHEA) had improved. Secretory IgA lines the mucosal cells of the body, including the gastrointestinal tract. At the time I wasn't sure if it was related to the nuts and seeds I was eating, but I ended up taking a break from them for a few months, and the secretory IgA normalized upon retesting.

Is it possible that this was a coincidence and the secretory IgA would have normalized regardless of whether I avoided the nuts and seeds? Perhaps, but there is no question that nuts and seeds can be harsh on the gut. Just to play it safe, I think it's best to avoid nuts and seeds when following a Level 3 Diet.

Once again, I share this story not to convince everyone with Graves' disease to follow a Level 3 Diet, as some of my patients have followed less restrictive diets and still restored their health. And perhaps if I had soaked and sprouted the nuts and seeds, or only ate ones lower in lectins and oxalates I wouldn't have hit this roadblock. I'm not sure, but the point is that I still showed some improvement when I was eating the nuts and seeds, but apparently had to give them up for awhile in order for my health to further improve.

Can You Combine a Level 3 Diet with Others?

I would recommend not combining this diet with other types of diets, unless absolutely necessary. The reason for this is that it's very restrictive, and I'd hate for anyone to have to give up even more foods. For example, in chapter 18 I discuss how if someone has Graves' disease and small intestinal bacterial overgrowth (SIBO), it might be best to first follow a SIBO-related diet (i.e., low FODMAP) and eradicate the SIBO. Then once this has been done, they can make the transition to the Level 3 Hyperthyroid Healing Diet.

Similarly, in Chapter 16 I discuss oxalates, and after reading that chapter you might be concerned about eating higher oxalate foods. While I would make an attempt to avoid foods that are extremely high in oxalates and have good substitutes (i.e. spinach), I wouldn't stress out about avoiding all of the higher oxalate foods…especially if you're following a Level 3 Diet. Once again, I'll discuss this more in Chapter 16.

Will Following a Level 3 Diet Cause Nutrient Deficiencies?

As a reminder, the Level 3 Diet isn't meant to be a long-term diet, but this isn't out of concern that people will become deficient in certain nutrients. Even though it's a restrictive diet, the allowed foods are nutrient dense. And while some of the excluded foods are also nutrient dense, such as eggs, nuts, and seeds, you can still get all the nutrients you need from the diet.

While meat is nutrient dense, especially when it is from a quality source, vegetables are also excellent sources of nutrients. One problem is that most people don't eat enough vegetables per day, and another problem is that many people who eat plenty of vegetables don't eat enough variety. I realize that for people who don't enjoy eating vegetables, this can be challenging, but one strategy is to "sneak" in some vegetables by adding them to a daily smoothie.

In addition, how you prepare your vegetables can make a huge difference with regard to taste. For example, I don't enjoy eating plain steamed broccoli. On the other hand, if I add garlic and olive oil to the broccoli, then I find that it tastes much better. You might prefer to add something else, and while I can't say that I'm very creative in the kitchen, that's what cookbooks are for!

Summary of What You Can Eat on a Level 3 Diet

So let's summarize the categories of foods that you can eat on a Level 3 Hyperthyroid Healing Diet:

- Meat (beef, lamb, pork, etc.)
- Poultry (chicken, turkey, duck, etc.)
- Organ meats
- Fish and other seafood low in mercury and not too high in iodine (i.e., wild salmon, sardines)
- Vegetables (excluding nightshades)
- Fruit (preferably lower in sugar, such as wild blueberries, strawberries, and cranberries)
- Mushrooms
- Cassava, green bananas, green mangos, green plantains, jicama, parsnips, rutabaga, sweet potatoes, taro, tiger nuts, turnips, and yucca
- Coconut products (unsweetened coconut yogurt, coconut milk, coconut kefir, etc.)
- Ghee
- Spices (excluding seed-based and nightshade-based spices such as cayenne, celery seed, chili powder, fenugreek, and paprika)
- Honey and pure maple syrup (in moderation)
- Certain flours in moderation (coconut flour, tapioca flour, cassava flour)
- Green tea in moderation (due to the caffeine), herbal teas
- Bone broth
- Kombucha

- Collagen powder
- Hydrolyzed beef powder

Level 3 Hyperthyroid Healing Diet Yes/No List

To make it easier to follow each diet, I have created a yes/no list of each one, which includes a comprehensive list of foods that you can and can't eat. To access the list for the Level 3 Hyperthyroid Healing Diet, visit the resources at **savemythyroid.com/HHDNotes**.

Chapter 5 Highlights

- The Level 3 Hyperthyroid Healing Diet is the most restrictive diet, and it's similar to an Autoimmune Paleo (AIP) Diet, also known as the Autoimmune Protocol.
- Ideally, those with Graves' disease should start with a Level 3 Diet.
- One purpose of the Level 3 Diet is to focus on eating nutrient-dense foods while at the same time avoiding inflammatory foods, including common allergens such as gluten, dairy, and corn.
- Another goal of the diet is to exclude foods higher in certain compounds that can have a negative effect on the gut.
- While following any of the three Hyperthyroid Healing Diets, you shouldn't be restricting calories.
- If you're a vegan or vegetarian, then you probably won't be able to get enough protein if you're following a Level 3 Diet.
- Whether you have Graves' disease, toxic multinodular goiter, or a different hyperthyroid condition, you might want to consider eating a low- to moderate-iodine diet while trying to restore your health.
- While it might be a good idea to increase your meat consumption in order to get sufficient protein, for all three Hyperthyroid Healing Diets I would try to eat at least five servings of vegetables per day.
- The Level 3 Diet isn't meant to be a long-term diet, although I would follow it for at least 30 days, and 90 days would be even better.
- If you have Graves' disease and feel stressed out about following a Level 3 Diet, then feel free to begin with a Level 2 or Level 1 Diet instead.

To access the book references and resources, visit SaveMyThyroid.com/HHDNotes.

CHAPTER
6

Hyperthyroid Healing Diet Level 2

n this chapter I will discuss the Level 2 Hyperthyroid Healing Diet. The Level 2 Diet is similar to a standard Paleo Diet. However, there are a few important variations, which I'll discuss in this chapter.

As for who should follow this diet, this is a good starting point for those with a non-autoimmune hyperthyroid condition, such as toxic multinodular goiter. It's also a good fit for those with Graves' disease who find the Level 3 Diet to be too challenging/restrictive to follow. If the latter describes you, keep in mind that you can always start with the Level 2 Diet and gradually transition to the Level 3 Diet. Or you can just stick with the Level 2 Diet and see how much your health improves.

Since the Level 2 Diet is similar to a Paleo Diet, I think it would be a good idea to discuss what the Paleo Diet entails. The Paleo Diet is based on the diet that our Paleolithic ancestors followed. As Dr. Loren Cordain mentioned in his book *The Paleo Diet*, there was no single Paleo Diet, as our ancient ancestors made the most of their environment. In other words, they ate what was readily available.

Whereas the ketogenic diet is a high-fat, low-carbohydrate, low- to moderate-protein diet, the Paleo Diet is a high-protein, low-carbohydrate, moderate-fat diet. Although I mention "low carbohydrate," the Paleo Diet usually isn't as extreme as the ketogenic diet when it comes to reducing carbohydrates, which is a big reason why the ketogenic diet can be more effective for people looking to lose weight. That being said, many people who follow a Paleo Diet for weight loss purposes also successfully shed unwanted pounds.

Here is a bulleted list of foods that are allowed on a standard Paleo Diet:

- Lean meats and poultry (beef, pork, lamb, chicken, turkey)
- Organ meats (liver, heart, kidney, etc.)
- Fish and other types of seafood (salmon, trout, sardines)
- Fruit
- Vegetables
- Mushrooms
- Eggs
- Nuts and seeds
- Healthy oils (olive oil, coconut oil, avocado oil)
- Spices (excluding nightshade-based spices such as cayenne, chili powder, and paprika)
- Honey and pure maple syrup (in moderation)
- Certain flours in moderation (coconut flour, tapioca flour, cassava flour)
- Green tea in moderation, herbal teas

Level 2 Hyperthyroid Healing Diet Variations

Some of the variations of the Level 3 Diet will also apply to the Level 2 Diet. You can refer back to chapter 5 for greater detail, but just to summarize, you'll want to consider following a low- to moderate-iodine diet (although make sure you read the rest of this chapter, as I expand on this), limit your consumption of seafood to three times per week, and eat a good variety of plant-based foods. There are also a few additional variations you will want to make:

- **Avoid nuts and seeds higher in lectins and oxalates.** This is based on the research of Dr. Steven Gundry and Sally K. Norton. Dr. Gundry is the author of the excellent book *The Plant Paradox*. While a standard Paleo Diet allows all nuts and seeds, certain nuts and seeds that are high in lectins should be avoided while restoring your health. You also want to be cautious about eating too many nuts high in oxalates.

  According to Dr. Gundry, raw almonds, cashews, and chia seeds are high in lectins, and Sally K. Norton, author of the fascinating book *Toxic Superfoods,* mentions how these are high in oxalates as well. However, there is a difference in opinion with other nuts and seeds. For example, Brazil nuts seem to be okay from a lectin standpoint, but not an oxalate standpoint. That being said, I think eating a couple of Brazil nuts per day is fine.

  Dr. Gundry recommends avoiding pumpkin seeds and sunflower seeds, but I haven't seen a source that shows that pumpkin seeds are high in lectins, and Sally Norton's research shows that they are low in oxalates, and she mentions that both sprouted pumpkin seeds and sunflower seeds are fine to consume. I would agree that sprouted pumpkin and sunflower seeds are okay to eat on a Level 2 Diet. Both Dr. Gundry and Sally Norton agree that flaxseeds are fine to consume. And even though peanuts are a legume and not a nut, I'll still let you know that both Dr. Gundry and Sally Norton feel that peanuts should be avoided as well.

  Walnuts and pecans are considered to be lower in lectins according to Dr. Gundry, and also don't seem to be too high in oxalates according to Sally K. Norton's book. However, I'll admit that there is some conflicting information. Under the Worst Offending Nuts, Sally lists in her book "almonds, cashews, pecans, pine nuts, and walnuts," but I wonder if this is mistake, as elsewhere it shows that seventeen pecan halves have only 18 mg of oxalates per serving, while fourteen walnut halves have only 16 mg of oxalates per serving. Therefore I think both of these are fine to consume. Macadamia nuts and pistachios are considered to be lower in lectins, according to Dr. Gundry, and moderate in oxalates, so I think these are also fine in moderation.

As I already mentioned, Brazil nuts seem to be okay from a lectin standpoint, and they are very popular for those who have thyroid conditions, as many are aware that they are high in selenium. While I do enjoy eating Brazil nuts, I wouldn't rely on them as your source of selenium when correcting a selenium deficiency. The reason for this is that you don't know how much selenium you'll be getting in a single nut. I discuss this in greater detail in chapter 25. Sally Norton says that Brazil nuts are higher in oxalates, but as I just mentioned, I think eating a couple of them per day is fine for most people.

To clear up any confusion, these are the nuts and seeds that should be fine to eat on a Level 2 Diet, although I would still limit your consumption to 1/2 cup per day:

Macadamia nuts
Pistachios
Walnuts
Pecans
Brazil nuts (two or three per day)
Flaxseeds
Sprouted pumpkin seeds
Sprouted sunflower seeds

I do want to add that after restoring your health, I think it's okay to eat some of the other nuts occasionally, but that's just my opinion. If you were to ask Sally Norton if it's okay for a person in good health to occasionally have almonds or cashews, my guess is that she would say no. But from a personal standpoint I can't say that I never eat those nuts, and I even eat peanuts a few times per year (which, once again, is a legume and not a nut).

Also, if you read the "Mold in Food" chapter (chapter 17), you'll notice that I mention some nuts are commonly contaminated with mold. This includes pistachios, walnuts, pecans, and Brazil nuts. The truth is that you can drive yourself crazy trying to eliminate everything that can be potentially harmful to your health. If you know or suspect that mold might be an issue, or if you hit a roadblock in your recovery, then I would try to avoid nuts that are more likely to be contaminated with mold, but otherwise I wouldn't be as concerned.

- **Avoid the nightshades.** Just a reminder that this includes tomatoes, eggplant, peppers, and white potatoes. Unlike an AIP Diet, nightshades are allowed on a standard Paleo Diet, and they do have some wonderful health benefits. That being said, if you have Graves' disease and choose to follow a Level 2 Diet because the Level 3 Diet is too restrictive, I would still try to avoid the nightshades for all the same reasons I mentioned in the previous chapter. Although you can't always go by symptoms, I will say that many people who react to nightshades do experience symptoms, including digestive symptoms, joint pain, and headaches.

- **Certain protein powders are allowed.** I understand the challenges some will have with getting enough protein through the diet, especially for those who don't want to eat a lot of meat. Hydrolyzed beef protein (from grass-fed cows) would be my first recommendation for those who want to use a protein powder as a supplemental form of protein. A good-quality bone broth or collagen protein powder are other options to consider. Even though I listed this under the Level 2 Diet, I don't see why these can't also be part of a Level 3 Diet, provided they are of good quality. For specific recommendations, check out the resources by visiting **savemythyroid.com/HHDNotes.**

How about pea protein? While peas are high in lectins, which is why they're excluded from both an AIP Diet and a standard Paleo Diet, some sources suggest that pea protein powder isn't as high in lectins. Quite frankly there's not a lot of research on this, but I can say that some other practitioners and I have recommended pea protein powder to our patients without a problem. I'm not suggesting that this would be my first choice of protein powder, but I wanted to bring it up for those who feel the need to get some extra protein in their diet and don't want to use an animal-based protein powder.

Can Dark Chocolate Be Eaten?

You'll notice that I didn't include dark chocolate as part of a Level 3 Hyperthyroid Healing Diet. The truth is that dark chocolate has some wonderful health benefits, as it contains several health-promoting factors (bioactive components—polyphenols, flavonoids, procyanidins, theobromines, etc., and vitamins and minerals) that positively modulate the immune system.[1] Dark chocolate is considered a functional food due to its anti-diabetic, anti-inflammatory, and anti-microbial properties.[1]

So why is dark chocolate excluded from an AIP/Level 3 Diet? In a 2017 article I wrote, I mentioned how dark chocolate has a high amount of phytic acid, which can prevent the absorption of certain nutrients. Cacao beans carry the highest amount of phytic acid, but even after refinement, some portion of this remains. According to Dr. Sarah Ballantyne, another reason why cocoa is excluded from an AIP Diet is that several studies show that cacao polyphenols suppress Th2 and increase Th1 helper T cell activity, which may or may not be helpful depending on the details of immune function in each individual.[2]

I should also mention that recently Consumer Reports revealed through their testing that a third of chocolate products are high in heavy metals . . . specifically lead and cadmium. This isn't the reason dark chocolate has been excluded from an AIP Diet in the past, although it, without question, is a reason for concern. In the resources, I'll include an article from Consumer Reports that lists the sources of dark chocolate that are considered to be safer choices, although keep in mind that these still aren't completely free of heavy metals.

In addition, dark chocolate is high in oxalates. And the higher the cacao content, the higher the oxalate content. According to the book *Toxic Superfoods* by Sally K. Norton, 1.75 ounces (50 grams) of 70 percent dark chocolate has 110 mg of oxalates per serving, while the same amount of 85 percent dark chocolate has 140 mg of oxalates. It's worth mentioning that most people don't eat 50 grams of dark chocolate per day, as one small square of dark chocolate equals approximately 10 grams. And so one square of dark chocolate will have approximately 28 grams of oxalates.

Now you know a few different reasons to consider excluding dark chocolate. Everything comes down to risks versus benefits, though, and while you certainly can completely eliminate dark chocolate from your diet permanently, I still have a small amount of dark chocolate on a regular basis, and I think it's fine for most people following a Level 2 or Level 1 Diet to also have a small amount of dark chocolate on a daily basis (i.e., 10 to 20 grams). With regard to the heavy metals, I would just make sure to stick with the safer choices, as well as continuously do things to support detoxification, which I discuss in chapter 24.

I also should mention that carob powder is a good substitute for chocolate, and is allowed on all three Hyperthyroid Healing Diets. While it doesn't taste exactly like chocolate, many people who are trying to avoid chocolate enjoy eating carob. And like dark chocolate, carob has numerous health benefits.

For Those with Toxic Multinodular Goiter

If you have toxic multinodular goiter, then you probably will need to make some slight modifications to this diet. The three main causes of toxic multinodular goiter include (1) problems with estrogen metabolism, (2) insulin resistance, and (3) an iodine deficiency. As for determining if you have an estrogen metabolism problem, you can consider doing a dried urine test to look at the estrogen metabolites, which I discuss in chapter 27. However, if in addition to thyroid nodules you also have a history of ovarian cysts, uterine fibroids, and/or endometriosis, then there is a very good chance that you have an estrogen metabolism problem.

From a food perspective, in order to support estrogen metabolism, I would make sure to eat plenty of cruciferous vegetables, especially broccoli. I would also encourage you to eat broccoli sprouts, which do a wonderful job of supporting estrogen metabolism. If you are unable to find broccoli sprouts locally at a health food store or farmer's market, you can either consider growing your own, or you can just focus on eating broccoli, Brussels sprouts, cauliflower, kale, etc.

As for insulin resistance, while many people with hyperthyroidism will get a fasting glucose done as part of a comprehensive metabolic panel, this isn't sufficient to confirm or rule out insulin resistance. Hemoglobin A1C is a marker I commonly recommend, although I would go a step further and also do a fasting insulin test. Fast for ten to twelve hours before the blood draw, and while ideally you want the fasting insulin to be below 5 μIU/mL, if it's above 7 μIU/mL, I'd be concerned, especially if the hemoglobin A1C is greater than 5.5 percent, although from an optimal standpoint you want the hemoglobin A1C to be 5 percent or less.

If insulin resistance is confirmed, then eating a low-carbohydrate, low-sugar diet is essential. Exercise can also be beneficial. However, eating well alone might not be enough to overcome insulin resistance. I discuss insulin resistance more in chapter 14, but I will say here that there usually is an inflammatory component that needs to be addressed, and diet and exercise alone might not be sufficient.

Should Phytoestrogens Be Avoided?

I probably should also briefly chat about phytoestrogens. Phytoestrogens are compounds that are derived from plants, and they have weak estrogenic or antiestrogenic activity.[3] There is a great deal of confusion as to whether phytoestrogens are safe to consume, or if they should be avoided.

The major groups of phytoestrogens include isoflavones, lignans, and coumestans. Isoflavones are mostly found in soy products, although some other foods have them as well. The most studied isoflavones include genistein and daidzein. Lignans are abundant in flax, although these compounds can be present in other foods as well, such as sesame seeds, grains, and even some fruits and vegetables.[4] For example, brassica vegetables (broccoli, cabbage, etc.) include high levels of lignans.[4] Coumestans are another type of phytoestrogen, and some food sources include split peas, pinto beans, and lima beans.

There are numerous studies that demonstrate the health benefits of phytoestrogens. For example, genistein inhibits the activity of protein tyrosine kinases in numerous tissues, including breast cancer cells. Phytoestrogens are also considered to be good antioxidants and anti-inflammatory agents. This is especially true regarding genistein and resveratrol.

Flaxseed is the richest source of lignans, and flaxseed lignans have been shown to reduce the risk of hormone-dependent cancers of the breast, uterus, and prostate.[5] One study showed that supplementation with flaxseed alters estrogen metabolism in postmenopausal women to a greater extent than supplementation with an equal amount of soy.[6] This caused increased concentrations of 2-hydroxyestrone, which is considered to be the "good" estrogen metabolite.

Overall I think that consuming food sources of phytoestrogens by adults can be beneficial. Of course cruciferous vegetables are very healthy, as are berries, and others such as flaxseed, curcumin, and resveratrol can have certain health benefits as well. Soy is more controversial, as while there are some health benefits of eating organic fermented soy, while healing, I recommend avoiding soy due to the reasons I mentioned in chapter 3.

The Iodine Controversy

I spoke about iodine in chapter 5, but I want to expand on this topic here. Iodine is controversial in the world of thyroid health, and it's no exception with toxic multinodular goiter. A few studies have shown that toxic multinodular goiter is more common in populations that are iodine deficient .[7,8] The latter study was interesting in that it showed that the incidence of Graves' disease was significantly higher in Iceland, where they had a high iodine intake.

Based on this, one can make the argument that those with Graves' disease should consider following a low iodine diet, while it might not be as big of a concern for those with toxic multinodular goiter. However, there is some evidence that too much iodine can be a factor in the formation of thyroid nodules,[9] so even if you have a toxic multinodular goiter I would still be cautious about consuming too much iodine. Again, it's controversial because an iodine deficiency can also be a factor when it comes to thyroid nodules, but there also are situations when too much iodine can be a factor in the formation of thyroid nodules.

But how much iodine is too much? This really does depend on the person, as in the previous chapter I mentioned how some practitioners recommend for those with thyroid conditions to limit their daily iodine intake to 200mcg.

While this might be necessary in some cases, I'd say that many people can exceed this (i.e., 500mcg), although more people will run into problems when they consume milligram doses.

This admittedly is more of a concern with iodine supplements, but in some people it can be problematic with foods high in iodine as well. Just to play it safe I would avoid sea vegetables while healing, along with seafood higher in iodine (refer back to chapter 5), and I'd also be cautious about taking separate iodine supplements, although I find that most people do fine taking a multivitamin that has iodine.

When Iodine Seems To Help

It's a challenging situation, as there are people who will notice an improvement when consuming foods higher in iodine, and even when taking iodine supplements. For example, while iodine can potentially worsen one's thyroid condition, I've had patients notice a decrease in their goiter when eating foods higher in iodine (or taking an iodine supplement). And so we can make the argument that you should listen to your body, as if you choose to experiment with higher iodine foods and notice positive benefits then why not continue eating them?

I think for some people with toxic multinodular goiter this is a valid argument, but there are still a few concerns. One is that in some cases iodine can worsen hyperthyroidism. Also, for those with Graves' disease, iodine can sometimes exacerbate the autoimmune response. And while sometimes this will result in a worsening of the person's symptoms, other times the only way to know is by seeing the thyroid stimulating immunoglobulins (TSI) increase on a blood test.

It's a bit of a tricky situation, as when I dealt with Graves' disease I didn't make an effort to follow a low-iodine diet, although I probably was doing so since

I wasn't eating a lot of iodine-rich foods. However, I actually supplemented with iodine, as back then it was common for people with both hyperthyroidism/Graves' disease and hypothyroidism/Hashimoto's to supplement with iodine. I did fine with iodine supplementation, but this isn't the case with everyone, which is why I don't encourage people to supplement with iodine while trying to restore their health.

I should mention that I discuss iodine in food in greater detail in the resources, which you can check out by visiting **savemythyroid.com/HHDNotes**.

Are Cruciferous Vegetables a Concern for Hyperthyroidism?

Since I encourage those with toxic multinodular goiter to increase their consumption of cruciferous vegetables, I figured I'd tackle the topic of goitrogenic foods here. Goitrogenic foods can potentially suppress the function of the thyroid gland, and they accomplish this by interfering with the uptake of iodine. This, in turn, can result in the formation of a goiter, which is an enlargement of the thyroid gland. There are also *environmental goitrogens*, which are certain substances or chemicals that can inhibit the production of thyroid hormone.

According to the literature, the following foods have been identified as being goitrogenic:[10]

- Broccoli
- Brussels sprouts
- Cabbage
- Cauliflower
- Mustard greens
- Radishes
- Millet
- Spinach

- Cassava
- Peanuts
- Soybeans
- Strawberries
- Sweet potatoes
- Peaches
- Pears
- Green tea

The focus here will be on cruciferous vegetables, although much of what I say will apply to other potentially goitrogenic foods as well. First of all, I just want to remind you that this is a book on hyperthyroidism, so even if goitrogens were to suppress thyroid hormone production, this wouldn't necessarily be a bad thing. In fact, I think most people would prefer to eat a lot of broccoli instead of taking methimazole!

But for those who are thinking about using cruciferous vegetables and other goitrogenic foods to manage their hyperthyroid symptoms, I'll say here that in most people, this won't be effective. And the reason I know this is because I tried this in the past with some of my hyperthyroid patients, specifically women with hyperthyroidism who were pregnant and didn't want to take antithyroid medication. Unfortunately, eating larger amounts of raw cruciferous vegetables didn't have much of an impact with regard to lowering thyroid hormone levels.

Can Soy Be Used to Lower Thyroid Hormones?

Some sources suggest that soy is more goitrogenic than cruciferous vegetables, but to be upfront, I've never had my hyperthyroid patients consume large amounts of soy in an attempt to lower their thyroid hormones. But before you give this a try, you might want to refer to a 2019 meta-analysis which showed that while soy supplementation modestly raises TSH levels, it has no effect on the thyroid hormones.[11] And there are reasons why I recommend that people avoid soy, which I discuss in chapter 3.

So I definitely encourage my patients to eat cruciferous vegetables, but it has nothing to do with their goitrogenic properties. The reason I recommend them is because they are very nutrient dense, are beneficial to the gut microbiome, and can support estrogen metabolism. Recent studies also show that a higher intake of cruciferous vegetables may benefit cardiovascular health by protecting against abdominal aortic calcification.[12]

For Those with Subacute Thyroiditis

If you have subacute thyroiditis, then I think a Level 2 Hyperthyroid Healing Diet is a good starting point. One thing to keep in mind is that viruses are the most common cause of subacute thyroiditis, so you almost have to look at this as more of an immune condition than a thyroid condition, which of course is also the case with Graves' disease. The reason for this perspective is that we all get exposed to viruses, but we don't all develop subacute thyroiditis.

So while this isn't an autoimmune condition like Graves' disease, I would still do everything you can to optimize your immune health. It wouldn't be unreasonable for people with subacute thyroiditis to follow a Level 3 Hyperthyroid Healing Diet initially. That being said, unless you have known gut issues, I think starting with a Level 2 Diet is perfectly fine for those with subacute thyroiditis.

For Those with Subclinical Hyperthyroidism

A Level 2 Hyperthyroid Healing Diet is also a good diet to follow for those with subclinical hyperthyroidism without an autoimmune component. For example, if someone has a low or depressed TSH in the presence of normal thyroid hormones, and if the thyroid antibodies are negative, then they should consider following a Level 2 Hyperthyroid Healing Diet. On the other hand, if someone has subclinical Graves' disease, where the thyroid hormones are normal but the thyroid antibodies are elevated, then they should follow a Level 3 Hyperthyroid Healing Diet.

Summary of What You Can Eat On a Level 2 Diet

Let's summarize the categories of foods you can eat on a Level 2 Hyperthyroid Healing Diet:

- Meat (beef, lamb, pork, etc.)
- Poultry (chicken, turkey, duck, etc.)
- Organ meats
- Fish and other seafood low in mercury and not too high in iodine (i.e., wild salmon, sardines)
- Vegetables (excluding nightshades)
- Fruit (preferably lower in sugar, such as wild blueberries, strawberries, and cranberries)
- Mushrooms
- Cassava, green bananas, green mangos, green plantains, jicama, parsnips, rutabaga, sweet potatoes, taro, tiger nuts, turnips, and yucca
- Eggs
- Nuts and seeds that aren't very high in lectins and oxalates (pistachios, macadamia nuts, walnuts, pecans, sprouted pumpkin seeds, sprouted sunflower seeds)
- Coconut products (unsweetened coconut yogurt, coconut milk, coconut kefir, etc.)
- Ghee
- Spices (excluding seed-based and nightshade-based spices such as cayenne, celery seed, chili powder, fenugreek, and paprika)
- Honey and pure maple syrup (in moderation)
- Certain flours (coconut flour, tapioca flour, cassava flour)

- Green tea in moderation (due to the caffeine), herbal teas
- Bone broth
- Kombucha
- Collagen powder
- Hydrolyzed beef powder
- Dark chocolate in moderation

Level 2 Hyperthyroid Healing Diet Yes/No List

To make it easier to follow each diet, I have created a yes/no list of each one, which includes a comprehensive list of foods that you can and can't eat. To access the list for the Level 2 Hyperthyroid Healing Diet, visit the resources at **savemythyroid.com/HHDNotes.**

Chapter 6 Highlights

- The Level 2 Hyperthyroid Healing Diet is similar to a Paleo Diet and is a good starting point for those with a non-autoimmune hyperthyroid condition, such as toxic multinodular goiter.
- It's also a good fit for those with Graves' disease who find the Level 3 Diet too challenging to follow.
- Hyperthyroid Healing Diet Level 2 variations include avoiding nuts and seeds higher in lectins and oxalates, avoiding or minimize the nightshades, the use of certain allowed protein powders.
- For those with toxic multinodular goiter, in order to support estrogen metabolism, I would make sure to eat plenty of cruciferous vegetables, especially broccoli, as well as broccoli sprouts.
- There are both benefits and risks when it comes to iodine, but just to play it safe, I would take a break from sea vegetables while healing, and I'd also be cautious about taking separate iodine supplements.
- Consuming goitrogenic foods such as cruciferous vegetables is fine, but they usually aren't effective in lowering thyroid hormone levels.
- If you have subacute thyroiditis, then I think a Level 2 Hyperthyroid Healing Diet is a good starting point.

To access the book references and resources, visit
SaveMyThyroid.com/HHDNotes.

Hyperthyroid Healing Diet Level 1

The Level 1 Hyperthyroid Healing Diet is the most basic diet for hyperthyroidism discussed in this book, although it still has some wonderful health benefits. As for who should follow this diet, while I recommend that most people with a non-autoimmune hyperthyroid condition start with a Level 2 Hyperthyroid Healing Diet, I think many people with hyperthyroidism would do fine starting with a Level 1 Diet. For example, if someone with Graves' disease finds both a Level 3 and Level 2 Diet to be too restrictive, they can always start with a Level 1 Diet and see how they progress.

Those who are vegans and vegetarians will probably want to follow a Level 1 Diet, as this offers a lot more flexibility than the Level 2 Diet. Just to clarify, the Level 1 Diet isn't a strict vegan or vegetarian diet, as it does include meat, fish, and poultry, but of course you can choose to exclude these. Whereas a Level 3 Diet is essentially a modified AIP Diet and a Level 2 Diet is a modified standard Paleo Diet, a Level 1 Diet is a modified Plant Paradox Diet.

While I'm sure many reading this book are familiar with a Paleo Diet, and many are familiar with an AIP Diet, not everyone will be familiar with the

Plant Paradox Diet. This is based on the research of Dr. Steven Gundry and is named after his excellent book *The Plant Paradox*. Like the AIP and standard Paleo Diets, Dr. Gundry recommends avoiding foods higher in lectins, although he makes certain exceptions.

For example, while legumes are excluded from both an AIP and standard Paleo Diet, properly prepared legumes are allowed on a Plant Paradox Diet. The reason is that properly preparing legumes through soaking or pressure cooking can greatly reduce the lectins. And for those concerned that this will decrease the nutrient content, studies don't seem to support this.[1]

Which Foods Can You Eat on the Plant Paradox Diet?

If you want a comprehensive list of everything Dr. Gundry allows, then I would read his book *The Plant Paradox*, but I'll also list some of the options in this chapter, and you can access a more comprehensive yes/no list by visiting the resources at **savemythyroid.com/HHDNotes**. Just keep in mind that I don't agree with everything he allows on his diet, at least concerning those who have hyperthyroidism. And of course that's perfectly fine, as there wouldn't be a reason for me to write this book if there weren't any modifications in any of the three diets (AIP, Paleo, Plant Paradox).

For example, Dr. Gundry includes many dairy products as part of the Plant Paradox Diet, and dairy is excluded in all of the three Hyperthyroid Healing Diets, with the exception of ghee. And there are other things that he allows that are excluded from all three Hyperthyroid Healing Diets. So next I'm going to list some of the foods that are permitted on a Plant Paradox Diet that I also recommend as part of a Level 1 Diet, and then I'll discuss the variations.

- **Most vegetables.** This, of course, is where your focus should be, as eating a good variety of vegetables is important with all three Hyperthyroid Healing Diets. Dr. Gundry does agree that nightshades should be avoided while trying to heal, so just as is the case with the Level 3 and Level 2 Hyperthyroid Healing Diets, I would recommend taking a break from tomatoes, eggplant, peppers, and white potatoes.

- **Fruit.** Dr. Gundry recommends limiting your fruit consumption to one small serving on weekends and only when that fruit is in season. He also highly recommends pomegranate and passion fruit seeds, followed by raspberries, blackberries, strawberries, and then blueberries, grapefruit, pixie tangerines, and kiwifruits. Although I think it's fine to follow his recommendations, in my opinion you don't need to limit your consumption of fruit to one serving per week. Also, since raspberries and blackberries are high in oxalates, I would focus more on wild blueberries, and cranberries are another great option.

How do you know which fruits are in season? If you purchase your fruit at a local farmer's market, then there is a good chance it is in season. Even if you purchase it at a local grocery store, you can usually tell if it is local. If you notice that the fruit is from a different country (i.e., Mexico) then you have no idea whether it is in season, no matter how fresh it looks. You might also be able to find a local produce chart that lists the fruits and vegetables that are in season.

For example, when doing an online search for "produce calendar North Carolina," I came across a PDF that shows the vegetables and fruit in season. According to the produce calendar, apples are in season from August through February, while blueberries are only in season from May through July. Ideally, you want to eat foods that are in season, although I'll admit that this is not something I've been recommending to my patients (and non-patients) over the years, and it hasn't seemed to affect people's overall progress.

- **Lean meats and poultry.** Dr. Gundry recommends limiting your consumption of meat and pastured poultry to four ounces per day each.

However, you want to make sure to get sufficient protein, so it's perfectly fine to exceed this while following any of the Hyperthyroid Healing Diets. As long as you are eating healthier types of meat (i.e., organic, grass-fed) I wouldn't worry about limiting your consumption of meat and poultry.

- **Wild seafood.** Dr. Gundry also recommends limiting your consumption of wild seafood to four ounces per day. As I mentioned in chapter 5, because of the environmental toxicants, I recommend limiting seafood to three times per week, and there are also some concerns with higher iodine seafood, which is why cod, lobster, and oysters are excluded from all three Hyperthyroid Healing Diets, even though they are allowed on a Plant Paradox Diet (not to mention an AIP and standard Paleo Diet). I just want to remind you that I discuss iodine in food in greater detail in the resources, which you can check out by visiting **savemythyroid.com/HHDNotes.**

- **Mushrooms.** Although some categorize mushrooms under "vegetables", they are actually part of the fungi family. Mushrooms are a great option for vegans and vegetarians, but of course omnivores can also enjoy the health benefits! Even though I didn't talk about mushrooms in Chapters 5 and 6 they are allowed on all three Hyperthyroid Healing Diets.

- **Certain nuts and seeds.** I discussed nuts and seeds in detail in chapter 6, but I'll briefly talk about them again here. Dr. Gundry recommends eating 1/2 cup of nuts per day, and I would agree that it's probably best not to exceed this. Some of the nuts he recommends include pistachios, walnuts, pecans, macadamia nuts, hazelnuts, and Brazil nuts in limited quantities. As for almonds, he only allows them blanched and doesn't allow cashews. He allows flaxseeds and hemp seeds but doesn't allow chia seeds, pumpkin seeds, and sunflower seeds. And while peanuts are a legume, I figured I'd mention here that he doesn't allow peanuts, and neither do I.

However, if you read chapter 6, then you're aware that I also recommend avoiding nuts and seeds that are higher in oxalates. I would focus on pistachios, macadamia nuts, walnuts, pecans, sprouted pumpkin and sunflower seeds, and flaxseeds. You'll notice that pumpkin seeds and sunflower seeds are allowed on a Level 1 Diet, even though they are excluded from a Plant Paradox Diet. I think having a couple of Brazil nuts is also fine.

- **Resistant starches.** Resistant starches are starches that are resistant to digestive enzymes and thus have some wonderful benefits to the gut microbiome. The fermentation products of resistant starch by gut bacteria include gases (methane, hydrogen, carbon dioxide) and short-chain fatty acids, which include acetate, propionate, butyrate, and valerate.[2] Some examples of resistance starches that Dr. Gundry recommends that are also allowed on all three Hyperthyroid Healing diets include cassava, green bananas, green mangos, green plantains, jicama, parsnips, rutabaga, sweet potatoes, taro, tiger nuts, turnips, and yucca.

After reading chapter 16 (on oxalates), you might question some of these foods because of their high oxalate content. All I'll say here is that over the years, I've had many people restore their health while eating these foods, and once again, you can drive yourself crazy if you try to eliminate all of the foods higher in oxalates, histamine, mold, etc.

- **Pressure-cooked lentils and other legumes.** According to Dr. Gundry, all beans and lentils are allowed if they are pressure-cooked, as well as pressure-cooked peas and chickpeas. It's worth mentioning that pea protein isolate is allowed, which is commonly used in vegan protein powders. He also allows properly prepared soy, but I would recommend avoiding soy for the reasons mentioned in chapter 3 unless you are 100 percent certain you don't have a soy allergy or sensitivity. However, after someone has restored their health, many people can eat organic fermented soy.

- **Pressure-cooked white basmati rice, millet, sorghum.** Grains are excluded from both an AIP Diet and a standard Paleo Diet, and most grains are also excluded from the Plant Paradox Diet, with the exception of these. The truth is that most of the research shows positive health benefits of whole grains, but the reason they are excluded from both an AIP and standard Paleo Diet is because of antinutrients such as phytates. Some argue that you need to eat grains to get sufficient fiber, but if you eat a wide variety of fruit and vegetables you can get enough fiber without eating grains.

Level 1 Hyperthyroid Healing Diet Variations

As is the case with the Level 2 and Level 3 Diets, you'll still want to consider following a low- to moderate-iodine diet, limit your consumption of seafood that's not too high in iodine to two to three times per week, and eat a good variety of plant-based foods. You'll also want to continue to avoid nuts and seeds higher in lectins and oxalates, and ideally avoid nightshades.

- **Only certain oils are allowed.** On the Plant Paradox Diet, organic, non-GMO canola oil is allowed, but the main reason I recommend avoiding canola oil is because it's high in omega-6 fatty acids, and too much omega-6 fatty acid results in an inflammatory state. This is the case with most other vegetable oils. Similarly, I don't recommend rice bran oil. I would try to stick with coconut oil, olive oil, avocado oil, and macadamia nut oil. Palm oil is also okay, depending on the source. (It should be sustainable and free from deforestation.)

- **No dairy products (with the exception of ghee).** Some of the dairy products allowed on a Plant Paradox Diet include goat's milk and cheeses, sheep's milk and cheeses, and goat and sheep yogurt. While these are healthier than dairy from a cow, I still recommend avoiding these sources while trying to restore your health. And if you're wondering about raw dairy, I discussed this in chapter 3.

- **Don't worry about restricting beef and poultry.** I realize that many vegans and vegetarians will choose to follow a Level 1 Diet, but if this doesn't describe you, then feel free to exceed the daily four-ounce limit that's on the Plant Paradox Diet. That being said, I would of course only recommend eating organic poultry (preferably pasture-raised) and 100 percent grass-fed and grass-finished meat. I also would try to have at least two thirds of your plate consist of vegetables.

- **Take a break from alcohol and coffee.** On the Plant Paradox Diet, Dr. Gundry allows six ounces per day of champagne and red wine, and he also allows coffee. These are controversial, as there are health benefits of both coffee and red wine. I think it's a good idea to take a break from most alcoholic beverages and coffee while healing . . . at least during the first few months.

- **More flexibility on polyphenol-rich fruits.** The Plant Paradox Diet recommends limiting fruit to one small serving on the weekends and only when that fruit is in season. I do think that people can overdo it when it comes to consuming fruit, and many people eat a lot more fruit than vegetables. That being said, I would say that most people will do fine eating two servings of fruit per day.

- **Limited or no grains.** Would it be the end of the world if you ate a small amount of the grains that Dr. Gundry allows (white basmati rice, millet, sorghum)? Just as is the case with legumes, if you properly prepare grains, it reduces the antinutrients. If you do this, then it might be okay to have a few servings of grains per week, but just to play it safe, I would say to take a break from grains, and then in the future you can reintroduce them, preferably after you have healed. That being said, if you're a vegan or vegetarian, I can understand if you choose to eat a few servings of properly prepared grains each week.

Additional Advice for Vegans and Vegetarians

As I mentioned earlier, you probably will want to follow a Level 1 Diet and just avoid meat, poultry, and fish if you're a strict vegetarian, and if you're a vegan, then you'll of course also avoid eating eggs. I would just make sure you're getting enough protein. You might need to supplement with a good quality protein powder, such as a clean organic pea protein. In many cases it's also a good idea to supplement with vitamin B_{12}, and some might also benefit from taking a good-quality multivitamin.

You might wonder if you can regain your health as a vegetarian or vegan. In many cases it is more challenging to restore one's health as a vegetarian or vegan, and there are a few reasons for this:

Reason #1: Most vegetarians/vegans don't consume enough protein. I mentioned this already, and in chapter 4 I mentioned how I recommend getting at least 75 percent of your ideal body weight in protein. For example, if your ideal weight is 120 pounds, you'd want to consume at least 90 grams of protein per day. This is challenging to do as a vegetarian or vegan, but certainly not impossible, especially if you supplement with a good-quality protein powder.

Reason #2: Nutrient deficiencies are more common. I already mentioned how a deficiency in vitamin B_{12} is common, and the same is true with iron. While it is usually safe to supplement with vitamin B_{12} even without testing, I still would consider testing for vitamin B_{12}. While serum B_{12} is an option, a better option to determine if someone has a vitamin B_{12} deficiency is urinary methylmalonic acid.

As for iron, I would never recommend supplementing with iron without first confirming that you have an iron deficiency. I would recommend a full iron panel, which includes serum iron, ferritin, iron saturation, and total iron binding capacity (TIBC). Also keep in mind that vitamin C and healthy stomach acid are important for optimal iron absorption.

Reason #3: Many vegetarians/vegans eat poor-quality foods. There are a lot of vegetarians and vegans who eat junk food on a daily basis. Obviously if someone eats a lot of refined foods and sugars, it will be difficult to restore their health, regardless of whether they're a vegetarian or not. As you know by now, a key piece to regaining your health is to eat an anti-inflammatory diet consisting of whole, healthy foods.

Reason #4: Grains and legumes can be harsh on the gut. This is why if you eat legumes and/or grains you want to make sure to properly prepare them. And even though Dr. Gundry allows pressure-cooked white basmati rice, sorghum, and millet, if you choose to eat these, I recommend limiting your consumption to two or three times per week.

Summary of What You Can Eat on a Level 1 Diet

So let's summarize the categories of foods that you can eat on a Level 1 Hyperthyroid Healing Diet:

- Meat (beef, lamb, pork, etc.)
- Poultry (chicken, turkey, duck, etc.)
- Organ meats
- Fish and other seafood low in mercury and not too high in iodine (i.e., wild salmon, sardines)
- Vegetables (excluding nightshades)
- Fruit (preferably lower in sugar, such as wild blueberries, strawberries, and cranberries)
- Mushrooms
- Cassava, green bananas, green mangos, green plantains, jicama, parsnips, rutabaga, sweet potatoes, taro, tiger nuts, turnips, and yucca

- Eggs
- Nuts and seeds that aren't very high in lectins and oxalates (pistachios, macadamia nuts, walnuts, pecans, sprouted pumpkin seeds, sprouted sunflower seeds)
- Coconut products (unsweetened coconut yogurt, coconut milk, coconut kefir, etc.)
- Ghee
- Spices (excluding seed-based and nightshade-based spices such as cayenne, celery seed, chili powder, fenugreek, and paprika)
- Honey and pure maple syrup (in moderation)
- Certain flours (coconut flour, tapioca flour, cassava flour)
- Green tea in moderation (due to the caffeine), herbal teas
- Bone broth
- Kombucha
- Collagen powder
- Hydrolyzed beef powder
- Dark chocolate in moderation
- Two to three times per week: a combination of pressure-cooked lentils and other legumes and the allowed grains mentioned in this chapter (pressure-cooked white basmati rice, millet, sorghum). So, for example, you can have pressure-cooked beans twice per week and pressure-cooked white basmati rice once per week. But as I mentioned in the chapter, if you're not a vegetarian or vegan, I would consider taking a break from grains for at least a couple of months.

Level 1 Hyperthyroid Healing Diet Yes/No List

To make it easier to follow each diet, I have created a yes/no list of each one, which includes a comprehensive list of foods that you can and can't eat. To access the list for the Level 1 Hyperthyroid Healing Diet, visit the resources at **savemythyroid.com/HHDNotes**.

Chapter 7 Highlights

- The Level 1 Hyperthyroid Healing Diet is the most basic diet for hyperthyroidism discussed in this book, although it still has some wonderful health benefits.
- The Level 1 Hyperthyroid Healing Diet is similar to the Plant Paradox Diet and is a good diet to follow for vegetarians and vegans.
- It's also a good fit for those with Graves' disease who find the Level 2 and 3 diets too challenging to follow.
- Hyperthyroid Healing Diet Level 1 variations include only certain oils are allowed, no dairy products (other than ghee), taking a break from alcohol and coffee, more flexibility on polyphenol-rich fruits, and limited or no grains.
- If you're a vegan or vegetarian, you want to make sure you're getting enough protein, and you might need to supplement with a good-quality protein powder.
- Here are a few reasons why it can be more challenging for a vegetarian or vegan to restore their health: most vegetarians/vegans don't consume enough protein, nutrient deficiencies are more common, many vegetarians/vegans eat poor-quality foods, and grains and legumes can be harsh on the gut.

To access the book references and resources, visit
SaveMyThyroid.com/HHDNotes.

CHAPTER

8

Healthy Beverages

Growing up I drank plenty of soda, fruit punch, and cow's milk. Of course, all of these are excluded from all three Hyperthyroid Healing Diets, but this doesn't mean that water is the only thing you can drink. That being said, if all you want to do is drink water, that's perfectly fine, as for the most part this is what I drink on a daily basis. However, I do drink some green tea and herbal tea as well, and there are other options to consider if you want to drink more than just water, which is what this chapter is all about.

So let's go ahead and take a look at some of the beverages you can drink:

Water. Although everyone knows that it's important to drink plenty of water each day, there is no consensus when it comes to the type of water someone should drink. I mostly drink reverse osmosis water, along with some spring water out of a glass bottle (Mountain Valley Springs). Others drink distilled water. Many of my patients have a different type of water filter.

The concern with reverse osmosis water and distilled water is that while they remove most of the environmental toxicants, they also remove the minerals.

When going through my master's in nutrition degree, I was taught that you rely on food for most of your minerals, and not water. That being said, if you want to drink reverse osmosis or distilled water to remove most of the toxicants but are concerned about the lack of minerals, you can either drink spring water out of a glass bottle or add minerals to the water.

As for how much water you should drink, many sources recommend drinking half your body weight in ounces. So, for example, if you weighed 150 pounds, you would want to drink approximately 75 ounces of water per day. I admit that I strive to do this on a daily basis, and I do count the water I drink in my herbal teas, smoothie, etc. But in addition to this I also drink water throughout the day.

Herbal teas. Tea is the most-consumed beverage worldwide, and it possesses significant antioxidative, anti-inflammatory, antimicrobial, anticarcinogenic, antihypertensive, neuroprotective, cholesterol-lowering, and thermogenic properties.[1] Teas prepared from different plants are referred to as *herbal teas*. Most herbal teas are fine to drink when dealing with hyperthyroidism. Some of my favorites include ginger, lemon balm, turmeric, peppermint, and rooibos. I usually drink a couple of cups of herbal tea each morning. And of course I highly recommend that any herbal teas you drink be organic.

Coconut milk. I can't say that I drink coconut milk on a regular basis, but I know some people will want to have options other than water and herbal teas. While it's more convenient to purchase coconut milk, you might want to try making it on your own so you can avoid the emulsifiers commonly added. I must admit I failed miserably when trying to make it on my own a few years ago, but this doesn't mean you can't be more successful than I was. Another option is to purchase a gizmo such as the Almond Cow, which makes it easier to make your own coconut milk and nut milks (more about nut milks shortly).

Non-dairy kefir. Kefir is a fermented drink with low alcohol content, acidic and bubbly from the fermentation carbonation of kefir grains with milk or water.[2] Consumption of this beverage is associated with a wide array of nutraceutical benefits, including anti-inflammatory, anti-oxidative, anti-cancer, anti-microbial, anti-diabetic, anti-hypertensive, and anti-hypercholesterolemic effects.[3] Drinking water and/or coconut kefir is fine, but you just want to be careful with the sugar content.

Kombucha. Kombucha is a fermented tea made from a symbiotic culture of bacteria and yeast (SCOBY). I love drinking kombucha, and if you also enjoy kombucha, then go ahead and drink some on a regular basis! Just be careful about brands that have added sugar, and you might even consider making your own. (I can't say that I've tried doing this as of writing this book.) One comprehensive study looked to characterize the microbial composition and biochemical properties of a specific brand of kombucha.[4] The study revealed a total of two hundred different species, including twenty dominant bacterial species and sixteen yeast species.[4]

Bone broth. Bone broth is made by boiling the bones of chickens, cows, fish, etc. in water for an extended period of time, and typically you'll also add some vegetables and herbs. Although you don't need to drink bone broth to support gut healing, it definitely can help with the healing process. In addition to supplying collagen, you also get amino acids such as glycine that support gut health, along with proline and hydroxyproline. While there are some companies that sell good-quality bone broth (organic, grass-fed, etc.), you of course can always make your own.

Smoothies. Some healthcare practitioners recommend not drinking smoothies because they feel you should eat your meals and not drink them. All I can say is that I've been drinking smoothies for many years, and I consider myself to be in an excellent state of health. There are many other natural healthcare practitioners who consume smoothies on a daily basis as well. I think smoothies are a great way to "sneak in" a lot of vegetables, although it's fine to start with one or two servings in your smoothie.

Oxalates are a concern if you stuff your smoothies with spinach or other high-oxalate veggies, but there are plenty of vegetables to choose from that are lower in oxalates. (I discuss oxalates in chapter 16.) If you experience a lot of gas and bloating with smoothies, this could mean that you have some overgrowth of bacteria in the small intestine (SIBO). This can be confirmed through a breath test, and I discuss SIBO in greater detail in chapter 18.

Controversial Beverages

Coffee. Over the years I have worked with many patients who were willing to give up just about anything . . . except for their morning cup of coffee. I've never been a coffee drinker, so I can't completely empathize with those who are unwilling to give up coffee. And of course there are worse things someone can do than drink a cup or two of coffee in the morning . . . especially if it's a good quality organic coffee.

The research actually shows that coffee has some pretty good health benefits. A literature review showed that coffee may contribute to the prevention of inflammatory and oxidative stress-related diseases, such as obesity, metabolic syndrome, and type 2 diabetes, as well as a lower incidence of several types of cancer.[5] These health benefits make me want to consider drinking coffee!

So why is coffee excluded from certain diets, including a Level 3 Hyperthyroid Healing Diet? The main reason is that coffee beans are used to make coffee, and they are actually seeds. (I know, weird, since regular beans are considered to be legumes, so why not just call them *coffee seeds*?) Seeds aren't allowed on a Level 3 Hyperthyroid Healing Diet.

Another concern is the caffeine content, as if someone has adrenal problems, then it probably is best to avoid caffeine while working on improving their adrenal health. And arguably, caffeine probably isn't a good idea for anyone with an elevated resting heart rate, which is common with hyperthyroidism, as caffeine ingestion has been demonstrated to increase circulating epinephrine and norepinephrine, elevate free fatty acids, and alter heart rate, blood pressure, and ventilation.[6]

If you're a coffee drinker, the good news is that most people don't have to wait until they completely regain their health to reintroduce coffee. If following a Level 3 Hyperthyroid Healing Diet, and/or if you have compromised adrenals, you'll want to avoid coffee for at least two months. If someone is following a Level 1 or 2 diet and their adrenals are in pretty good shape, they might be able to reintroduce a cup of organic coffee after thirty days.

Black tea. Although black tea has certain health benefits, it also has caffeine. And while it's in lower amounts than coffee, it's still high enough that I would recommend avoiding it while in the initial phases of restoring your health. Just as is the case with coffee, if you're following a Level 3 Hyperthyroid Healing Diet and/or you have compromised adrenals, you'll want to avoid black tea for at least two months. If you're wondering how much caffeine is in black tea when compared to coffee, the mean values per cup of black tea is 28 to 46 mg of caffeine, while for brewed coffee it is 107 to 151 mg.[7]

Green tea. You might be surprised that I included green tea under the "controversial" beverages. There is no question that green tea has some wonderful health benefits. The main concern I have with my hyperthyroid patients is the caffeine. And once again, the primary reason for this concern is the impact of the caffeine on the adrenals.

Even though the caffeine content is lower than in coffee and black tea, if someone has compromised adrenals, I recommend that they avoid green tea. Otherwise I think it's fine to drink a cup or two per day. If you do have compromised adrenals, then decaffeinated green tea is an option to consider, as there are a couple of brands of organic decaf green tea to choose from.

Nut milks. If you're following a Level 3 Hyperthyroid Healing Diet, then nut milks aren't allowed, as nuts are excluded from a Level 3 Diet. On the other hand, if someone is following one of the other diets discussed in this section, then it's okay to drink certain types of nut milks, avoiding those high in lectins and/or oxalates. For example, I would recommend avoiding drinking almond and cashew milk while healing. Just as is the case with coconut milk, it's best to make your own nut-based milks to avoid the extra ingredients commonly found in pre-packaged nut milks you purchase at the grocery store.

Oat milk. Unfortunately, oat milk isn't allowed on any of the Hyperthyroid Healing Diets, and the reason for this is that it is made from grains. This doesn't mean that you can't drink some oat milk every now and then after you have regained your health, but until then I would avoid it.

Alcohol. While restoring your health I think it's a good idea to completely avoid all alcohol. An exception would be taking herbal extracts that use ethanol, as these include such a small amount that it rarely causes a problem. And while there are alcohol-free extracts that use glycerin, you need to keep in mind that ethanol is a better solvent and therefore does a better job of extracting the phytochemicals from the herb, which is why when recommending liquid extracts, I usually recommend alcohol-based herbs.

One of the main problems with alcohol is that it can increase the permeability of the gut.[8,9] But is this true with healthier types of alcohol, such as red wine? Well, in the past, I would cite evidence that red wine can increase gut permeability, but while doing research for this book, I actually came across a more recent study showing that red wine extract preserves tight junctions in intestinal epithelial cells.[10] Another study showed that red wine polyphenols significantly increased the number of fecal bifidobacteria and lactobacillus (intestinal barrier protectors) and butyrate-producing bacteria (*Faecalibacterium prausnitzii* and *Roseburia*) at the expense of less desirable groups of bacteria such as LPS producers (*Escherichia coli* and *Enterobacter cloacae*).[11]

There is concern that consuming alcohol can lead to bacterial overgrowth. And while this is true in some cases, for many people, drinking one or two small glasses of red wine per week (i.e., five ounces) probably isn't going to cause any issues. However, if you're following a Hyperthyroid Healing Diet, you might want to avoid it for at least a couple of months just to play it safe. And if someone already has a condition such as SIBO, then it probably is best to refrain from red wine.

I should also remind you that if you're taking a liquid herbal extract that has alcohol, such as bugleweed or motherwort, it is usually fine. It's such a tiny amount, and of course everything comes down to risks versus benefits. While using a non-alcoholic liquid extract with glycerin is an option, I mentioned earlier that glycerin is not as good of a solvent as ethanol, so you might not get the same benefits using an extract with glycerin when compared to ethanol.

Raw dairy. While there is no question that drinking raw milk is a healthier option when compared to commercialized milk, unfortunately dairy isn't allowed on any of the Hyperthyroid Healing Diets (with the exception of ghee). This is also true with milk from a goat or sheep. The reason is that many people will still react to dairy proteins, specifically casein and whey.

While you might be able to tolerate these healthier milks after you have regained your health, it really does depend on the person. Some people have no problem reintroducing certain forms of dairy, while others do better when eliminating them permanently. Since being in remission from Graves' disease in 2009, I've enjoyed dairy on an occasional basis, although I usually consume it in the form of cheese, as rarely do I drink milk of any kind.

A2 milk. It's also worth mentioning that there are different types of casein in dairy cows. The most common forms of beta-casein in dairy cattle breeds are A1 and A2. It is thought that beta-casein variant A1 yields the bioactive peptide beta-casomorphin-7 (BCM-7), which may play a role in the development of certain human diseases, such as diabetes mellitus and ischemic heart disease. There also might be a relationship of BCM-7 to sudden infant death syndrome.[12] So just to clarify, BCM-7 can lead to the development of numerous chronic health conditions and is found in beta-casein A1.

It's also important to understand that some people react to beta-casein A1 but do perfectly fine when consuming beta-casein A2. That being said, not everyone will tolerate A2 milk. Because of this, while healing, I usually recommend avoiding all forms of dairy, including A2 milk.

In summary, while you want to drink plenty of water each day, you can also drink other beverages. As for some of the controversial beverages, ultimately it's up to you whether you choose to drink coffee, black tea, oat milk, alcohol, etc. But while trying to restore your health, I would recommend taking a break from these.

Chapter 8 Highlights

- It's important to stay well hydrated and make sure you drink plenty of water each day.
- Many sources recommend drinking half your body weight in ounces each day.
- While lemon balm is a popular herbal tea to drink for those with hyperthyroidism, most other herbal teas are also fine to drink.
- Drinking coconut milk is okay, although you might want to try making it on your own to avoid the emulsifiers commonly added.
- Other beverages to consider include non-dairy kefir, kombucha, bone broth, and smoothies.
- Oxalates are a concern if you stuff your smoothies with spinach or other high-oxalate veggies, but there are plenty of vegetables to choose from that are lower in oxalates.
- Avoid coffee and black tea for at least two months if following a Level 3 Diet, and at least thirty days if following a Level 1 or 2 Diet.
- Nut milks are allowed on a Level 1 or 2 Diet, but be careful about drinking nut milks higher in oxalates, such as almond and cashew milk.
- While restoring your health, I would avoid all alcohol with the exception of taking herbal extracts that use ethanol.
- Raw milk is a healthier option than commercialized milk, but it's still not allowed on any of the three diets.

To access the book references and resources, visit
SaveMyThyroid.com/HHDNotes.

CHAPTER
9

The Fermented Foods Chapter

was debating whether I should include a separate chapter on fermented foods, and the reason for this is that when I dealt with Graves' disease, I admittedly didn't eat fermented foods on a daily basis. I can't even say that I eat a lot of fermented foods these days, so I'm definitely not a fermented foods guru. That being said, the more you can do for your gut microbiome, the better, not only when it comes to regaining your health, but also for achieving optimal health in the future.

This chapter isn't just based on my opinion, as I did a good amount of research. In fact, after going through the research, it reminded me of all of the health benefits of fermented foods. And while I've been in remission from Graves' disease since 2009, it's not as if I haven't had any health concerns since then, as in 2016 I had shingles, in 2018 I was diagnosed with chronic Lyme disease, and in 2022 I got hit hard with the SARS-Cov-2 virus. And while eating more fermented foods may not have prevented these health issues from occurring, whenever you have an opportunity to improve the health of your gut, it's a good idea, as doing so will also improve your immune system health, making you less susceptible to viruses and other infections, not to mention also benefiting the autoimmune component in those with Graves' disease.

While I'll be discussing some of the different fermented food options in this chapter, if you currently don't eat fermented foods, please don't think you need to add all the ones I mention. In fact, I would say to pick one to start with. If you already eat fermented foods, then perhaps add another. And if you eat a lot of fermented foods and even make your own fermented foods, then send me an email so I can hop into my time machine and have you help me write this chapter! Seriously, though, even if you eat a lot of fermented foods, you still can benefit from the information in this chapter.

Why Fermented Foods Can Benefit Your Health

Raw cultured vegetables have been around for thousands of years. Here are some of the many benefits they offer: [1,2]

- Antiobesity effects
- Antidiabetic effects
- Antihypertensive effects
- Anticarcinogenic properties
- Anti-inflammatory and immunomodulatory functions
- Rich source of nutrients, phytochemicals, and bioactive microbes

Hopefully you understand that fermented foods don't just offer benefits to the gut microbiome, but they have many other potential health benefits as well. And while some of this is attributed to the direct effect of the microorganisms, fermentation also increases the peptides, amino acids, vitamins, minerals, and antioxidant contents of foods.[3]

Raw vs. Pasteurized Fermented Foods

If you prefer not to make your own fermented foods but are willing to purchase them at a local health food store, it's best to try to get them unpasteurized. However, while the pasteurization process will eradicate some of the micro-organisms, there are still health benefits of eating pasteurized fermented foods. In fact, one study involving pasteurized versus unpasteurized sauerkraut intake in IBS patients showed significant improvements in symptoms and a significant change in the composition of the gut microbiota in both groups, although the unpasteurized group showed significantly greater numbers of sauerkraut-associated lactobacillus (*Lactobacillus plantarum* and *Lactobacillus brevis*) than their pasteurized counterparts.[4] So if you have been eating pasteurized fermented foods (i.e., sauerkraut) up until this time, it's not like you haven't received any health benefits, but unpasteurized is even better.

Which Fermented Foods Should You Consume?

What I'd like to do now is briefly discuss some of the different fermented foods. Keep in mind that some of these were mentioned in chapter 8 where I discussed beverages, but I'd like to dive even more into the research, and do it in a way I think you'll find interesting. After all, during my research for this chapter, I came across a few health benefits related to fermented foods that I didn't know, and I'm guessing you might not know them either.

Also, I'm only going to discuss fermented foods that can be included in any of the three Hyperthyroid Healing Diets. So, for example, when I discuss kefir or yogurt, I'll only discuss non-dairy forms, such as coconut yogurt. And while I can't deny that sourdough bread is healthier than most other breads you can buy at your grocery store, for numerous reasons it's not part of any of the diets. This doesn't mean that in the future you can't eat healthier types of bread, especially on an occasional basis, but while trying to restore your health, I would recommend refraining from eating bread.

So let's go ahead and look at some of the different fermented foods you can enjoy:

Sauerkraut. I can't say that I love the taste of sauerkraut, but I eat it occasionally because the health benefits are amazing. Sauerkraut is produced from a combination of shredded cabbage and 2.3 percent–3.0 percent salt, which is left to undergo spontaneous fermentation. Culture-dependent techniques show that sauerkraut can contain *Bifidobacterium dentium, Enterococcus faecalis, Lactobacillus casei, Lactobacillus delbrueckii, Staphylococcus epidermidis, Lactobacillus sakei, Lactobacillus curvatus, Lactobacillus plantarum, Lactobacillus brevis, Weissella confusa, Lactococcus lactis* and Enterobacteriaceae.[5,6,7]

Although the microbial composition of sauerkraut can vary during the initial stages of fermentation, when done appropriately you should expect lactic acid bacteria to be the dominant microorganisms in the final fermented product.[8] And you can see this listed previously, as the majority of the species were from the *Lactobacillus* genus. These lactic acid bacteria produce the organic acids, bacteriocins, vitamins, and flavor compounds responsible for many of the characteristic sensory qualities of fermented foods, including extended shelf life, flavor, and nutritional content.[9,10,11]

In addition to helping to support the gut microbiome, eating sauerkraut can provide other health benefits. One study showed that oral administration of sauerkraut juices (in rats) increased glutathione S-transferase levels.[12] Just a reminder that glutathione is the master antioxidant that plays a role in phase 2 detoxification. Another study showed that some of the bacteria in sauerkraut can generate conjugated linolenic acid,[13] which potentially has anti-carcinogenic and anti-atherosclerotic activity.[14,15]

Kimchi. Kimchi originates from Korea and consists of Chinese cabbage and/or radishes and various flavoring ingredients (e.g., chili, pepper, garlic, onion, ginger), seasonings (e.g., salt, soybean sauce, sesame seed), and other additional foods (e.g., carrot, apple, pear, shrimp).[16,17] The fermentation occurs spontaneously by the microorganisms naturally found on the cabbage and foods included in the mixture, although starter cultures may be used for commercial production of kimchi.[17] Once fermentation has started, the bacterial diversity decreases and the bacterial community is rapidly dominated by the genus *Leuconostoc* within only three days of fermentation.[18] A few different archaea and yeast genera have also been identified in commercially available kimchi.[19]

Although kimchi can have some amazing health benefits, keep in mind that it commonly includes red peppers. These are part of the nightshade family and thus are excluded from all of the Hyperthyroid Healing Diets. However, you can make non-spicy kimchi without the peppers, which is called *baek-kimchi* or *white kimchi*. And of course in the future, as your health improves, you can try to reintroduce nightshades, and very well may be fine making kimchi with peppers.

H. pylori can be a potential trigger of Graves' disease, and there was a small study that looked at the effects of kimchi on the stomach and colon health of people with an *H. pylori* infection.[20] The results of the study showed that consuming kimchi didn't show any therapeutic effect on *H. pylori* in the stomach, although it was good for colon health. That being said, you'll see shortly that other fermented foods might actually help with the eradication of *H. pylori*.

Kefir. Traditional kefir involves adding kefir grains to milk. Kefir grain, as a natural starter culture, contains numerous lactic acid bacteria, acetic acid bacteria, and yeasts within a polysaccharide structure.[21] Studies show that kefir has more than fifty species of probiotic bacteria and yeast and has been demonstrated to have multiple properties conferring health benefits, including antiobesity, anti-hepatic steatosis, antioxidative, antiallergenic, antitumor, anti-inflammatory, cholesterol-lowering, constipation-alleviating, and antimicrobial properties.[22] As a bacteria- and yeast-containing food, kefir can modulate both the gut microbiota and mycobiota.[22]

Even though milk-based kefir has many health benefits, since dairy isn't part of the Hyperthyroid Healing Diets, I recommend consuming non-dairy forms of kefir while restoring your health. This includes water kefir or coconut kefir. Water kefir is a sparkling, slightly acidic fermented beverage produced by fermenting a solution of sucrose, to which dried fruits have been added, with water kefir grains.[23] Lactic acid bacteria, yeast, and acetic acid bacteria are the primary microbial members of the sugary kefir grain.[23]

One study looked at the differences and similarities between water kefir grain and milk kefir grain.[24] The study showed that milk kefir grain has more nutritional content compared to water kefir grain. However, it did mention that water kefir grain is a good source of minerals and health-friendly microorganisms such as lactic acid bacteria and yeasts.[24]

Earlier I mentioned how kimchi was shown not to be effective in eradicating *H. pylori*, but the same might not be true with kefir. One randomized, double-blind study examined the effect of combining triple therapy with kefir.[25] This was carried out on eighty-two people with symptoms of dyspepsia and *H. pylori* infection confirmed by the urea breath test.

Patients were given a two-times-a-day, fourteen-day course of lansoprazole (30 mg), amoxicillin (1,000 mg), and clarithromycin (500 mg) with either 250 mL of kefir twice daily or 250 mL of milk containing a placebo. Upon doing a follow-up urea breath test forty-five days after beginning treatment, significantly more people who had the triple therapy combined with the kefir successfully eradicated the *H. pylori* (78.25 versus 50 percent).

Of course this doesn't prove that consuming kefir alone will successfully eradicate *H. pylori*, but it might help those who choose to take a more natural approach to eradicating *H. pylori*. And perhaps drinking kefir regularly, along with consuming some of the other fermented foods discussed in this chapter, might be a way to prevent *H. pylori* from becoming a problem in the future.

Kombucha. I briefly discussed kombucha in chapter 8. Kombucha tea originated in China two thousand years ago, and it is a non-alcoholic or low-alcoholic functional beverage obtained by the fermentation of sweetened tea by a symbiotic culture of bacteria and yeasts (SCOBY).[26] It includes organic acids, minerals, and vitamins originating mainly from tea, amino acids, and biologically active compounds such as polyphenols.[27] Although it usually is prepared using black tea, other types of teas can be used. In fact, one study showed that green tea and red tea are more prominent sources of antioxidants,[27] and another study confirmed that green tea had the strongest antioxidant properties when compared to other tested teas.[28]

This is why you might want to consider making your own kombucha, as most of the products on the market use black tea. And if you drink one with green tea, you ideally want it to be organic. That being said, I can't say that I'm an expert when it comes to making kombucha, as I mentioned in chapter 8 that I have never made my own kombucha.

Pre-clinical studies conducted on kombucha revealed that it has desired bioactivities such as antimicrobial, antioxidant, hepatoprotective, anti-hypercholesterolemic, anticancer, and anti-inflammatory properties, to name a few.[29] The SCOBY includes a mixture of bacteria, especially from the Acetobacteraceae family (*Acetobacter aceti, A. estunensis, A. pasteurianus, Gluconobacter oxydans, Komagataeibacter kombuchae, K. rhaeticus,* and *K. xylinus*) and *Lactobacillus* as well as osmophilic yeasts (*Brettanomyces/Dekkera, Candida, Saccharomyces, Schizosaccharomyces, Starmerella, Torulopsis, Pichia,* and *Zygosaccharomyces*).[29,30] The low pH of kombucha, owing mainly to the production of a high concentration of acetic acid, has been shown to prevent the growth of pathogenic bacteria such as *Helicobacter pylori, Escherichia coli, Salmonella typhimurium,* and *Campylobacter jejuni.*[31]

Fermented pickles. Fermented pickles are yet another great source of probiotic bacteria. Significant lactic acid bacteria responsible for traditional pickle fermentation include *Lactobacillus plantarum, L. brevis, Leuconostoc mesenteroides, Pediococcus cerevisiae, Pediococcus pentosaceus,* and *Enterococcus faecalis.*[32,33]

There are two types of fermented pickles:[33]

1. Sour fermented pickles: Made by submerging raw materials in a dilute brine (2–5 percent salt), and then naturally occurring bacteria grow over one to two weeks to produce lactic acid, which then prevents the growth of food poisoning bacteria and other spoilage microorganisms
2. Sweet fermented pickles: Preserved by a combination of lactic or acetic acid, sugar, and spices. Although cucumbers are the main vegetables used in the production of pickles, other vegetables can be used.

Non-dairy yogurt. Conventional yogurt is made through the fermentation of cow's milk by *Streptococcus thermophilus* and *Lactobacillus delbrueckii* (subsp. *bulgaricus*) until a pH lower than 4.5 and final lactic acid bacteria density higher than 8 log10 cfu/g are reached.[34] Fortunately there are plenty of dairy-free alternatives. The problem is that most of the products out there have too much sugar. And of course, just because it's dairy-free doesn't mean it's included in any of the Hyperthyroid Healing Diets.

Unsweetened coconut yogurt is a safe bet with all of the different Hyperthyroid Healing Diets recommended in this book. Certain nut-based yogurts are also an option with the Level 2 and Level 3 Hyperthyroid Healing Diets, although the most common nut-based yogurt is almond yogurt, and almonds are excluded from all three diets. But since coconut yogurt is low in oxalates

(I discuss oxalates in chapter 16), if you enjoy coconut yogurt, I recommend choosing this. This is also something you can make on your own.

What's the Deal with Fermented Soy?

Although there is no question that fermented soy has some great health benefits, soy isn't allowed on any of the Hyperthyroid Healing Diets. One reason is because soy is a common allergen. Soy also is high in phytates, lectins, and trypsin inhibitors,[35] although the fermentation process greatly reduces these compounds.[36,37]

Unfortunately, most soy is genetically modified. One of the main concerns is that genetically modified soybeans contain high residues of glyphosate.[38,39] Of course, this can be avoided by eating organic soy. Speaking of which, as one's health improves, I do think it's fine to eat some organic fermented soy products, including tempeh, natto, and miso.

How to Make Your Own Fermented Foods

Although I've made some of my own fermented foods (i.e., sauerkraut, unsweetened coconut yogurt), I can't say that I'm creative enough to make my own recipes! So rather than list the recipes of others here, if you want to learn how to prepare your own fermented foods, I'll refer you to some resources at **savemythyroid.com/HHDNotes**.

Chapter 9 Highlights

- If you currently don't eat fermented foods, please don't think you need to add all of the ones I mention in this chapter.
- Some of the benefits of fermented foods include antiobesity effects, antidiabetic effects, antihypertensive effects, anticarcinogenic properties, and anti-inflammatory and immunomodulatory functions.
- Fermented foods don't just offer benefits to the gut microbiome, but they have many other potential health benefits as well.
- If you prefer not to make your own fermented foods but are willing to purchase them at a local health food store, it's best to try to get them unpasteurized.
- Some of the different fermented foods you can enjoy include sauerkraut, non-spicy kimchi, non-dairy kefir, kombucha, and coconut yogurt.

**To access the book references and resources, visit
SaveMyThyroid.com/HHDNotes.**

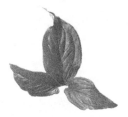

Additional Hyperthyroid Healing Diet Tips

CHAPTER
10

Hyperthyroid Healing Diet Troubleshooting

Whﬁle some people will follow one of the Hyperthyroid Healing Diets without a problem, for others it won't go as smoothly. For example, someone might have problems with high-histamine foods, and while I do have a separate chapter that focuses on histamine (chapter 15), I realize that not everyone will read the book from cover to cover, so I thought it would be a good idea to have a separate "troubleshooting" chapter. If you experience any bumps in the road while making dietary changes, then this chapter is a good starting point.

I'll add that keeping a food and symptom diary can be a good idea when starting the diet. This can come in handy if you experience any negative reactions to a food you eat, as you can refer back to this diary and determine if there are any obvious connections between the food you eat and the symptoms you develop. The only downside I can think of is that people can have delayed reactions to foods, and when this is the case, it can be challenging to make the connection between a specific food and any symptoms.

Loose stools/diarrhea. Many people with hyperthyroidism experience loose stools due to the increase in thyroid hormone, but if you don't experience loose stools until you change your diet, or if you *are* experiencing loose stools and it worsens upon changing your diet, then chances are you are reacting to something you reintroduced. It's also possible that your body isn't used to eating so many vegetables, so you might have to back off. For example, if before reading this book you were eating two servings of vegetables per day but then started eating eight servings per day, your body might not be ready for this. Everyone is different, so if this describes you, then you might want to scale back to four or five servings per day and then gradually increase.

If someone experiences loose stools or diarrhea upon incorporating one of the Hyperthyroid Healing Diets is it possible that it's just a coincidence and that something else is causing it? Without question this is possible. For example, people can get parasites from salads, so if someone starts eating more vegetables, there is the possibility that their body doesn't have a problem with eating more vegetables, but they just happened to get exposed to parasites upon increasing their vegetable consumption. Or it could also be a case of food poisoning. While this is more likely when someone goes out to eat, it doesn't mean it can't happen in your own home.

If you have persistent diarrhea that lasts for more than a few days, it's a good idea to schedule an appointment with your primary care doctor. In the meantime you will want to stay well hydrated, and taking some electrolytes would also be a good idea. I'll include some suggestions for pre-packaged electrolytes in the resources (**savemythyroid.com/HHDNotes**), or you can also make your own electrolyte drink.

Sometimes, taking a probiotic supplement can be beneficial for cases of diarrhea. The research shows that *Lactobacillus rhamnosus GG* and *Saccharomyces boulardii* might be beneficial to take.[1] Eating fermented foods might also help with diarrhea.[2]

Activated charcoal can also be considered on a short-term basis, but just keep in mind that if you were to take it, you want to do so away from meals and supplements, as it will affect their absorption. One study compared activated charcoal with other common anti-diarrheal treatments and mentioned that activated charcoal has exceptionally fewer side effects.[3] Some might be wondering about bismuth subsalicylate, also known as Pepto-Bismol. Although it's not my first choice, it definitely can help in some cases of diarrhea. You just need to keep in mind that the goal shouldn't be to only cover up the symptoms, but to try to find out why someone is experiencing the loose stools or diarrhea.

Constipation. Although loose stools are more common with hyperthyroidism, there can be many reasons why someone experiences constipation. Three factors include (1) taking antithyroid medication, (2) not being well hydrated, and (3) being sedentary. Of course there is a time and place for taking antithyroid medication, but if you begin experiencing constipation after taking antithyroid medication, then it makes sense that this can be the culprit. As for staying hydrated, I would try to drink at least half your body weight in ounces of water each day. And with regard to regular movement, while you don't want to overexert yourself, especially if you have an elevated resting heart rate, taking regular light walks is usually fine for someone with hyperthyroidism.

What happens if someone is having daily bowel movements without straining, but then their bowel pattern changes when changing their diet? There is no question that in some people, eliminating grains and legumes can sometimes be a factor in developing constipation. This doesn't mean that you can't stay regular without these foods, but what happens many times is that people will stop eating these foods and not get enough fiber from other sources.

If you experience constipation upon eliminating grains and/or legumes, many times increasing your fiber intake by eating more vegetables can help. This isn't always the case, and I realize that some people are unable to eat larger quantities of vegetables without experiencing gas and bloating, which means we need to work on improving their digestion. But if you are able to tolerate more veggies, then I do think this is a good place to start.

Magnesium citrate is also something worth trying if someone is doing everything they can (without reintroducing the "forbidden" foods) and remains constipated. Start with 200 to 400 mg before going to bed, but keep in mind that some people might need to go up to 1,000 mg, sometimes even a little higher.

Certain probiotics might help with constipation. One study showed that *Bifidobacterium lactis* HN019 ameliorates chronic idiopathic constipation.[4] Another study showed that probiotics significantly ameliorated stool consistency in patients with chronic constipation, and it mentioned how the beneficial effect of *Lactobacillus plantarum* LRCC5193 on stool consistency remained after the probiotic supplementation was discontinued.[5]

If you experience constipation, you might wonder if taking an herbal laxative supplement can be of benefit. Rhubarb, senna leaf, and aloe are three frequently used herbal remedies for achieving regular bowel movements.[6] Triphala can also benefit the GI tract and in some cases can help with constipation.[7] Once again, I think there's a time and place for herbs, and I'd rather take herbs instead of over-the-counter laxatives. But I also wouldn't want to rely on herbs for having daily bowel movements, so I look at this as a temporary solution.

Bloating. There can be numerous causes of abdominal bloating, including gut hypersensitivity, impaired gas handling, altered gut microbiota, and abnormal abdominal-phrenic reflexes.[8] If you experience bloating with or without pain upon incorporating one of the Hyperthyroid Healing Diets, then I'd be leaning toward a problem with gut hypersensitivity, or more likely an altered gut microbiota. Small intestinal bacterial overgrowth (SIBO) is something to consider if you have bloating upon eating high-FODMAP foods. FODMAP stands for *fermentable oligosaccharides, disaccharides, monosaccharides and polyols*, and I discuss the benefits of a low-FODMAP diet in chapter 18.

So what can be done for bloating? Of course you want to address the cause of the problem, and if eliminating certain foods doesn't provide quick relief, there are a few things you can do on a temporary basis to get relief while doing this. Taking activated charcoal might help to absorb some of the gas. There is also an herbal formula I sometimes recommend as a prokinetic to SIBO patients called Iberogast (I'll discuss prokinetics in Chapter 18), but even if you don't have SIBO it might provide relief from bloating. Once again, if someone has SIBO they would want to address this, and of course the same is true with other potential causes.

Acid reflux. While many medical doctors would consider acid reflux to be a problem of having too much stomach acid, this isn't always the case. And while there is a time and place for taking acid blockers (i.e., proton pump inhibitors [PPIs]) on a short-term basis, the research shows that chronic PPI therapy can lead to hypergastrinemia, increased bacterial colonization of the stomach and small intestine, and deficiencies in nutrients such as iron and vitamin B_{12}.[9]

Taking one teaspoon of baking soda can often provide immediate relief, but if low stomach acid is the cause of the acid reflux, then doing things to increase stomach acid can obviously help. One thing you can do is mix one tablespoon of apple cider vinegar in a glass of water and take it before meals and see if this helps. Herbal bitters can also have a similar effect. Something else that can benefit some people is taking betaine HCL supplements with meals high in protein, although if you experience any heartburn, you should either decrease the dosage or discontinue it, and if necessary take one teaspoon of baking soda mixed with water.

It's also worth mentioning that *H. pylori* can cause acid reflux, and if you have Graves' disease it's important to know that in some cases, *H. pylori* can be a potential trigger. But even if you have a non-autoimmune hyperthyroid condition, it might still be worth testing for *H. pylori* if you're experiencing acid reflux.

Sugar cravings. For those who have a sweet tooth, I definitely can relate, as I grew up eating plenty of sugar. Even after graduating from chiropractic school, I ate more sugar on a daily basis than I'd like to admit. The first three to five days of reducing your sugar intake are usually the most challenging, although some people still experience strong sweet cravings even weeks after making this change.

First of all, I suggest trying your best to keep sweets out of your home, as it will be more challenging to avoid foods higher in sugar if you have them readily available. If necessary you can use monk fruit as a sugar substitute, but make sure to avoid all artificial sweeteners, as some (i.e., saccharin and sucralose) can have a negative effect on the gut microbiome.[10] Having a couple of servings of fruit is okay for most people, and also consider sweet-tasting vegetables such as carrots and butternut squash. Drinking certain herbal teas such as rooibos might help, or even drinking water with freshly squeezed lemon or lime juice.

It's also worth mentioning that having a candida overgrowth can cause sugar cravings. There are a few different ways to test for a candida overgrowth, including blood testing for antibodies, stool testing, and a urinary organic acids test. I find the latter to be more accurate, but either way, if you know or suspect you have a candida overgrowth it can be beneficial to follow a diet lower in carbohydrates and sugars. Probiotics can offer some benefit, include Saccharomyces boulardii, which is a beneficial yeast. And sometimes taking herbal or prescription antifungals can be beneficial as well.

Caffeine withdrawal. For many people, giving up coffee is the biggest challenge. If someone is drinking three or more cups of coffee per day, then it might be best to gradually decrease the amount you drink on a daily basis. You can do this by reducing the number of cups you drink each day, or another strategy is to combine caffeinated coffee with decaf. For example, if you drink three cups of coffee per day, you can try reducing it to two cups per day, or you can continue drinking three cups per day, but each cup would consist of 75 percent caffeinated coffee and 25 percent decaffeinated coffee. Then after a week you can reduce it to 50/50, and then continue to reduce the amount of caffeinated coffee until you are only drinking decaf.

Another approach is to try replacing the caffeinated coffee with organic green tea, which still has caffeine but not as much as coffee. So once again, if you drink three cups of caffeinated coffee per day, you can drink two cups of coffee and one cup of green tea, and then after one week drink one cup of coffee and two cups of green tea, and then eventually stop drinking coffee altogether and exclusively drink green tea. While some people should take a break from caffeine altogether while improving their adrenal health, it arguably is better to drink a few cups of green tea than a few cups of coffee (even though coffee does have some health benefits as well). I would also make sure that you drink plenty of water throughout the day.

General indigestion. There can be many reasons for general indigestion. If this happens immediately after eating, then you might be low in stomach acid. On the other hand, if you notice it an hour or two after eating, it might be related to low digestive enzymes. If you experience nausea, you might find ginger to be helpful, either as a supplement (i.e., capsule or extract) or as a tea. But once again, you want to address the cause of the problem.

Another thing to keep in mind is that some people will experience some of these symptoms temporarily as they "adjust" to the Hyperthyroid Healing Diet they're following, but then eventually these symptoms will subside. I wouldn't panic if you experience some of the symptoms discussed in this chapter for a few days after making changes to your diet. But if the symptoms persist after three or four days, then you might want to start incorporating some of the tips discussed in this chapter.

Cross-contamination. I decided to include this in the troubleshooting chapter just because there have been situations where someone was having issues with an allergen such as gluten, and they thought they had been avoiding it as part of their elimination diet, but there was some cross contamination occurring. This is more common if the person continues to eat out on a regular basis, as even if you order gluten-free items, if the restaurant doesn't have a dedicated gluten-free kitchen then cross contamination is very possible. And while many people aren't sensitive to the point where a small amount of gluten from cross contamination will result in symptoms, everyone is different, and some people experience symptoms even when exposed to very small amounts of gluten.

Herxheimer reaction. A Jarisch-Herxheimer reaction, also known as "die-off," is quite common when you start utilizing certain modalities to address microbes such as bacteria, fungi (i.e., yeast, mold), parasites, and even viruses. These symptoms are usually temporary, but at times can be extreme, as some of the more common symptoms include fatigue, headaches, brain fog, gastrointestinal symptoms, and even skin rashes. While these symptoms usually start decreasing and often disappear completely within seventy-two hours, in some cases they can persist for longer.

As for what causes this, when trying to eradicate microbes, they will release cellular debris and sometimes biotoxins, and as a result, there is an increase in proinflammatory cytokines, and the body does what it can to detoxify the cellular debris and biotoxins from the body. Having healthy liver and kidney function is essential, and supporting the lymphatics can also help reduce any "herx" symptoms. I talk more about supporting the liver and lymphatics in chapter 24.

Having regular bowel movements and staying well hydrated are both essential, and this can help to minimize "die-off" effects. But you might need to do other things to lessen the symptoms if they are severe. You can always back off on any antimicrobial supplements or medications you're taking (under the guidance of the prescribing doctor), as well as support the lymphatics.

In summary, while many people with hyperthyroidism will follow one of the Hyperthyroid Healing Diets without any issues, this isn't the case with everyone. If this describes you, then hopefully you have found this chapter helpful, as I discussed some of the more common symptoms people may experience when following one of the diets and what can be done to help.

Chapter 10 Highlights

- While some people will follow one of the Hyperthyroid Healing Diets without a problem, for others it won't go as smoothly.
- Many people with hyperthyroidism experience loose stools due to the increase in thyroid hormone, but if you don't experience loose stools until you change your diet, or if you are experiencing loose stools and it worsens upon changing your diet, then chances are you are reacting to something you reintroduced.
- Three factors that can cause constipation include (1) taking antithyroid medication, (2) not being well hydrated, and (3) being sedentary.
- Increasing one's fiber intake, taking magnesium citrate, and/or certain probiotics can help with constipation.
- There can be numerous causes of abdominal bloating, including gut hypersensitivity, impaired gas handling, an altered gut microbiota, and abnormal abdominal-phrenic reflexes.
- Although too much stomach acid can cause acid reflux, in some cases low stomach acid can also be a cause.
- For many people, giving up coffee is the biggest challenge. If this describes you, then you might need to gradually decrease the amount you drink each day, or you can try replacing it with organic decaffeinated coffee or organic green tea.
- If you experience indigestion immediately after eating, then you might have low stomach acid, but if you notice it an hour or two after eating, it might be related to low digestive enzymes.
- Having healthy liver and kidney function is essential to reduce any Herxheimer symptoms, and supporting the lymphatics can also be beneficial.

To access the book references and resources, visit
SaveMyThyroid.com/HHDNotes.

Detecting and Removing Specific Food Triggers

Although changing one's diet alone usually isn't sufficient to reverse hyper-thyroidism, eating well is definitely an important piece of the puzzle. And while you know that you need to avoid common food allergens (i.e., gluten) and other inflammatory foods, the truth is that different people have different food triggers. But how can you identify *your* specific food triggers?

There are two main methods most natural healthcare practitioners use to determine whether someone is reacting to a specific food. One method is an elimination diet, where the person eliminates certain foods for a period of time and then slowly reintroduces foods to see which ones they react to. The second method is food sensitivity testing, and there are a few different options that fall under this category. I'd like to discuss these methods of detecting food triggers separately, including the pros and cons of each, and I'll also discuss a third method to consider: the pulse test.

How Can Food Be a Trigger?

Before comparing the elimination diet with food sensitivity testing, I'll discuss how food can be an inflammatory trigger in the first place. Certain foods, such as gluten, can cause an increase in proinflammatory cytokines, as well as a decrease in regulatory T cells.[1,2,3] As I mentioned in an earlier chapter, regulatory T cells (Tregs) help to keep autoimmunity in check, so you want to have an abundance of these cells.

Molecular mimicry can also play a role, as this is when the peptide sequences of certain foods (i.e., milk and wheat) are similar to those of human molecules. This similarity can result in cross-reactivity that leads to food autoimmunity and even autoimmune disorders.[4]

In addition, certain food allergens can result in a decrease in oral tolerance. This, in turn, triggers an immune system response against various components of food proteins, and cross-reaction with B-cell molecules may trigger autoimmunity.[5] In other words, eating certain foods will result in the immune system attacking the food proteins, and, in the case of mistaken identity, the immune system can also attack body tissues with a similar amino acid sequence.

In addition to causing an increase in proinflammatory cytokines or resulting in a molecular mimicry mechanism, certain food allergens can also cause an increase in intestinal permeability, which is the medical term for a leaky gut. And for those with Graves' disease, according to the triad of autoimmunity discussed in chapter 2, a leaky gut is one of three factors required for the development of an autoimmune condition. It can also lead to food sensitivities through a loss of oral tolerance.

What Is Oral Tolerance?

Oral tolerance plays a key role in preventing our immune system from attacking dietary proteins. Regulatory T cells (Tregs) play a big role in preventing our immune system from reacting to food antigens, as well as from attacking the commensal bacteria. Commensal bacteria (and other microbes) live in harmony with us. Breastfeeding helps the baby to develop oral tolerance, although other factors can also activate Tregs earlier in life. I'm very thankful for these other factors since I wasn't breastfed as a baby!

Having a decrease in Tregs can cause a loss of oral tolerance. This loss of oral tolerance can set the stage for an increase in intestinal permeability, which, in turn, can lead to food sensitivities. While food sensitivities won't always lead to an autoimmune condition such as Graves' disease, having a loss of oral tolerance can increase the likelihood of certain foods becoming an autoimmune trigger. And even if you have a non-autoimmune hyperthyroid condition, it still isn't a good thing to have a loss of oral tolerance, as this can make you more susceptible to health issues in the future.

What Are the Most Common Allergens?

While it is possible to have a sensitivity to any food, the following are the most common food allergens:

- Gluten
- Dairy
- Corn
- Soy
- Eggs
- Shellfish
- Peanuts

In addition, the following foods are commonly problematic in some people:

- Beef
- Pork
- Coffee
- Tea
- Citrus fruits
- Chocolate

Three Ways of Detecting Food Triggers

There are three different methods of detecting specific food triggers, which we'll discuss now.

Food Trigger Detection Method #1: Elimination and Reintroduction Diet. I've been recommending an elimination diet in my practice for many years, and I wouldn't continue to do so if I didn't have success with it. Any of the Hyperthyroid Healing Diets can serve as an elimination diet, although a "true" elimination diet will usually eliminate some of the foods allowed in a Level 1 or Level 2 Hyperthyroid Healing Diet. If you want to be super strict, then it probably is best to go with a Level 3 Hyperthyroid Healing Diet.

For example, most elimination diets will exclude eggs, yet eggs are allowed on both a Level 1 and Level 2 Hyperthyroid Healing Diet. The main reason eggs are excluded is because even though they are nutrient dense, they are also a common allergen. And I as I mentioned in chapter 5, they are also excluded from a Level 3 Hyperthyroid Healing Diet because there are compounds in the egg whites which can have a negative effect on the health of the gastrointestinal tract.

The Benefits of an Elimination Diet

There are a few reasons why I like to have my patients do an elimination diet initially. First, I find that many patients can identify their food triggers if they follow this type of diet carefully. Essentially, you want to follow an elimination diet for a minimum of thirty days, and then after thirty days, you can choose to reintroduce certain foods one at a time, every three days, paying close attention to symptoms.

That being said, I usually try to encourage my patients to follow such a diet for at least ninety days. For many people this will sound too challenging, and from a mental perspective it might be best to set your mind to follow an elimination diet for thirty days, and then if all goes well in those thirty days, you can always continue for another thirty days, etc.

Another benefit of the elimination/reintroduction diet is that it is more cost-effective than doing food sensitivity testing. Testing for food allergens can cost a lot of money, which wouldn't be a problem if the information provided was completely accurate. However, food sensitivity testing is far from perfect, and I'll discuss this in further detail shortly.

The Flaws of an Elimination Diet

Although I have most of my patients initially follow an elimination diet, I'll admit that this does have some limitations. One limitation is that while many people are able to identify foods they are sensitive to, this doesn't always happen. For example, a person with hyperthyroidism might follow an elimination diet, and then upon reintroducing a certain food, they might experience obvious symptoms, such as bloating and gas, headaches, an increase in fatigue, brain fog, or other symptoms. However, some people don't experience any symptoms upon reintroducing foods, and the lack of symptoms doesn't always rule out a food sensitivity.

I will add that the majority of people will notice symptoms upon reintroducing foods they are sensitive to if they pay close attention. And you don't just want to focus on digestive symptoms, as other symptoms can develop as well. Examples of other symptoms people can experience include fatigue, headaches, and rashes, although there can be other symptoms. How can you know for certain if a specific symptom you experience is related to the food you just introduced? As an example, if someone reintroduces egg yolks and they experience a headache, how do they know if the headache was caused by the egg yolks?

It very well could be a coincidence and the person might have experienced the headache regardless. This can be challenging at times, but in a situation where you are unsure if the symptom experienced was a result of the food that was reintroduced, you would stop eating that food for at least two or three additional weeks, and then you can reintroduce the food again. If you experience the same symptom, then you can almost be certain that the food is responsible for that specific symptom.

Another limitation of an elimination/reintroduction diet is that it is possible for someone to be sensitive to one or more of the "permitted" foods. For example, someone can be sensitive to foods that are not normally part of an elimination diet, such as broccoli, asparagus, lettuce, avocados, chicken, blueberries, etc. This can be another major limitation of the elimination diet, and it is a good argument for at least considering food sensitivity testing and/or the pulse test.

How to Reintroduce Foods

After someone has gone on an elimination diet for thirty to ninety days, the next step is to consider the reintroduction of foods. Before I discuss this, I will add that some people thrive on a strict version of the Hyperthyroid Healing Diet (i.e., Level 3), and if this is true with you, then please feel free to stick with the diet for a longer period. For example, if you experience a tremendous improvement in your symptoms upon following a Level 3 Hyperthyroid Healing Diet for ninety days, and if following such a restrictive diet isn't stressful, then it might make sense to continue with the diet for a few additional months. However, I'll add that many people are ready to reintroduce foods after ninety days of a Level 3 Hyperthyroid Healing Diet, and some choose to reintroduce foods sooner than this.

How should you go about reintroducing foods? First of all, you should reintroduce one new food at a time. The obvious reason for this is that if you were to reintroduce multiple foods simultaneously and have a negative reaction, there would be no way to know which food was responsible.

Some suggest that you should eat the food you reintroduce a couple of times on the same day, starting with a smaller serving the first time and then a full serving the second time. This isn't necessary for most people, but some people might have a negative reaction with a small serving and a worsening of symptoms with a larger portion, so it makes sense to start small. After reintroducing the food, you should wait at least an additional two days before reintroducing the next food because it is possible to have a delayed reaction. If everything goes well with the reintroduction, then you can continue eating that food regularly and can then reintroduce the next food.

Just to make sure you understand this process, I'd like to give an example. Let's say you followed a Level 3 Hyperthyroid Healing Diet for ninety days, and on day ninety-one, you decide to reintroduce egg yolks and have half of a scrambled egg yolk for breakfast and an entire egg yolk with lunch. If by the end of day ninety-three (the third day after reintroducing the food) you experience no negative symptoms, then on day ninety-four you can reintroduce a new food. However, if you did experience a negative reaction to the eggs, then you would wait until the symptoms subsided before reintroducing the next food.

Which Foods Should You Reintroduce First?

While some healthcare practitioners recommend that their patients reintroduce foods in a specific order, others don't take this approach. I fall somewhere in between, as while I would never have someone initially reintroduce common allergens (i.e., gluten, dairy), I don't think everyone has to reintroduce the same foods in a specific order. One of the main reasons for this is because not everyone likes to eat the same foods. For example, for those following a Level 3 Hyperthyroid Healing Diet, I commonly recommend that they reintroduce egg yolks first, but some people don't like eggs, and if someone is a vegan, this also wouldn't be an ideal first food to reintroduce.

What I usually do is ask my patients the following question when they are ready to reintroduce foods: "If you had to choose three to five healthy foods to reintroduce, which ones would you choose?" Some of the common responses include foods such as eggs, nuts and seeds, dark chocolate, and nightshade vegetables (i.e., tomatoes). Others want to know if they can reintroduce legumes and gluten-free grains.

For those looking for a specific order of foods to reintroduce, Dr. Sarah Ballantyne, author of the excellent book *The Paleo Approach* recommends reintroducing foods in four different stages. Ideally, you would want to start with the foods in stage #1, and this is the order she has the foods listed in her 2022 update to the Autoimmune Protocol:[6]

Stage #1:

- Egg yolks
- Fruit- and berry-based spices
- Seed and nut oils
- Ghee from grass-fed dairy
- Occasional coffee

- Cocoa or chocolate
- Peas and legumes with edible pods
- Legume sprouts

Stage #2:

- Seeds
- Nuts
- Chia seeds
- Coffee on a daily basis
- Egg whites
- Grass-fed butter
- Alcohol in small quantities

Stage #3:

- Eggplant
- Sweet peppers
- Paprika
- Peeled potatoes
- Grass-fed dairy
- Lentils, split peas, and garbanzo beans (aka chickpeas)

Stage #4:

- Chili peppers and nightshade spices
- Tomatoes
- Unpeeled potatoes
- Alcohol in larger quantities
- Gluten-free grains and pseudo grains
- Traditionally prepared or fermented legumes
- White rice
- Foods you are allergic to or have a history of strong reactions to

I can't say I have all of my patients with hyperthyroidism follow these stages strictly. For example, I usually recommend that my patients reintroduce nuts before legumes. Also, while Dr. Sarah doesn't recommend reintroducing nightshades until stage #3, some of my patients reintroduce nightshades sooner than later. Now to be fair, if you read her 2022 update (which I'll include in the resources), Dr. Sarah does admit that "the AIP dietary framework is not a one-size-fits-all-diet", and I'll add that there is no right or wrong way to choose what foods to reintroduce first. Her suggested order is based on the likelihood that someone will react to a certain food, along with the inherent nutritional value of the food.

I should also mention that it's entirely possible that Dr. Sarah's recommendations have changed since updating this list. Since then she has done a ton of research related to **www.Nutrivore.com**, as well as her new Nutrivore book. And in fact, in November 2023 she conducted a webinar entitled "The Truth about Food Toxins," where she spoke positively about some of the foods that have been excluded from autoimmune protocols.

Symptoms You Might Experience When Reintroducing Foods

If all goes well, then you won't experience a negative reaction when reintroducing a specific food. However, if you do have a negative reaction, then some of the symptoms you may experience can include gas, bloating, abdominal pain, headaches, a decrease in energy, muscle and/or joint pain, insomnia, skin issues, sinus congestion, etc. One question you might have is, "If I experience a specific symptom, how do I know for certain it's related to the food I reintroduced?"

I briefly mentioned this earlier, but it's worth repeating. As another example, if you reintroduce a new food and shortly thereafter you experience severe gas and bloating, then there is a good chance the symptoms are related to the food. However, if you experience a headache or an increase in fatigue, then these symptoms might be related to the food, but there is also a chance that they aren't related.

If you're not certain if a symptom is related to the food being reintroduced, then I would recommend that you stop eating the food for a few weeks and then reintroduce it again in the future. If you do this and experience the same symptoms again, then chances are the specific food is responsible for the symptoms.

Food Trigger Detection Method #2: Food Sensitivity Testing. Although I've recommended IgG food sensitivity testing to some of my patients over the years, through 2022 I honestly wasn't a big fan of IgG food sensitivity testing. However, I started to incorporate more food sensitivity testing into my practice in 2023, although it's still not something I recommend to everyone. What I'd like to do now is discuss the pros and cons of food sensitivity testing:

The Benefits of Food Sensitivity Testing

Perhaps the main benefit of food sensitivity testing is that it can potentially identify specific foods you are reacting to that might be allowed on an elimination diet (i.e., Level 3 Diet). Although over the years I haven't been a big fan of such testing due to some of the limitations I'll discuss shortly, I have had some patients successfully identify foods that were causing problems. In some of these cases, the foods were permitted on an elimination/ reintroduction diet.

Another advantage of food sensitivity testing is that it might prevent the person from having to eliminate certain foods. However, we also need to keep in mind that false negatives are possible with this type of testing. In addition, there are other reasons for avoiding certain foods. For example, I recommend that my patients avoid gluten and dairy while restoring their health, regardless of what a food sensitivity panel shows. With regard to some of the other "excluded" foods, we need to keep in mind that some foods are excluded not because they are common allergens but because they have compounds that can affect the healing of the gut.

Nightshades represent an example of this, as they are excluded from certain diets due to the compounds that can result in inflammation and/or an increase in intestinal permeability in some people. Solanine is a glycoalkaloid found in the nightshade foods, especially eggplant and white potatoes, although it's also found in tomatoes and peppers. However, if someone does a food sensitivity panel and tests negative for eggplant, white potatoes, tomatoes, and peppers, this doesn't mean that these foods won't cause problems.

One additional benefit of food sensitivity testing is that if someone tests positive and if it is a "true" positive, then this serves as a baseline reading. In other words, if someone tests positive for one or more foods, and if they decide to reintroduce the food in the future when their gut is healed and immune tolerance has been restored, they have the option of doing another food sensitivity test after reintroducing the food to see if they are still reacting to that specific food.

The Disadvantages of Food Sensitivity Testing

While it might sound great to do food sensitivity testing to determine the specific foods you are reacting to, unfortunately, this type of testing has some disadvantages as well. Here are a few of the main ones:

- **False results are possible.** This is a big deal, as you can test negative for a specific food on some panels, and it very well might be a false negative. This means that you might continue to eat foods you are sensitive to because they showed up as negative on a food sensitivity test. As for false positives, this also can happen, and it is common to test positive for dozens of foods when someone has a leaky gut, but this doesn't mean that you have "true" food sensitivities to all of these foods. You might just need to focus on healing your gut, which I discuss in chapter 21.

- **With IgG testing you need to have recently eaten the foods you're testing for.** With certain types of food sensitivity tests (i.e., IgG food sensitivity testing), you need to either be eating the foods, or have recently eaten the foods you're testing for to get an accurate result. The reason for this is that IgG food sensitivity testing measures antibodies associated with an immune reaction to foods, and you won't produce antibodies to a food if you have avoided it for a few months.

- **Most food sensitivity panels are incomplete.** By this I mean that most panels don't test for all of the foods a person eats. Even the more comprehensive panels that test for close to two hundred foods commonly omit some common ones, which means that even if the test were accurate, there would be no way to know if you had a sensitivity to the foods it doesn't test for.

- **Doing this type of testing can be expensive.** The truth is that a lot of different tests are expensive, and this shouldn't be the primary reason not to do a certain test. In other words, if food sensitivity testing was pretty accurate, I would recommend it a lot more frequently than I do now, regardless of the cost, and then if the patient wasn't able to afford it, that would be fine. But it's still something to consider, as if someone is on a very tight budget, I'd rather them do other testing I consider to be more important (and more accurate).

- **There can be differences between raw and cooked foods.** This is one of the advantages of Cyrex Labs Multiple Food Immune Reactivity Screen (Array #10), as it measures some foods both raw and cooked. Some of the foods it tests for both raw and cooked include broccoli, cabbage, carrots, garlic, and mushrooms. I don't know of any other food sensitivity test that does this.

Comparing the Different Types of Testing for Food Allergens

Now that you know some of the pros and cons of food sensitivity testing, let's look at some of the different types of testing available for food allergens.

IgE testing. This relates to food allergies, which usually result in immediate symptoms. Skin-prick testing is still used initially by many doctors to determine the presence of an IgE allergy. This test involves introducing a needle into the upper layers of the skin and using a drop of the allergen, and then the release of histamine from mast cells will lead to the development of a wheal greater than 3 mm in diameter if the person is sensitive to the allergen.[7,8] However, the research shows that there is the possibility of false positive results with this test.[9,10] Serum IgE testing (through the blood) can also be used in some cases to detect food allergies.[11] Although this also has some limitations, this does seem to be more accurate than the skin-prick test.

IgG testing. Serum IgG testing is commonly used by practitioners to determine whether someone has a food sensitivity. Unlike IgE food allergies, which involve an immediate response, IgG testing for food sensitivities involve a delayed response. In other words, the person with one or more IgG sensitivities might not experience symptoms for a few hours or, in some cases, a few days after eating a certain food.

This type of testing is available from many different companies. However, just as is the case with IgE testing for food allergies, IgG testing for food sensitivities has the potential of giving a false negative or a false positive result. It's also important to keep in mind that an increase in intestinal permeability (leaky gut) can increase the incidence of food sensitivities. As a result, if someone has many food sensitivities on a panel, then this is good indication of an increase in intestinal permeability, along with a loss of oral tolerance. Therefore, if someone has many food sensitivities, then it makes sense to take measures to heal the gut and restore oral tolerance, which I discussed earlier in this chapter.

How to Choose a Company for Food Sensitivity Testing

When choosing a company for food sensitivity testing, keep in mind that they are testing food proteins, and the purity and quality of these purified proteins are very important because if there are any contaminants, then it's possible for a positive reading to be false due to the contaminant and not the food protein.

In addition, some people might react to a certain food when eaten raw, but they might do fine when eating that same food cooked. I mentioned this earlier when I discussed one of the advantages of the Multiple Food Immune Reactivity Screen from Cyrex Labs (Array #10), as this panel tests a number of different foods both raw and cooked. I have run this test on some of my patients and have seen some people test positive for a raw food and negative for the same food when cooked, and vice versa.

If you choose IgG food sensitivity testing you ideally want to choose a lab that runs every sample through twice, as it's important for the results to be reproducible. There have been some cases with certain labs when two separate blood samples from the same person were submitted and the two reports gave different findings.

Although I like Cyrex Labs a lot and recommend their panels at times due to some of the reasons discussed here, some other food sensitivity tests from different companies can also be valuable. If your doctor is using a specific company and has been doing so for a long time, chances are they are doing so because they are getting good results with their patients. I admit that I have used other labs for food sensitivity testing as well such as Alletess Medical Laboratory.

Mediator release testing (MRT). This is a blood test that determines how you react to 170 different foods and food chemicals, and according to their website has 93.6 percent split sample reproducibility. The way it works is by measuring the size of your white blood cells before and after they are exposed to each food and food chemical. Essentially, the more your white blood cells decrease in size, the more pro-inflammatory chemicals they have released, which in turn means that you have a stronger food sensitivity.

So unlike IgG food sensitivity testing, which measures antibodies, MRT measures the release of mediators, which are inflammatory chemicals. An example of a mediator is histamine, although there are many more. Once someone receives their MRT results, they are put on a LEAP (Lifestyle Eating and Performance) elimination diet, which can be combined with any of the Hyperthyroid Healing Diets discussed earlier. I'll talk more about my experience with MRT shortly.

Leukocyte activation testing. The ALCAT test from Cell Science Systems utilizes this technology, and, as mentioned on their website, "The ALCAT test measures food/immune reactions through stimulation of leukocytes. The leukocytes, which comprise five classes of white blood cells, including monocytes, lymphocytes, eosinophils, basophils, and neutrophils, can be challenged with individual food or chemical extracts."[12] The patient's unique set of responses helps to identify substances that may trigger potentially harmful immune system reactions.

This is different than IgG testing, but is it more accurate? Some healthcare professionals question whether leukocyte activation testing is reproducible. Many healthcare professionals use other labs for IgG testing and receive great results with their patients, although some healthcare professionals have successfully used leukocyte activation testing in their practice for many years.

Can You Do Both Food Sensitivity Testing *and* Follow an Elimination Diet?

I briefly mentioned this in my book *Hashimoto's Triggers*, which was published in 2018. This is what I said back then: Since neither an elimination diet nor food sensitivity testing is a perfect method for detecting food sensitivities, in some cases, it might make sense to combine both. You can choose to do a food sensitivity panel initially, and combine this with an elimination diet.

So before starting an elimination diet, the person would get the blood draw for the food sensitivity panel. Then, while waiting for the results, they can go ahead and follow the elimination diet for thirty days, and then upon receiving the results of the food sensitivity test, they would stop eating any foods they test positive for. For example, if they test positive on the food sensitivity panel for broccoli, carrots, and a few other "allowed" foods, they will not only stop eating these foods, but they won't reintroduce these foods until their gut has healed.

Even though I mentioned this in my book *Hashimoto's Triggers*, I didn't think of incorporating it until I interviewed Elizabeth Yarnell and Dr. Anshul Gupta on the *Save My Thyroid* podcast. I met Elizabeth at a retreat in Tampa, Florida, in November of 2021, and she was using mediator release testing (MRT) as a tool to help her autoimmune patients. (Elizabeth herself was diagnosed with multiple sclerosis and was thriving.) I had heard of MRT, and actually had some patients do this testing through other practitioners over the years, but I never really considered using it in my practice.

However, shortly after interviewing Elizabeth I also interviewed Dr. Anshul Gupta, as during a podcast episode (**www.savemythyroid.com/28**) we were discussing the different autoimmune thyroid triggers. When the topic of food came up, I asked Dr. Gupta if he uses an elimination diet, or food sensitivity testing to detect food triggers. He responded by saying "both," and then I asked him what he uses for food sensitivity testing, and he mentioned IgG food sensitivity testing and MRT.

I found this interesting, and I asked which of the two he prefers, and he said MRT is his first choice. It was at this point when I decided that I would start incorporating MRT into my practice, although I admittedly didn't do it frequently until later interviews I had on my podcast with other practitioners who mentioned that they used MRT. And even currently I can't say that it's a test I recommend to every patient.

My Experience with Mediator Release Testing

So I admittedly remained skeptical about MRT initially, even after chatting with Elizabeth Yarnell and Dr. Gupta, and when I did bring it up to patients I was upfront and let them know that I had just started recommending this type of test and wasn't sure if I would continue to do so in the future. It of course would depend on the results people received, as I already had a lot of success in my practice without using any type of food sensitivity testing. But just like any other natural healthcare practitioner, I'm always looking for ways to get even better results, and with some clients it's been more challenging to find their triggers, and I figured that MRT could be another tool to help with this.

Fast-forward to the second half of 2023, and I started recommending mediator release testing more frequently (although still not to everyone), along with still recommending one of the Hyperthyroid Healing Diets as well. Has this led to better outcomes with my patients? Although it might have resulted in slightly better outcomes overall, I have gotten great results with many patients throughout the years without taking this approach. Many people are able to find their food triggers with an elimination diet alone, but combining this with MRT, or even Cyrex Labs Array #10, will make it even more likely that you will find any food triggers that may be present.

I still recommend an elimination diet initially to most patients, and at times will recommend food sensitivity testing if the person isn't progressing as expected. If someone absolutely wants a food sensitivity test when I consult with them initially, I'll order it for them, but I currently prioritize other testing.

Testing for Chemicals

It's also worth mentioning that some of these food sensitivity tests not only test for foods, but also measure reactivity to chemicals commonly found in food. For example, MRT tests for over two dozen non-food ingredients, including potassium nitrite and nitrate, aspartame, MSG, acetaminophen, FD&C blue #1, FD&C yellow #5, and FD&C red #40, as well as others. The Multiple Food Immune Reactivity Screen from Cyrex Labs tests for carrageenan, food coloring, guar gum, locust bean gum, and xanthan gum. Of course it would be great if there were a single test that measured the reactivity to all of these, as it's not practical for most people to do multiple food sensitivity tests.

Food Trigger Detection Method #3: The Pulse Test. Although I had heard of the pulse test many years ago, I can't say that I have consistently used it in my practice. Part of the challenge is that most people with hyperthyroidism have an elevated resting heart rate, and many take antithyroid medication and/or beta blockers, which can also influence the heart rate. However, I still wanted to mention the pulse test here as an option to detect food triggers, as it still might be something you want to try, perhaps in combination with an elimination diet or food sensitivity testing.

The pulse test is based on the premise that being exposed to allergens will speed up your pulse rate shortly after they are eaten. So essentially you test foods individually to determine which ones speed up the pulse. If you really want to learn more about this, I recommend reading the book *The Pulse Test* by Dr. Arthur Coca.

But this is essentially how it works:

- Take your pulse in the morning before getting out of bed, and again right before your first meal.
- Limit the meal to a single, simple food (i.e., egg, plain piece of chicken, avocado, plain steamed broccoli).
- Check your pulse again thirty minutes after the meal, and then again sixty minutes after the meal.
- After checking your pulse at the sixty-minute mark you can eat another single food and repeat the procedure.
- Repeat this throughout the day.

According to the author, "any count above 84 beats per minute (BPM), in children or adults, if taken when the patient is quiet and has no infection such as a cold, has usually been a sign of allergy." But once again, the problem is that many people with hyperthyroidism have an elevated resting heart rate that exceeds 84 BPM. If this describes you, then you might not be a good candidate for the pulse test. On the other hand, if your hyperthyroidism is more subclinical and your resting heart rate is in the 50s, 60s, or 70s (without taking antithyroid agents), then this is something you might want to look into.

Chapter 11 Highlights

- While you need to avoid common food allergens (i.e., gluten) and other inflammatory foods, the truth is that different people have different food triggers.
- Certain foods, such as gluten, can cause an increase in proinflammatory cytokines, as well as a decrease in regulatory T cells (Tregs).
- Oral tolerance plays a key role in preventing our immune system from attacking dietary proteins, and having a decrease in Tregs can cause a loss of oral tolerance.
- The most common food allergens include gluten, dairy, corn, soy, eggs, shellfish, and peanuts.
- Three ways to detect food triggers include (1) an elimination and reintroduction diet, (2) food sensitivity testing, and (3) the pulse test.
- Any of the Hyperthyroid Healing Diets can serve as an elimination diet, although a "true" elimination diet will usually eliminate some of the foods allowed in a Level 1 or Level 2 Hyperthyroid Healing Diet. If you want to be super strict, then it probably is best to go with a Level 3 Hyperthyroid Healing Diet
- Although I have most of my patients initially follow an elimination diet, I'll admit that this does have some limitations.
- After someone has gone on an elimination diet for thirty to ninety days, the next step is to consider the reintroduction of foods.
- Perhaps the main benefit of food sensitivity testing is that it can potentially identify specific foods you are reacting to that might be allowed on an elimination diet.
- Here are a few disadvantages of food sensitivity testing: false results are possible, with IgG testing you need to eat the foods you're testing for, most food sensitivity panels are incomplete, doing this type of testing can be expensive, and there can be differences between raw and cooked foods.
- The pulse test is based on the premise that eating foods you are allergic to will speed up your pulse rate shortly after you eat them.

To access the book references and resources, visit
SaveMyThyroid.com/HHDNotes.

Hidden Sources of Common Allergens and Other Ingredients to Avoid

W hile many people reading this will make an effort to avoid the common allergens, for some it can be challenging to completely avoid these. One reason is because of the "hidden" sources of these common allergens. For example, someone might think it's perfectly safe to eat deli meat, only to find that it isn't completely free of these allergens. Or they might eat out and order something they think is free of these allergens, only to realize (or perhaps not realize) that there is cross contamination.

It's amazing how many foods contain gluten, not to mention dairy, corn, soy, etc. Because of this, you really do need to carefully read the labels on any packaged foods. You also need to understand that companies may change their ingredients, so just because something is allergen-free today doesn't mean it will remain allergen-free.

In this chapter I will discuss some of the most common hidden sources of gluten, dairy, corn, and soy. Then I will discuss other ingredients you will want to try your best to avoid. Of course the best way to avoid these allergens and other ingredients is to prepare your own meals and focus on eating whole, healthy foods.

But just a reminder that even packaged whole foods can have "hidden" ingredients at times, which is why you want to carefully read the label of any food that comes in a package. An example of this is deli meat, as some might consider sliced chicken or turkey to be a healthy option. But if you purchase sliced chicken or turkey, you want to carefully read the label, especially if it's not organic, as you might find ingredients such as corn syrup and nitrites.

Reminder: Gluten-Free Isn't Always Healthy

There are a lot of gluten-free options available these days, especially when compared to ten to twenty years ago. But remember that just because something is gluten-free doesn't mean it's healthy. For some this will be obvious, especially when it comes to foods such as gluten-free pizza. Others will gravitate toward gluten-free cookies, crackers, and cereals.

Of course, the same is true with some organic foods, as just because something is "organic" doesn't mean it's healthy. There is plenty of organic junk food in health food stores. Now, to be completely upfront, I can't say that I never eat gluten-free and organic junk food, but I don't eat it regularly, and I definitely didn't eat it when I was dealing with hyperthyroidism back in 2008/2009 and trying to get into remission.

Is Gluten Free *Really* Gluten Free?

Even if you purchase a processed food which is gluten-free, it still might have traces of gluten in it. According to the US Food and Drug Administration, one of the criteria proposed is that foods bearing the claim gluten-free cannot contain 20 parts per million (ppm) or more gluten.[1] I once attended a seminar where the presenter spoke about some people with a gluten sensitivity problem reacting if the food contained as low as 5 ppm. I wasn't able to find any studies showing this, but if someone is trying to avoid gluten, it's important to realize that many packaged foods that are labeled as being gluten-free might still contain trace amounts of gluten, and in some cases this can cause problems. The obvious solution to this is to ditch the processed foods, even the "healthier" ones, and stick with whole, healthy foods.

It's also important to understand that gluten-free certification is different from general gluten-free labeling, as if a company is *certified gluten-free*, it means that this is confirmed by an independent third-party organization. There are currently three different agencies that certify foods as being gluten-free, and they each have different standards. For example, the Gluten-Free Certification Program (GFCP) requires the gluten levels to be less than 20 ppm, while the Celiac Support Association (CSA) only certifies foods containing less than 5 ppm of gluten.[2]

Hidden Sources of Gluten

Once again, if you are focusing on eating naturally gluten-free foods such as meat, fish, fruits, and nuts, you will greatly minimize your exposure to gluten. But in addition to packaged foods that may include gluten (even if they have a gluten-free label), here are some other potential sources of gluten:

- Broth/stock
- Eggs (at some restaurants)
- Certain marinades
- Certain medications
- Certain nutritional supplements
- Licorice and other candy
- Non-certified oat products
- Processed lunch meats and deli meats

- Salad dressings
- Some alcoholic beverages (i.e., beer, ale)
- Some cosmetics
- Some flavored coffees and teas
- Some potato chips and French fries
- Soups and gravies

If you have any doubts as to whether something has gluten in it, even after reading the ingredients, I recommend avoiding it. Just focus on eating naturally gluten-free foods that you know are safe to eat (meat, fish, poultry, fruits, and vegetables). But just remember what I said earlier: if any food is packaged, you want to carefully read the label.

Hidden Sources of Dairy

Now let's focus on some of the hidden sources of dairy. Once again, I would make sure you carefully read the ingredients of anything you consume.

- Certain medications (including methimazole and PTU, which have lactose)
- Certain nutritional supplements
- Lactose-free products
- Some brands of dark chocolate
- Some gravies
- Some salad dressings
- Some soups

I want to expand on lactose-free products, as while lactose is a sugar found in milk, there are other ingredients in dairy as well, including whey and casein. As a result, just because something is labeled as lactose-free doesn't mean that it's completely dairy-free. While I'm sure many people reading this are aware of this, I'm also sure there are some people who don't know this.

You might have also noticed that antithyroid medication is on the list, as both methimazole and PTU have lactose. First of all, I'm honestly more concerned about casein than lactose when it comes to a dairy sensitivity. Many people have a lactose "intolerance" which is related to a deficiency in the enzyme lactase, and isn't related to an allergy or sensitivity. And second, everything comes down to risks vs. benefits, and so while I chose not to take antithyroid medication when I dealt with Graves' disease, some people do need to take it…hopefully on a temporary basis while trying to restore their health.

Hidden Sources of Corn

Obviously, anything that has the word corn in it (i.e., corn syrup) has corn. But there are many other foods and products that can have corn:

- Ascorbic acid
- Caramel
- Confectioners' sugar
- Hydrolyzed vegetable protein
- Maltodextrin
- Modified food starch
- Xanthan gum
- Xylitol
- Vegetable oil (may contain corn or soy)
- Certain medications (including methimazole and PTU, which have corn starch)
- Certain nutritional supplements

Not all of these ingredients include corn. For example, maltodextrin may be tapioca-based, but if it just says "maltodextrin," then I would assume it's corn-based. The Gluten Free Society has a comprehensive list of possible ingredients that may have corn, which you can check out by visiting the following link: **www.glutenfreesociety.org/hidden-corn-based-ingredients**.

Once again, antithyroid medication is listed here, as both methimazole and PTU have corn starch. This can be more of a concern than the lactose I mentioned earlier, and this is especially true if someone has a sensitivity to corn. So while everything comes down to risks vs. benefits, if someone is taking antithyroid medication and at the same time is trying to restore their health, but they don't seem to be improving, there is always the chance that one or more of the ingredients in the antithyroid medication is the culprit. This doesn't mean you should abruptly stop taking it, but I just want to make you aware of this possibility, even if it is an unlikely scenario.

Hidden Sources of Soy

Just as is the case with corn, anything that has the word *soy* in it (i.e., soy protein isolate) has soy. But here are some of the foods and products that may also have soy:[3]

- Kinako flour
- Kyodofu (freeze-dried tofu)
- Natto
- Lecithin (may be derived from soy)
- Mono & diglycerides
- Monosodium glutamate (or MSG)
- Tamari
- Teriyaki
- Textured vegetable protein (or TVP)
- Vegetable oil (may contain corn or soybean oil)
- Vegetable starch
- Tofu
- Yuba
- Edamame
- Natural flavoring

Not all of these ingredients include soy. For example, if you purchase vegetable oil, you need to read the label and see if it includes soy. Natural flavors may include soy on the label, although in some cases you may need to contact the manufacturer.

Other Ingredients to Avoid

There are many other ingredients you should avoid, and I won't be listing all of these in this chapter. I will focus on what I consider to be some of the main ingredients to avoid, but this doesn't mean that there aren't others. While I would try your best to avoid the ingredients I'll be listing, I would get in the habit of looking up any other ingredients you're unsure of.

Here are some of the main ingredients to avoid:

- Artificial coloring (i.e., Blue 1, Red 40, Yellow #5)
- Artificial flavors and sweeteners
- BHA (butylated hydroxyanisole) synthetic preservative
- BHT (butylated hydroxytoluene) synthetic preservative
- Caramel color
- Carrageenan (thickener and emulsifier)
- Citric acid: preservative and flavor
- Corn syrup and high fructose corn syrup: heavily processed form of sugar made from corn
- Hydrolyzed protein: monosodium glutamate
- Maltodextrin: heavily processed starch used as a filler, thickener, preservative and sweetener
- Monosodium glutamate (MSG): artificial flavor enhancer
- Natural flavors: flavors made from a proprietary mixture of chemicals derived from anything in nature
- Sodium benzoate or potassium benzoate
- Sodium nitrate or sodium nitrite
- Titanium dioxide: food color used to brighten and whiten

Once again, there are many more ingredients you should avoid that aren't listed here, but these are some of the more common ones you're likely to find, even in some foods that are allowed on the Hyperthyroid Healing Diets. For example, coconut milk is allowed, but you might find one or more of the ingredients I just listed in some brands of coconut milk. However, one way around this is to make your own coconut milk.

Once again, focusing on eating whole, healthy foods and preparing your own foods is the best way to avoid common allergens, along with these potentially harmful ingredients. As soon as you purchase something prepackaged and/ or eat out at a restaurant, you greatly increase your chances of being exposed to one or more of these ingredients.

Should You Avoid Thickening Gums?

Some products include thickening gums, such as xanthan, guar gum, and locust bean gum. These are important to avoid if you have an autoimmune condition such as Graves' disease. The Multiple Food Immune Reactivity Screen from Cyrex Labs actually measures reactivity to the different gums commonly found in products, including guar gum, locust bean gum, mastic gum, and xanthan gum.

How to Become an Expert in Reading and Understanding Food Labels

One of the best books out there to help you read and understand what's on the label is *The Pantry Principle* by Mira Dessy. You can also check out the interview I did with her on the *Save My Thyroid* podcast (**www.savemythyroid.com/104**). While reading her book is highly recommended and will greatly increase your knowledge when it comes to the different ingredients you should avoid, the very best way to become an expert is to apply what you learn. In other words, after you read her book, start carefully reading labels every time you visit the grocery store!

Chapter 12 Highlights

- In order to avoid common allergens such as gluten, dairy, corn, and soy, you need to carefully read the labels on any packaged foods.
- Remember that just because something is gluten-free doesn't mean it's healthy, and the same is true with some organic foods.
- If you purchase a processed food that is gluten-free, it still might have traces of gluten in it.
- Hidden sources of gluten include broth, eggs, marinades, medications, nutritional supplements, processed lunch meats, salad dressings, some alcoholic beverages, some flavored coffees and teas, soups and gravies.
- Hidden sources of dairy include medications, nutritional supplements, dark chocolate, gravies, salad dressings, soups.
- Just because something is labeled as lactose-free doesn't mean that it's completely dairy free.
- Hidden sources of corn include ascorbic acid, caramel, confectioners' sugar, hydrolyzed vegetable protein, maltodextrin, modified food starch, xanthan gum, xylitol, medications, and nutritional supplements.
- Hidden sources of soy include edamame, kinako flour, lecithin, mono and diglycerides, MSG, tamari, textured vegetable protein, vegetable oil, and natural flavoring.
- Other ingredients to avoid include artificial colors, flavors, and sweeteners, BHA and BHT, carrageenan, citric acid, corn syrup, high fructose corn syrup, MSG, sodium nitrate and nitrite, and titanium dioxide.

To access the book references and resources, visit
SaveMyThyroid.com/HHDNotes.

CHAPTER
13

Weight Loss and Weight Gain Concerns

W hen I dealt with Graves' disease in 2008, I lost a lot of weight. Forty two pounds to be exact. That being said, some people with hyperthyroidism gain weight due to numerous factors, and in this chapter I will cover both scenarios. First I will discuss the concerns related to weight loss during hyperthyroidism, and then I will discuss how some people with hyperthyroidism gain weight and what they can do about it.

Obviously the primary (or even secondary) goal of any of the diet options I discussed in this book isn't to lose weight. The primary goal is to eat an anti-inflammatory, gut-healing diet that is packed with nutrients. Caloric restriction isn't required, but some weight loss is common when following this diet because people are reducing the carbohydrates and inflammatory foods.

The Number One Reason People with Hyperthyroidism Lose Weight

The main reason many people with hyperthyroidism lose weight is because of the elevated thyroid hormone levels, which in turn increases the metabolism. As a result, it makes sense that in order to gain weight, you need to do things to lower the thyroid hormones. While the goal is to try to address the underlying cause of the condition, initially you might choose to take antithyroid medication such as methimazole, or perhaps natural agents that can lower thyroid hormones such as bugleweed, higher doses of L-carnitine, or lithium orotate.

Without question, antithyroid medication is more potent, so if someone is able to tolerate the medication, they are more likely to gain weight quicker when compared to someone who is managing their symptoms naturally. In my situation I took the herb bugleweed (along with motherwort), and while I eventually gained weight, it was a slow process. And in many cases it's the same situation with the patients I work with.

Another Reason People Commonly Lose Weight

While the number one reason people with hyperthyroidism lose weight is related to elevated thyroid hormone levels, this doesn't mean there can't be other factors. Malabsorption is another reason why some people lose weight. In fact, if someone's thyroid hormone levels are decreasing and they still aren't gaining weight within a reasonable amount of time, then it's very possible that they have some type of malabsorption issue.

So how can someone with hyperthyroidism have a malabsorption problem? Well, there are a few different ways:

1. **Elevated thyroid hormones.** It's known that the acceleration of intestinal transit can increase nutrient malabsorption, and hyperthyroidism can increase intestinal transit. So while the increased metabolism associated with hyperthyroidism can be a big factor when it comes to losing weight, we can't ignore the impact of high thyroid hormone levels on the gastrointestinal tract.

2. **Celiac disease.** Celiac disease is defined as an autoimmune disorder originating from an aberrant adaptive immune response against

gluten-containing grains in susceptible individuals.[1] In those with this condition, the ingestion of gluten leads to an enteropathy with an impairment of the mucosal surface and, consequently, abnormal absorption of nutrients.[1] The research shows that those with thyroid autoimmunity are more likely to develop celiac disease, and one study showed that those with hyperthyroidism were more likely to develop it than those with hypothyroidism.[2]

3. **Bile acid malabsorption.** This probably isn't a common cause, although there is a case study that shows an association between bile acid malabsorption and Graves' disease.[3]

4. **Small intestinal bacterial overgrowth (SIBO).** To some people this might not make sense, as whereas hyperthyroidism speeds up the intestinal transit, a delayed small intestinal transit can cause SIBO. Obviously I'm not suggesting that hyperthyroidism is a cause of SIBO, but people with hyperthyroidism can have SIBO for other reasons. I discuss SIBO in greater detail in chapter 18.

5. **Other causes.** Some other potential causes of malabsorption include inflammatory bowel disease (Crohn's disease, ulcerative colitis), chronic pancreatitis, cystic fibrosis, and even certain infections of the gut, including parasites.

For those who have Graves' disease, part of the triad of autoimmunity involves an increase in intestinal permeability, or a leaky gut. Some will assume that if they have a leaky gut that this will cause malabsorption, and thus can be a reason behind one's weight loss. Although some of the factors that can cause a leaky gut can also cause malabsorption (i.e., inflammatory bowel disease), this doesn't mean that everyone with a leaky gut will experience malabsorption. Even though I've mentioned leaky gut numerous times throughout this book, I talk more about what a leaky gut is in chapter 21.

Are There Foods You Can Eat to Gain Weight?

While people with hyperthyroidism commonly ask me what foods they can eat to gain weight, you really need to address the underlying cause of the weight loss. For example, if someone is losing weight because of elevated thyroid hormone levels, eating certain foods is unlikely to cause them to gain a significant amount of weight, and the same is true if someone has a separate malabsorption problem (i.e., not caused by hyperthyroidism). That being said, I would of course make sure to eat nutrient-dense foods consisting of healthy fats and sufficient protein, which I discussed in chapter 4.

Some people will do the opposite and will load up on carbohydrates. While it's probably okay to increase the amount of healthy carbohydrates you consume on a temporary basis (i.e., sweet potatoes), if the ultimate goal is to regain your health, then you don't want to binge on processed and packaged carbohydrates. And while there are healthier versions of these foods (i.e., sweet potato chips with coconut oil), I still wouldn't recommend indulging too much just for the purpose of gaining weight.

When Should Weight Loss Be a Concern?

Just as a reminder, when I was dealing with Graves' disease I had lost 42 pounds. Initially I weighed 182 pounds, so I dropped down to 140 pounds, which definitely was a lot less than it should have been for my height. I'd be lying if I told you there was no concern, but it wasn't like it would have been an emergency situation if I lost another 5 to 10 pounds. Of course there are women who are very petite who lose a lot of weight, and I understand the concern here.

For example, if someone normally weighs 120 pounds and drops down to 95 pounds, then this could be very stressful. I have worked with a lot of patients in this situation, and it's very common for them to tell me that they can't afford to lose any more weight. The truth is that most of these people wouldn't be in a dire situation if they lost a few more pounds, but of course my goal is to help them address the cause of the weight loss (usually by addressing the hyperthyroidism).

As for when weight loss is a concern, if you do some research you might find sources that state if you lose more than 5 percent of your weight over six to twelve months, then this is a reason for concern. Of course, with hyperthyroidism many people lose well beyond 5 percent in a much shorter time span. So the real question should be, "When is weight loss a dire concern?" In other words, how much weight loss is considered to be an emergency situation?

The truth is that everyone is different, and if someone drops from 120 pounds to 95 pounds, then this would be considered losing slightly more than 20 percent of their body weight. Once again, in most situations this is a concern, but not necessarily a dire concern. On the other hand, if someone loses 30 percent or more weight, then I'd say this is definitely a more urgent situation.

But once again, every situation is different, so if someone loses 10 to 15 percent of their weight in a short period of time, I don't want them to think there is absolutely no concern, as in any of these scenarios I would recommend doing everything you can to lower the thyroid hormones and address any other potential causes discussed earlier in this chapter. And of course I also need to mention here that you need to use your own judgment, and if necessary, don't hesitate to consult with your primary care doctor.

Weight Gain Challenges and Hyperthyroidism

Although weight loss is a classic symptom of hyperthyroidism (which is why it was discussed first), there are some people with hyperthyroidism who struggle to lose weight. Here, I cover the more common reasons why some people with hyperthyroidism gain weight.

Reason #1: Taking antithyroid agents. It should be obvious why this would cause weight gain, as the goal of both prescription and natural antithyroid agents is to lower thyroid hormone levels. And while the perfect scenario would involve someone taking the antithyroid agent and having optimal thyroid hormone levels, many times this isn't the case. This is especially true when taking antithyroid medication such as methimazole. In fact, it's not uncommon for someone to become hypothyroid while taking the antithyroid medication, and this definitely can cause unwanted weight gain. But at times it can also happen with natural antithyroid agents such as bugleweed.

Reason #2: Chronic stress and high cortisol. In many cases chronic stress is a big factor in the development of hyperthyroidism. And when cortisol remains elevated for a prolonged period of time, it is likely to result in weight gain. In fact, the research shows that chronic stress and cortisol imbalances can play a role in obesity.[4,5] You and I know that we can't eliminate all of our stressors, but most people can do things to improve their stress-handling skills. After all, our perception of stress is usually a bigger factor than the stressor itself.

Reason #3: Insulin resistance. With insulin resistance there is plenty of insulin, but it doesn't get into the cell. While eating a healthy diet consisting of whole foods while minimizing carbohydrate intake can help with some cases of insulin resistance, inflammation is also associated with insulin resistance.[6,7] In order to overcome many cases of insulin resistance, the inflammation needs to be addressed.

Reason #4: Leptin resistance. Leptin is an adipocyte-secreted hormone that regulates the appetite and represents a key factor in the development of obesity.[8] Just a small increase in leptin causes a reduction of appetite. But just as is the case with insulin resistance, leptin resistance involves higher concentrations of leptin in the blood, which results from problems with the leptin receptor and/or decreases in leptin transport across the blood-brain barrier.[8,9]

Reason #5: Inflammation. I mentioned inflammation earlier when I discussed insulin resistance. And there can be many different causes of inflammation, including food sensitivities, chemicals, and infections. There are plenty of studies that show a connection between inflammation and obesity.[10,11,12]

Reason #6: Estrogen metabolism problems. Just a reminder that estrogen isn't a "bad" hormone, and in fact, it's important to have healthy levels of estrogen. There are multiple reasons why many women (and even men) have estrogen metabolism problems. Unfortunately, one of the main reasons is our exposure to xenoestrogens, which are endocrine-disrupting chemicals that are also referred to as *obesogens*.[13]

How Do Obesogens Cause Weight Gain?

Obesogens cause metabolism changes due to the effects they have on hormones in the body. For example, these chemicals can affect thyroid hormone production, which in turn will lower the metabolic rate and lead to weight gain. Obesogens can also affect other hormones, including resistin and leptin, which affect insulin sensitivity and satiety respectively. This shows that the effects of exposure to these chemicals can be adverse. Scientists are worried about obesogens because even the slightest exposure can have adverse effects.

We interact with these chemicals frequently, and while it's impossible to completely avoid them, limiting exposure to them can be an effective way to combat obesogenic effects. When doing research, I came across a journal article that classified arsenic as an obesogen. And while arsenic is harmful in other ways, it also has been shown to impair white adipose tissue metabolism,[14] which plays a big role in the onset of obesity. Some of the sources of arsenic include pesticides, herbicides, chicken, brown rice, and drinking water can also be a potential source.

When you are following a weight loss plan strictly and you continue to gain weight, you could be facing the wrath of these notorious chemicals. Apart from the universally known role of storing and releasing energy, scientists have also unearthed another role of fat tissue: playing the role of releasing appetite and metabolism hormones. As a result, an effect on either the performance or nature of this cell is bound to cause adverse effects in the body.

So far, research has shown that this can happen in the following ways:

- Transformation of normal cells to fat cells
- Increased population of fat cells in body
- Higher fat content in fat cells
- Altered metabolic rate leading to more storage of calories

How to Overcome Unwanted Weight Gain with Hyperthyroidism

I just discussed six factors that can make it challenging for anyone to lose weight, and not just those with hyperthyroidism. For those with hyperthyroidism who struggle with unwanted weight gain, in order to lose weight you obviously want to find the cause of the weight gain and then address it. You might want to refer to some of the other chapters where I discuss these factors in greater detail (i.e., chronic stress, insulin resistance), but here are a few quick tips to help get you started with shedding unwanted pounds:

- **If you're taking antithyroid medication, check with the prescribing doctor to make sure you're not taking too high of a dosage.** Truth be told, you probably don't need to check with the prescribing doctor to know if you're taking too high of a dosage, but I still need to mention it here. If you experience hypothyroid symptoms and/or your thyroid panel is on the hypothyroid side, then it doesn't take a rocket scientist to figure out that you need to ask the prescribing doctor to decrease the dosage. And if you're not taking medication but instead are taking natural antithyroid agents (i.e., bugleweed, higher amounts of L-carnitine) and your thyroid hormones are on the hypothyroid side, then you should also consider lowering the dosage.

- **Eat healthier and be more active.** You'll notice that I didn't include poor diet and lack of movement as causes of weight gain, but of course everyone knows that they are factors. I decided not to include these because just about everyone knows that eating healthily and exercising regularly are important, so I wanted to focus on other factors. However, I figured I'd briefly mention it here just in case you're still eating like crap and are sedentary most of the time. If you're nervous about exercising because of your hyperthyroid condition, I completely understand, and I cover exercise in chapter 23.

- **Block out time for stress management . . . *every day*.** I discuss this in chapter 20, but it's worth mentioning it here, as most people don't do enough to decrease their perception of stress. Please make sure you block out at least five minutes per day to work on your stress-management skills.

- **Do everything you can to reduce inflammation.** Admittedly this is easier said than done, as there can be many different sources of inflammation. Changing one's diet alone can greatly reduce inflammation in the body, but of course there can be other factors. Insomnia can cause inflammation,[15] so getting sufficient sleep is important. Exposure to environmental toxicants and infections can also cause inflammation.

- **Support estrogen metabolism.** If someone has a problem with estrogen metabolism, then this needs to be addressed. This might mean doing a dried urine test to look at the estrogen metabolites, or if someone has an elevated beta glucuronidase marker on a comprehensive stool panel, then this could be an indication of problems with estrogen metabolism. It's important to understand that genetics can play an important role when it comes to estrogen metabolism, so if someone has certain genetic variations, then they very well might need continuous support.

For example, both the COMT and MTHFR enzymes support methylation, which helps to detoxify estrogens. If you have a genetic variation in either

COMT or MTHFR (or both), then this can have a negative effect on methylation, which in turn can cause problems with the metabolism of estrogen. On a dried urine test this might present with elevated 4-OH-E1 metabolites.

Is Intermittent Fasting an Option?

Intermittent fasting is a popular strategy for losing weight. For example, someone might fast for sixteen hours and then have an eight hour window to eat. There are different variations of this, and I must admit that I personally incorporate intermittent fasting these days, as I commonly fast for fourteen to sixteen hours, and sometimes longer than this.

However, this isn't something I did while I was dealing with hyperthyroidism. Of course, in my situation I lost forty-two pounds, so it definitely wouldn't have made sense for me to have fasted for long periods of time. But how about those with hyperthyroidism who aren't losing weight and/or struggle with weight gain? If someone has hyperthyroidism and insulin resistance, then perhaps intermittent fasting is something they can consider.

One concern I have is the effect of intermittent fasting on adrenal health. Should someone incorporate intermittent fasting if they have depressed or elevated cortisol levels? There isn't a lot of research on this topic, but one study showed that there is a risk of complications in those who have adrenal insufficiency.[16] However, in the medical world, "adrenal insufficiency" is the medical term for Addison's disease, which is a more serious adrenal disorder. When I was dealing with Graves' disease I had depressed morning cortisol levels, but this doesn't mean that I had Addison's disease.

A few other studies have shown that intermittent fasting can cause an increase in cortisol.[17,18] Does this mean that if someone has elevated cortisol that intermittent fasting should be avoided? If so, should it be indicated in those with low cortisol levels? I really think it depends on the person. One problem is that most people who practice intermittent fasting don't do any adrenal testing, so the average person who incorporates intermittent fasting probably doesn't know for certain whether or not they have high or low cortisol levels.

Intermittent Fasting vs. Time-Restricted Eating

You might have also heard of the term *time restricted eating* (TRE), which shares some similarities with intermittent fasting. In fact, intermittent fasting falls under the category of TRE, but whereas intermittent fasting usually involves some caloric restriction, with TRE you're not modifying the quality and quantity of food. For example, with TRE you're only eating within a certain time period, but you essentially can eat as much food as you want during this time, and you're also not paying attention to the quality of the food.

Concerns with Getting Enough Protein

A big concern with intermittent fasting is that many people don't get enough protein. This is especially true for someone who only eats one meal per day, but even if you eat two meals per day you might not get enough protein. Remember that in chapter 4 I discussed how a good goal is to aim for a protein intake that's at least 75 percent of your ideal body weight in pounds. For example, if your ideal body weight is 120 pounds, you should aim for at least 90 grams of protein per day.

And you ideally want to spread this out throughout the day to get maximum benefits. So if you eat only two meals per day and are aiming for 90 grams of protein per day then you would look to get approximately 45 grams of protein per meal. But from a muscle mass perspective it might be best to spread this out to 30 grams of protein for three daily meals. This admittedly is easier to accomplish with a 14-hour fast compared to a 16-hour fast, but even with a 16-hour fast it's doable.

Intermittent Fasting vs. Eating Regularly

If you have visited my website **www.naturalendocrinesolutions.com** and read some of my early articles and blog posts, you might wonder why I'm bringing up fasting. After all, years ago I would encourage all of my patients to eat every two to three hours to keep their blood sugar levels stable. While I don't think everyone needs to do this, some practitioners still recommend this approach to all of their patients.

I do think that most people with hyperthyroidism can benefit by eating regular meals. This is what I did when I dealt with Graves' disease. In fact, with as strong of an appetite as I had, I couldn't imagine not eating regular meals throughout the day. And I think many of my hyperthyroid patients would struggle if they didn't eat every two to three hours. On the other hand, if someone with hyperthyroidism is struggling to lose weight due to insulin resistance or other factors that result in weight gain, then it might be a good idea for them to incorporate intermittent fasting.

And even though I incorporate intermittent fasting into my life, I do usually eat three meals per day. So while these days I don't eat breakfast early in the morning and then eat every two to three hours thereafter, I'm also not going extremely long periods of time without eating throughout the day. I want to emphasize the word "extremely", as since I do incorporate intermittent fasting I will frequently go sixteen hours without eating, but approximately half of those hours are when I'm asleep. And I usually stop eating three to four hours before going to bed, and so the next morning I might go five hours before eating my first meal, which isn't too extreme for most people.

I realize there is a lot of conflicting information out there, but most people with hyperthyroidism probably shouldn't be fasting for long periods of time, and eating regularly throughout the day is fine. Once you have restored your health, you might choose to incorporate some intermittent fasting into your life, but even if this is the case, you don't want to be too extreme.

Restore Your Health First and Fast Later?

So just to summarize, I think in many situations it would be wise for those with hyperthyroidism to refrain from longer fasts until they have greatly improved their health, although there definitely are exceptions. In most cases fasting for twelve to fourteen hours probably won't be too big of a deal while working on restoring your health, although this of course depends on the person. For example, if someone is hypoglycemic, they probably won't want to fast for twelve to fourteen hours.

If you're thinking about incorporating intermittent fasting, I think it's a good idea to work with a natural healthcare practitioner. This way they not only can do some blood work to see if insulin resistance is a factor, but they can also run a saliva panel or a dried urine test to look at the circadian rhythm of cortisol and evaluate the health of the adrenals. Then they can put everything together and discuss whether you would be a good candidate to incorporate intermittent fasting, or if you should refrain from doing this until you are in a better state of health.

The Carbohydrate Conundrum

Many weight loss diets recommend minimizing one's carbohydrate intake. If you're losing weight you might wonder if you should eat more carbohydrates, while if you're gaining weight you might wonder if you should restrict carbohydrates. I definitely don't recommend extremely limiting one's carbohydrate intake when dealing with hyperthyroidism, but if someone with hyperthyroidism has problems losing weight and they are also dealing with insulin resistance, then keeping the carbohydrate intake to 150 grams or less is something to consider doing.

On the other hand, if you're losing weight I wouldn't worry too much about restricting carbohydrates as long as you are eating healthy sources of these . . . mostly in the form of vegetables and fruits. This doesn't mean that you should eat five sweet potatoes daily, but eating one per day is fine in most cases, along with consuming other healthier forms of carbohydrates.

In summary, while a lot of people with hyperthyroidism lose weight, some people with hyperthyroidism actually struggle to lose weight. So the goal of the Hyperthyroid Healing Diets isn't to help someone gain or lose weight, and of course whether someone is losing or gaining weight, the goal should always be to address the cause of the weight loss or weight gain. For those people losing weight, addressing the hyperthyroidism and improving the health of the gut will almost always help. With weight gain and hyperthyroidism, it can sometimes be more complex, but it still comes down to finding and addressing the underlying causes.

Chapter 13 Highlights

- Although weight loss is a classic symptom of hyperthyroidism, many people with hyperthyroidism gain weight.
- The main reason why many people with hyperthyroidism lose weight is because of elevated thyroid hormone levels.
- Two ways people with hyperthyroidism can gain weight are to (1) lower thyroid hormones and (2) heal the gut.
- Some of the causes of malabsorption include hyperthyroidism, celiac disease, bile acid malabsorption, and SIBO.
- Common causes of weight gain in those with hyperthyroidism include taking antithyroid agents, chronic stress and high cortisol, insulin resistance, leptin resistance, inflammation, and estrogen metabolism problems.
- Obesogens cause metabolism changes due to the effects they have on hormones in the body.
- In order to overcome unwanted weight gain (1) make sure you're not taking too high of a dosage of antithyroid agents, (2) eat healthier and be more active, (3) practice stress management daily, (4) reduce inflammation, and (5) support estrogen metabolism.
- Intermittent fasting is something to consider if you're struggling to lose weight and/or dealing with insulin resistance, but not everyone should incorporate intermittent fasting, so I would recommend working with a healthcare practitioner if you want to try it.

To access the book references and resources, visit
SaveMyThyroid.com/HHDNotes.

Addressing Blood Sugar Imbalances

Blood sugar imbalances are very common in this day and age in the general population, and many people with hyperthyroidism are impacted as well. I'll be talking about both hypoglycemia and hyperglycemia, as well as insulin resistance in this chapter, and while many assume that insulin resistance is associated with obesity, this isn't always the case. In other words, if someone has hyperthyroidism and is underweight due to weight loss, this doesn't necessarily rule out insulin resistance or other blood sugar imbalances.

What Is Insulin?

Insulin is a peptide hormone secreted by the beta cells of the pancreatic islets of Langerhans. It plays a role in maintaining normal blood glucose levels by facilitating cellular glucose uptake; regulating carbohydrate, lipid, and protein metabolism; and promoting cell division and growth through its mitogenic effects.[1] Just like all hormones, insulin binds to specific receptors. Insulin receptors have been located in different parts of the body, including the brain, pancreas, pituitary, kidney, ovaries, and even osteoblasts and osteoclasts of the bone.[1]

With insulin resistance, the insulin levels stay persistently high due to down-regulation of the insulin receptors. Although the focus of this chapter is the relationship of blood sugar imbalances to hyperthyroidism, insulin resistance has actually been linked to many different health conditions, including high blood pressure, non-alcoholic fatty liver disease, PCOS, and perhaps even cancer.[2,3]

The Role of Thyroid Hormone

The research shows that thyroid hormones have a significant effect on glucose metabolism and the development of insulin resistance.[4] However, while insulin resistance can develop in those with both hyperthyroidism and hypothyroidism, the mechanisms appear to be different, as in hyperthyroidism, impaired glucose tolerance may be the result of mainly hepatic insulin resistance, whereas in hypothyroidism the available data suggests that the insulin resistance of peripheral tissues prevails.[4] Another study mentioned how excess thyroid hormone causes mitochondrial dysfunction, which can also represent the link between hyperthyroidism and the development of insulin resistance and diabetes.[5]

Insulin Resistance vs. Hypoglycemia

Glycemia refers to the presence of glucose in the blood. As the name implies, hypoglycemia is a condition characterized by low blood sugar levels, whereas insulin resistance is more characteristic of hyperglycemia, which of course involves high blood sugar levels. I already spoke about how insulin resistance involves too much insulin, so with the next few paragraphs I'd like to focus on hypoglycemia.

Hypoglycemia refers to low blood sugar levels, typically less than 70 mg/dL. What happens is that either the body's glucose is used up too quickly, the body's glucose is released into the bloodstream too slowly, or too much insulin is released into the bloodstream. Some of the causes of hypoglycemia include alcohol consumption, an infection, hypothyroidism or hypoadrenalism, and severe heart, kidney, or liver failure.[6] Some of the common symptoms associated with low blood sugar levels include weakness, fatigue, sweating, disorientation, and shakiness.[7]

Reactive hypoglycemia is an exaggerated fall in the blood glucose levels and is due to excessive insulin secretion in response to a meal. Dr. Alan Gaby has dedicated a chapter to reactive hypoglycemia in his excellent book *Nutritional Medicine*, discussing how if the blood glucose levels fall too rapidly, then the body compensates by releasing adrenaline, as well as other compounds that raise blood glucose levels. This in turn results in fight-or-flight symptoms such as anxiety, panic attacks, hunger, palpitations, tachycardia, tremors, sweating, and even abdominal pain.

Dr. Gaby also talks about the symptoms presented when the blood glucose levels fall slowly over a period of hours, as this can lead to symptoms such as headaches, fatigue, blurred vision, mental confusion, impaired memory, and even seizures. These symptoms usually are worse before meals and frequently are relieved by eating.

What you need to understand is that people with hyperthyroidism can experience either hyperglycemia/insulin resistance or hypoglycemia. And these conditions can play a big role in the development of different hyperthyroid conditions. I'll explain some of the mechanisms, and by the time you're done reading this chapter, I hope you'll understand why it's important to have healthy blood sugar levels.

Can Insulin Resistance Trigger Graves' Disease?

While insulin resistance plays a role in many cases of toxic multinodular goiter (I'll discuss this in greater detail soon), I want to point out a study that evaluated insulin sensitivity and beta-cell function in those with Graves' disease, including the changes that took place when taking antithyroid medication.[8] As I mentioned earlier, beta cells are located in the islets of Langerhans in the pancreas, and they synthesize and secrete the hormone insulin. Anyway, the study showed that abnormal glucose tolerance is a significant metabolic consequence in patients with Graves' disease, and there is decreased beta-cell function.[8]

While abnormal glucose tolerance can be a consequence of Graves' disease, it's also possible for insulin resistance to be a factor in the development of different hyperthyroid conditions. With Graves' disease I think it's safe to say that in most cases insulin resistance isn't the main trigger, but since insulin resistance usually involves an inflammatory process,[9] at the very least it can be a contributing factor. And if you have both Graves' disease and insulin resistance, you might not be able to get into remission without balancing your blood sugar levels. This is why diet is important, but many times diet alone isn't sufficient to reverse insulin resistance. More on this later in this chapter.

Insulin Resistance and Thyroid Nodules

A number of studies show that insulin resistance can potentially increase thyroid proliferation, nodule volume, and nodule formation.[10] One of these studies mentioned how the increased vascularization of thyroid nodules may be what contributes to the growth and progression of thyroid nodules.[11] Another study showed that there is an association between insulin resistance and benign thyroid nodules,[12] while yet another study showed that those with type 2 diabetes are more likely to develop thyroid nodules, and suggested that insulin resistance might be involved in thyroid nodule development.[13]

But it's not just the thyroid nodules that increase in association with insulin resistance, but the thyroid gland itself can also potentially increase. In other words, insulin resistance can be a factor in the development of multinodular goiter. Polycystic ovary syndrome (PCOS) is associated with insulin resistance, and one study demonstrated that thyroid volume and frequency of nodular goiter were increased in patients with PCOS, and the result was related to insulin resistance.[14] Another study demonstrated that insulin-like growth factor–binding proteins (IGFBPs) might be responsible for the development of a goiter.[15]

Leptin Resistance vs. Insulin Resistance

Leptin is a hormone which is produced by adipocytes, also known as *fat cells*. This hormone is very important when it comes to regulating food intake and energy storage. It actually helps to suppress appetite, and this helps one to maintain a healthy weight.

Insulin and leptin work together, as if leptin does its job and suppresses our appetite, then insulin drops, which can help us maintain a healthy weight. On the other hand, if someone develops insulin resistance, this will signal the body to keep storing fat, and this in turn causes leptin to stay persistently high. So essentially someone who develops insulin resistance is likely to develop leptin resistance.

The good news is that if you address insulin resistance this also should help with leptin resistance. I'm getting ready to discuss some things you can do to balance blood sugar levels and address insulin resistance. While you can do a lot through diet and lifestyle, there is a time and place for nutritional supplements and herbs, so I'll discuss both here.

Solutions to Balance Blood Sugar Levels

Eat a healthy diet. This one is obvious, but while simply eating a healthy diet consisting of whole foods might be sufficient to prevent the development of insulin resistance, it might not be enough to overcome it. In other words, if someone already has insulin resistance, then they very well might need to do more than just eat a healthy diet. Many recommend a low carbohydrate diet for insulin resistance.

In fact, many practitioners recommend a ketogenic diet for helping with insulin resistance. When following such a diet, the person will typically consume 20 to 50 grams of carbohydrates per day. It usually consists of 70 percent fat, 20 percent protein, and 10 percent carbohydrates, although there is also a variation called the *high-protein ketogenic diet*, where the ratio is around 60 percent fat and 30–35 percent protein. Following a ketogenic diet causes glucose reserves to decrease, and ketones are used as an alternative source of energy, which is referred to as *ketosis*.

While a ketogenic diet can help with many cases of insulin resistance, following one of the Hyperthyroid Healing Diets can potentially help as well. While I agree that you don't want to eat an excess of carbohydrates, most people with insulin resistance don't need to limit their carbohydrate consumption to 20 to 50 grams per day, though it might be a good idea not to exceed 150 grams of carbohydrates on a daily basis.

But it's not just about restricting carbohydrates, as with insulin resistance there is an inflammatory component that also needs to be addressed. I'll discuss this shortly, but I also wanted to mention it here so you don't think carbohydrate restriction is the key to overcoming insulin resistance.

Is Intermittent Fasting Something to Consider?

I already spoke about this in chapter 13, so I won't get into great detail here. The truth is that intermittent fasting can help with many cases of insulin resistance. If someone has compromised adrenals, there might be a concern with incorporating longer fasting windows (i.e., greater than fourteen hours), but it really depends on the person. And you want to make sure to consume sufficient protein. I will say that while I didn't incorporate intermittent fasting while I was dealing with Graves' disease, I do utilize it these days while maintaining a state of wellness.

Exercise regularly. Numerous studies show that exercise increases insulin sensitivity.[16,17] It seems that a combination of aerobic exercise and resistance training can be effective in helping with insulin resistance.[18] High-intensity interval training can also be effective, although one study I came across showed that when compared to moderate-intensity continuous training, high intensity interval training isn't superior at reducing insulin resistance.[19]

I discuss exercise and hyperthyroidism in greater detail in chapter 23. In the chapter I mention how many people with hyperthyroidism want to be cautious about overexerting themselves when doing continuous aerobic exercise, and it's probably a good idea for most people with hyperthyroidism to avoid high-intensity interval training while trying to restore their health. That being said, doing some resistance training can be beneficial for those with hyperthyroidism, and regular movement is also important.

Decrease inflammation. With insulin resistance, there usually is an inflammatory process that needs to be addressed. The challenge is that there are many factors that can cause inflammation. As you know, the focus of this book is to give you guidance with regard to diet, so you already know you should eliminate any inflammatory foods, regardless of whether you're dealing with insulin resistance or not. Other causes of inflammation are discussed in different chapters throughout this book, but I'll also list some of them here:

- Food allergens (i.e., gluten, dairy, corn)
- Chronic stress
- Lack of sleep
- Increased toxic burden

- Infections (i.e., viruses, Lyme disease)
- Toxic mold
- Gut microbiome disruption

Unfortunately, I can't discuss all of these topics in this book in great detail, but I can point you toward a couple of free resources. My first recommendation is to check out the *Save My Thyroid* podcast, which you can find by visiting **www.savemythyroid.com,** or simply visit your favorite podcast platform. While most of the guest interviews will benefit people with both hyperthyroidism and Hashimoto's thyroiditis, there are many solo episodes that focus exclusively on hyperthyroidism. You also might want to check out the third edition of my other book on hyperthyroidism, *Natural Treatment Solutions for Hyperthyroidism and Graves' Disease.*

Improve the health of the gut microbiome. I'm not going to go into great detail about improving the health of the gut microbiome in this chapter, as I discuss this in great detail in chapter 21. While having a healthy gut is essential for a healthy immune system, which is of course essential for someone with Graves' disease, the truth is that having a healthy gut is important for so many other reasons. This includes having healthy blood sugar, as there are many studies that show a relationship between an unhealthy gut microbiome and insulin resistance.[20,21,22]

Supporting Blood Sugar Imbalances Through Nutritional Supplements and Herbs

Although diet and lifestyle play an important role in balancing blood sugar levels, taking certain nutritional supplements and herbs can also be beneficial. Some of the nutritional supplements and herbs that can address blood sugar imbalances include chromium, magnesium, berberine, gymnema, alpha-lipoic acid, cinnamon, and American ginseng. Remember that I have a bonus chapter where I discuss nutritional supplements and herbs that can support different areas of the body, including blood sugar. So for more information on these, including suggested doses, visit **savemythyroid.com/HHDNotes**.

Is There a Time and Place for Metformin?

Just as is the case with hyperthyroidism, there is a time and place for medication to help with blood sugar imbalances. Metformin is still commonly given to those with type 2 diabetes, which is characterized by insulin resistance. Metformin has been shown to improve whole-body sensitivity to insulin in a number of different studies.[23,24] It's worth mentioning that berberine has many of the same aspects as metformin when it comes to its actions and mechanisms.[25] And since there are side effects of metformin, including an increased risk of a vitamin B_{12} deficiency,[26] berberine might be a better first option for some people.

Should You Invest in a Continuous Glucose Monitor?

A continuous glucose monitor (CGM) is a device that measures blood glucose on a continuous basis (throughout the day and night). The way it works is that a tiny sensor is inserted under your skin (i.e., on your arm), and the sensor measures the glucose every few minutes. Even though I do think that many people can benefit from using a CGM, it can be especially helpful for someone who has blood sugar imbalances. This is particularly true for those with insulin resistance or diabetes (both type 1 and type 2), but it can also play a role in preventing hypoglycemia.[27]

That being said, anyone can use a CGM to determine which foods spike up their blood sugar. While it shouldn't be surprising that refined sugars will spike someone's blood glucose, everyone is different, and in some cases certain foods will spike the blood glucose levels in one person, whereas the same food might not spike another person's blood glucose. An example is a banana, as some people will eat a banana and notice a big increase in their blood glucose levels, whereas someone else might eat a banana and not have a significant increase in their blood glucose levels. In this scenario, the person whose blood glucose greatly increases when eating a banana will probably want to be cautious about eating bananas on a regular basis, and the same would apply to other foods that result in a large increase in their blood glucose levels.

In summary, blood sugar imbalances, including insulin resistance, can impact those with both hyperthyroidism and hypothyroidism, although the mechanisms appear to be different. Insulin resistance can be a potential cause of thyroid nodules. While eating well and exercising regularly can help address blood sugar imbalances, other factors may be necessary, including reducing inflammation, improving the health of the gut microbiome, and certain nutritional supplements. At times a continuous glucose monitor may also be helpful.

Chapter 14 Highlights

- If someone has hyperthyroidism and is underweight due to weight loss, this doesn't necessarily rule out insulin resistance or other blood sugar imbalances.
- With insulin resistance, insulin levels stay persistently high due to down-regulation of the insulin receptors.
- Insulin resistance plays a role in many cases of toxic multinodular goiter, and it can be a contributing factor in the development of Graves' disease.
- A number of studies show that insulin resistance can potentially increase thyroid proliferation, nodule volume, and nodule formation.
- Insulin and leptin work together, as if leptin does its job and suppresses our appetite, then insulin drops, which can help us maintain a healthy weight
- Solutions to balance blood sugar levels include eating a healthy diet, exercising regularly, decreasing inflammation, improving the health of the gut microbiome, and certain nutritional supplements
- A continuous glucose monitor (CGM) is a device that measures blood glucose on a continuous basis (throughout the day and night).

To access the book references and resources, visit
SaveMyThyroid.com/HHDNotes.

CHAPTER
15

The Hyperthyroid-Histamine Connection

hile it would be great if everyone could simply choose one of the Hyperthyroid Healing Diets and live happily ever after, unfortunately this isn't always the case. One reason is because some people are unable to tolerate certain foods, and there could be numerous reasons for this. Having a histamine intolerance is one of those reasons.

Although I assume that many people reading this are familiar with histamine, it's also probably safe to assume that some people are unfamiliar with it. *Histamine* is a chemical messenger that is synthesized from the amino acid *histidine*, and it mediates several cellular responses. It plays a role in the inflammatory process and in allergic reactions, and it's also important for stomach acid secretion. Histamine receptors are found in just about all of the tissues in the body. Histamine is stored in granules in mast cells, and it is released in response to tissue injury.

Histamine Metabolism Basics

A histamine intolerance develops when there is an imbalance between levels of released histamine and the ability of the body to metabolize it. There are a couple of enzymes that play a role in the metabolism of histamine. The most well known one is diamine oxidase (DAO), which is the first-line defense against extracellular histamine (i.e., histamine ingested through the diet or released within the gut). Vitamin B_6 is a cofactor of DAO, along with vitamin C and copper. So if you are deficient in any of these nutrients, then this can also affect histamine metabolism.

N-methyl transferase (HNMT) is another enzyme that can play a role in the breakdown of histamine . . . mainly intracellular histamine. In other words, it doesn't seem to play a major role in degrading histamine from food, or even histamine produced by the gut microbiome.

Methylation is necessary for most of the body's systems. It is involved in the repair of DNA, it helps to prevent the overproduction of homocysteine, and it's important when it comes to detoxification. If someone has problems with methylation, and many people do, then they will have a greater risk of developing certain chronic health conditions. I'm bringing it up here because inactivation of intracellular histamine is mediated by methylation of the imidazole nucleus.[1] All you need to understand is that if you don't have healthy methylation, this can affect the degradation of histamine.

More about Mast Cells

I mentioned how histamine is stored in granules in mast cells. But what exactly are mast cells? *Mast cells* are our front-line defending and sensing cells of the immune system. They're in almost every tissue in the body, and they sense every molecule of air, food, water, supplement, medication, anything you put in your mouth, and anything you smell and touch. They even sense stressors.

They also sense what's happening inside our bodies. They line the blood vessels and sense the blood going through the vessels. They have hormone receptors for things like estrogen, progesterone, and thyroid hormones. Speaking of the thyroid, I should mention that thyroid tissue has mast cells. Mast cells also sense for pathogens, viruses, bacteria, parasites, molds, and yeasts. There are all kinds of sensors for different types of medications, even vitamin D.

What they do is mobilize an immune response if it's needed. For example, if you cut your finger and don't get the bacteria cleaned out, it starts to get red and puffy. That is the mast cells creating local inflammation as a protective mechanism. If we get surgery, we get local inflammation around the surgical site afterward. Part of that inflammation is the mast cells protecting us. If we get sick and we get sinus congestion and a sore throat, it is not a result of the virus itself, it is our immune system launching a protective attack.

So mast cells are releasing these inflammatory mediators to protect us and then restabilizing themselves. In mast cell activation syndrome (MCAS), the mast cells have become dysregulated for a variety of reasons, but really, it boils down to an overload of pathogens, toxins, and other stressors. Stressors could be related to emotional trauma, injuries, surgeries, etc.

Histamine Intolerance Symptoms

There are many potential symptoms associated with a histamine intolerance. I'll list some of the more common ones here, but just keep in mind that some people with such an intolerance will only have a few of these symptoms, while others will have what seem to be most, if not all, of them.

- Heart palpitations
- Tachycardia
- Headaches
- Itching

- Swelling
- Hives
- Abdominal pain
- Gas/diarrhea/bloating
- Hypo/hypertension
- Fatigue
- Anxiety
- Insomnia

One thing you'll notice is that some of these symptoms overlap with those of hyperthyroidism. For example, with hyperthyroidism it is very common to experience tachycardia, heart palpitations, and anxiety. The difference is that with hyperthyroidism, these symptoms are usually consistent for as long as the thyroid hormones remain elevated, whereas with a histamine intolerance the symptoms may vary, especially when eating certain types of foods (i.e., those high in histamine).

I also want to mention a questionnaire I came across in a study that revealed that bloating was the most common and most severe symptom indicated by more than 90 percent of histamine intolerance patients.[2] According to the questionnaire, other commonly related GI symptoms included postprandial fullness and diarrhea (both in >70 percent of patients), abdominal pain (>65 percent), and constipation (55 percent).[3]

Reasons Why Some People Develop a Histamine Intolerance

Reason #1: Genetics. Some people have genetic variations in the genes that break down histamine. For example, having a genetic variation in the DAO gene can lower DAO activity, thus affecting the breakdown of histamine. What makes it challenging is that there are fifty known non-synonymous single-nucleotide polymorphisms for the gene that codes DAO[4] and the histamine receptors.[5] It's also possible to have a genetic variation in the HNMT gene, although as I mentioned earlier, this doesn't seem to play a role in the breakdown of histamine from food or produced by the gut microbiome.

Reason #2: Impairment of DAO activity. While genetics can play a role in the breakdown of histamine, there are other factors that can impair DAO activity. Some of these factors include drinking alcohol, taking certain medications, and certain gastrointestinal conditions. For example, while antihistamines block DAO activity, other medications that can do this include analgesics, antidepressants, antirheumatics, antiarrhythmics, and mucolytics.[6]

Reason #3: Gut dysbiosis. Speaking of the gut, having imbalances in the gut flora can lead to a histamine intolerance. One study showed alterations in the gut flora and an elevated stool zonulin test in those with histamine intolerance, suggesting that dysbiosis and intestinal barrier dysfunction may play a role.[7] Elevated zonulin is indicative of a leaky gut, so this is essentially saying that there might be a relationship between having a leaky gut and a histamine intolerance. Another journal article concluded that histamine intolerance seems to play a more significant role in GI disorders and complaints.[8]

Reason #4: Methylation problems. As I mentioned earlier, the enzyme HNMT is dependent on methylation. If methylation is impacted, it can affect this enzyme, which in turn can have a negative effect on histamine degradation.

Reason #5: Estrogen dominance. Too much estrogen can downregulate DAO activity, which can contribute to an intolerance of histamine. Estrogen also sensitizes the mast cells, and this in turn causes more histamine to be released. Estrogen dominance not only refers to high levels of estrogen, but can also mean there are low levels of progesterone. It's worth mentioning that having healthy levels of progesterone is necessary to upregulate DAO. It's also important to know that taking hormonal birth control can result in a histamine intolerance by increasing estrogen levels, thus causing more histamine to be released.

Reason #6: Medications. Certain medications have an inhibitory effect on the DAO enzyme, which can lead to a histamine intolerance. If this is the case, then asking the prescribing doctor to change to a different medication very well may help. Some examples of medications that can have an inhibitory effect on the DAO enzyme include cimetidine, verapamil, isoniazid, metamizole (not to be confused with methimazole), acetyl cysteine, and amitriptyline.[9]

Other factors. There can be other factors that can increase the sensitivity of individuals to histamine, including alcohol (blocks DAO and can also release endogenous histamine), and even malnutrition, which can cause a deficiency of the important cofactors (vitamin C, copper, vitamin B_6).

High Histamine Foods vs. Histamine Liberators

While some foods are high in histamine, other foods are labeled as *histamine-liberators*, as they can trigger the release of endogenous histamine. Some of the foods that have been shown to have the ability to release histamine include citrus fruits, seafood, papaya, tomato, nuts, pineapple, spinach, chocolate, and strawberries.[10]

Tests Related to Histamine

The testing options aren't great when it comes to determining if someone has a histamine intolerance. You can measure plasma levels of histamine, but the accuracy of the testing is questionable. The most studied but still controversial laboratory diagnostic approach is the analysis of DAO enzyme activity in serum.

The test measures the amount of histamine that degrades over a specified time in a blood sample, using enzyme-linked immunosorbent assay (ELISA) or radioimmunoassay (RIA). The company Precision Point Diagnostics offers an Advanced Intestinal Barrier Assessment, which is a blood test that measures

DAO, plasma histamine, zonulin, and lipopolysaccharides (LPS), the latter two which play a role in the permeability of the gut.

What Can You Do If You Have a Histamine Intolerance?

If you have a histamine intolerance, there are a few different things you can do:

1. **Follow a low-histamine diet.** This isn't addressing the cause of the histamine intolerance, but initially you want to avoid foods that contain a high amount of histamine. The challenge is that studies show that there is variability when it comes to the foods that are recommended. You might even want to avoid the histamine liberators I listed earlier.

2. **Supplement.** There are a few supplements that can be helpful with a histamine intolerance. One is quercetin, which is a naturally occurring polyphenol flavonoid rich in antioxidants, and it has anti-allergic functions that are known for inhibiting histamine production.[11] Taking a DAO supplement can also be very helpful in many cases. The dosage form must be gastro-resistant in order to deliver the enzyme undamaged to the place of presumed effect (small intestine). It has been demonstrated that DAO exogenous supplementation has improved the symptoms in clinical practice.[12]

3. **Use antihistamines.** In most cases, H1 antihistamines are prescribed for a histamine intolerance, although H2 blockers might be a better option if the person has a lot of gastrointestinal symptoms (i.e., hyperacidity and reflux). This of course also should be a short-term solution, as you don't want to rely on taking these on a long term basis.

4. **Correct gut dysbiosis**. I mentioned how gut dysbiosis can be a factor in histamine intolerance, so it makes sense to do things to optimize the health of your gut. For more information on how to optimize the health of the gut, refer to chapter 21.

5. **Improve methylation.** I also mentioned earlier that methylation plays a role in the degradation of histamine, so if you have problems with methylation, then this can be a factor. But how can you (1) determine if you have a methylation problem, and (2) correct it? I won't get into great detail about this, but I will say that an elevation in homocysteine can sometimes indicate problems with methylation, and this marker can be tested at most labs.

This was the case with me, as years ago I tested for homocysteine and saw that it was elevated, and through genetic testing I eventually discovered that this was related to a homozygous MTHFR C677T genetic polymorphism. There is of course nothing I can do to change my genetics, so I have taken methylation support on a daily basis since then. Nutrients that can support methylation include vitamin B_{12}, folate, vitamin B_6, and riboflavin.[13]

It's also worth mentioning that a dried urine test I sometimes recommend to my patients called the DUTCH Complete can help determine someone's methylation status. The reason for this is that methylation plays a role in the phase 2 metabolism of estrogens, as both 4-OH-E1 and 2-OH-E1 estrogens can be deactivated and eliminated by methylation. In addition to MTHFR, earlier I also mentioned COMT, which is another enzyme that plays a role in methylation. You can also have a genetic variation in this gene.

6. **Address estrogen imbalances.** Since too much estrogen can downregulate DAO activity as well as sensitize the mast cells, it makes sense to address higher levels of estrogen and/or problems with estrogen metabolism. Although you can test for the different estrogens (estradiol, estrone, estriol) in the blood, urine is the only place where you can look at the metabolism of estrogen.

In summary, histamine plays a role in the inflammatory process and in allergic reactions, and a histamine intolerance develops when there is an imbalance between levels of released histamine and the ability of the body to metabolize it. Some of the more common histamine intolerance symptoms overlap with hyperthyroid symptoms, including heart palpitations, tachycardia, and anxiety. While genetics can be a factor in a histamine intolerance, gut dysbiosis, methylation problems, estrogen dominance, and certain medications can also be causes or contributing factors. So while following a low histamine diet and/or taking certain supplements can help, if possible you want to address the underlying cause.

Chapter 15 Highlights

- Histamine is a chemical messenger that plays a role in the inflammatory process and in allergic reactions. It's also important for stomach acid secretion.
- A histamine intolerance develops when there is an imbalance between levels of released histamine and the ability of the body to metabolize it.
- DAO and HNMT are enzymes that play a role in the breakdown of histamine.
- Some histamine intolerance symptoms include heart palpitations, tachycardia, headaches, itching, swelling, hives, gas/diarrhea/bloating, fatigue, anxiety, and insomnia.
- Six reasons why some people develop a histamine intolerance include (1) genetics, (2) impairment of DAO activity, (3) gut dysbiosis, (4) methylation problems, (5) estrogen dominance, and (6) certain medications.
- If you have a histamine intolerance, you can follow a low-histamine diet, take certain supplements such as quercetin or a DAO supplement, take antihistamines, correct gut dysbiosis, improve methylation, and address estrogen metabolism.

To access the book references and resources, visit
SaveMyThyroid.com/HHDNotes.

CHAPTER
16

Are There Concerns with High-Oxalate Foods?

B efore I go into detail about oxalates, I just want to begin this chapter by letting you know that I'm not recommending for everyone with hyper-thyroidism to completely avoid high-oxalate foods, let alone some of the other foods discussed in this book. In fact, some foods high in oxalates (i.e., sweet potatoes) are allowed on all three levels of the Hyperthyroid Healing Diet. That being said, you don't want to go overboard with high-oxalate foods, and certain people will need to stick with lower-oxalate foods. If you're not sure if it's okay for you to eat some higher-oxalate foods I'm confident you will know after reading this chapter.

So what are oxalates, and why are they a potential concern? Oxalates are small molecules that have the ability to form crystals, which in turn can deposit in different areas of the body, including the thyroid gland. In fact, these oxalates can form just about anywhere in the body, and when they do, they can impair the function of the organ or gland. Some of the most common areas where they accumulate include the bones, blood vessels, central nervous system, peripheral nervous system, retina, skin, and thyroid gland.

There is also a relationship between oxalates and kidney stones. When someone develops a kidney stone, this usually is caused by high oxalates. This doesn't mean that everyone with high oxalates will develop kidney stones. But if someone tests positive for high oxalates, then they have a much greater chance of developing kidney stones when compared with someone with low oxalates.

What Causes Elevated Oxalate Levels?

Here are three main reasons why some people have elevated oxalate levels:

1. **Eating foods high in oxalates.** For years I used to load my smoothies with spinach and berries, which are very high in oxalates. These days I still have smoothies on a daily basis, but I've eliminated the spinach and replaced it with other green leafy vegetables lower in oxalates (i.e., arugula, collard greens), and I only add a small amount of organic berries to my smoothies (raspberries and blackberries are higher in oxalates). However, two of my main indulgences are dark chocolate and nuts, and both of these are high in oxalates. I just make sure not to eat large amounts of these foods.

2. **Overgrowth of fungi/yeast.** Candida, aspergillus, and some other types of yeast and mold produce oxalic acid. As a result, if someone has a yeast or mold overgrowth along with high oxalates, taking antifungal herbs or medications might help to lower the oxalate levels. Speaking of mold, in chapter 17 I discuss mold in food.

3. **Having problems with oxalate metabolism.** Some people have a genetic predisposition for developing higher amounts of oxalates. The organic acids test from Mosaic Diagnostics tests for the metabolites oxalic acid and glycolic acid. While elevated oxalic acid levels are usually related

to dietary intake of oxalates or yeast overgrowth, elevated glycolic acid levels can be an indicator of genetic disease of oxalate metabolism called hyperoxaluria type 1, and elevated glyceric acid levels can be related to hyperoxaluria type 2.[1]

What Are Some Common Symptoms of High Oxalate Levels?

I'd like to briefly list some of the more common symptoms of having high levels of oxalates. Keep in mind that many people who have elevated levels of oxalates on an organic acids test don't have these symptoms. But if someone has one or more of these symptoms for a prolonged period of time, then they might want to consider testing for oxalates:

- Sandy stools
- Bladder irritability
- Pain on urination
- Urethral irritation
- Eye pain
- Body aches, burning feeling in muscles
- Fibromyalgia-like discomfort
- Moodiness and irritability
- Tendon pain
- Trigger point tenderness

What Foods Are High in Oxalates?

Many foods are high in oxalates. And I realize it can become challenging to try to minimize your exposure to high-oxalate foods, especially when trying to follow one of the Hyperthyroid Healing Diets. For example, while some foods high in oxalates are excluded from the Level 3 Hyperthyroid Healing Diet (i.e., nuts, seeds, soy), other foods, such as spinach, sweet potatoes, and blackberries, are included.

For those looking for more comprehensive information related to high-oxalate foods I would check out Susan Owens's Facebook group, Trying Low Oxalates, and/or read Sally Norton's excellent book, *Toxic Superfoods*. Here are some of the foods that have high levels of oxalates:

- Spinach
- Swiss chard
- Nuts (especially almonds and cashews)
- Soy
- Peanuts
- Raspberries and blackberries
- Beets
- Sweet potatoes
- Chia seeds
- Collagen (contains hydroxyproline, which is converted into oxalate in your body)

Once again, you'll notice that many of these are allowed on the different Hyperthyroid Healing Diets. The good news is that there are adequate substitutes for some of these (i.e., spinach), but for other foods (i.e., sweet potatoes) it can be more challenging to find a good replacement. You'll notice that collagen is listed, as it's an oxalate precursor. Collagen is allowed on all three Hyperthyroid Healing Diets, and I still add collagen to my smoothies, but if you have a known oxalate problem, then it might be best not to consume it.

Say What . . . I Have to Avoid Sweet Potatoes?

Unfortunately, sweet potatoes are considered to be a high-oxalate food, which might cause some people to want to quit reading this book. But before you do, please hear me out, as I'm not necessarily recommending that everyone avoid eating sweet potatoes. For years I've had patients regularly eat sweet potatoes and still restore their health, and while this doesn't mean it can't lead to other problems in the future, everything comes down to risks versus benefits.

If you're following a Level 3, or even a Level 2 Hyperthyroid Healing Diet and you find it too much of a struggle to avoid sweet potatoes, you can always eat them while trying to restore your health, and then cut back once you have accomplished this. I'm pretty sure that Sally K. Norton wouldn't agree with this, but ultimately it's your hyperthyroid healing journey. I will add that if for any reason you continue eating them and aren't progressing as expected, then perhaps you should take a break from them and see if this helps.

Please Pass on the Almond Milk, Almond Butter, etc.

While having a small sweet potato each day or a few times per week might be okay, for those following a Level 1 or Level 2 Hyperthyroid Healing Diet, I would be cautious about overloading on almond-based products. Almonds themselves are high in oxalates, so it's not surprising that almond milk, almond butter, almond yogurt, and almond baked goods are also high oxalates. And while I can't deny eating a chocolate chip almond cookie every now and then, the problem is that some people eat these almond-based foods throughout the day.

So for example, someone might add almond milk to their smoothies (like I used to do), have a rice cake with almond butter for a mid-afternoon snack, and then after dinner eat almond yogurt or some almond-based cookies. Once again, this described me, as while I can't say I had rice cakes with almond butter regularly, in addition to adding almond milk to my smoothies, I also ate dark chocolate–covered almonds frequently as well as cookies with almond flour. Coconut milk and unsweetened coconut yogurt are great alternatives, and you can use coconut flour instead of almond flour for baking.

Foods That Are Lower in Oxalates:

- Meat and poultry
- Seafood
- Eggs
- Flaxseeds
- Sprouted pumpkin and sunflower seeds
- Arugula
- Collard greens
- Cauliflower
- Lettuces (romaine, green leaf, red leaf)
- Mushrooms
- Apples
- Blueberries
- Cranberries
- Coconut
- Herbal teas
- Coconut milk

How to Determine If You Have High Oxalate Levels

The urinary organic acids test from Mosaic Diagnostics (formerly Great Plains Laboratory) measures three specific oxalate metabolites. This includes gylceric, glycolic, and oxalic. The one most commonly high on an organic acids test is oxalic, but I'd like to briefly discuss the other two metabolites.

Glycolic relates to primary hyperoxaluria type 1, which is caused by a deficiency of the enzyme alanine glyoxylate aminotransferase (AGT). This enzyme breaks down oxalates. It's important to keep in mind that AGT is dependent on vitamin B_6, which means that if someone is deficient in vitamin B_6, it can sometimes be a factor in high oxalates. Some people with high oxalates can benefit from taking 100 mg of vitamin B_6 daily, although it might be a good idea to start with lower doses (i.e., 10 to 20 mg per day) and then gradually increase. Children with high oxalates might also require vitamin B_6, but should take lower doses than adults.

High glyceric levels on an organic acids test usually relate to primary hyperoxaluria type 2. In this condition there is a deficiency of glyoxylate reductase/hydroxypyruvate reductase (GRHFR). Whereas primary hyperoxaluria type 1 can lead to kidney failure, primary hyperoxaluria type 2 is more likely to cause the formation of kidney stones.

Of course neither one of these conditions is good to have, and while there is a genetic component, you can support these conditions by making sure you have healthy vitamin B_6 levels. If you have either primary hyperoxaluria type 1 or type 2 you also want to make sure you're not eating a lot of high-oxalate foods.

Earlier I mentioned that a candida overgrowth and/or mold exposure can also cause an increase in oxalates. The good news is that the organic acids test from Mosaic Diagnostics not only tests for oxalate metabolites, but also is a wonderful test for determining if someone has certain yeast in their body, along with mold exposure. And while you can test for a candida overgrowth in the stool and/or blood, I find the organic acids test to be more reliable. In addition, the organic acids test not only looks at metabolites related to candida, but other fungi that can produce oxalates. For example, *Aspergillus niger* is a fungus that can lead to black mold, and the research shows that it can produce oxalates.[2,3]

What Is Oxalate Dumping?

Dumping is the excretion of stored oxalates from the tissues of the body into the bloodstream. They are eliminated through the urine, stool, tears, and sweat. Certain symptoms associated with oxalate dumping can occur when you abruptly reduce your dietary oxalates, and this is a reason why it's wise to reduce them slowly. Keep in mind that not everyone experiences dumping symptoms, as when I found out I had high oxalates, I abruptly cut out spinach from my diet and didn't experience any symptoms.

That being said, if you are looking to reduce the oxalates from your diet, it really is a good idea to go about this slowly. So for example, if you have a daily smoothie and you currently add one cup of spinach to it and want to replace it with a lower oxalate green leafy vegetable (i.e., arugula, lettuce), then you might want to start by reducing it to 3/4 of a cup of spinach for one week, and then the next week reduce it to 1/2 cup of spinach and so on. You'd take the same approach with other high-oxalate foods.

If you want to learn more about oxalate dumping, I highly recommend joining the group Trying Low Oxalates, and then visiting the "Guides" section. Under this section there are many other free resources where you can learn about oxalates. This combined with reading the book *Toxic Superfoods* will greatly expand your knowledge when it comes to oxalates. And if you listen to *Toxic Superfoods* on audio, make sure you get the PDF handout, as there is plenty of information pertaining to high- and low- oxalate foods.

How Can You Lower Oxalate Levels?

If you find out that you have high oxalate levels, here are a few things you can focus on to help lower them:

1. **Reduce your intake of high-oxalate foods.** If you test high for oxalates, then I think reducing your intake of the high-oxalate foods I mentioned earlier is a good starting point. Just remember that this doesn't mean that you need to completely eliminate these foods, although if you have high oxalates it probably would be wise to greatly reduce your consumption of spinach and decrease your consumption of other foods that are very high in oxalates. And as I just mentioned, you'll want to gradually reduce your oxalate consumption.

2. **Address yeast/fungi overgrowth.** Having a yeast overgrowth or mold issue can lead to high oxalates, so if this is the case with you, then it makes sense to address this problem. And of course this can relate to one's diet, as if someone consumes a lot of sugar, then this can either cause or exacerbate a yeast overgrowth. As I discuss in chapter 17, mold in food can also be problematic.

3. **Supplement with vitamin B$_6$.** An enzyme I mentioned earlier called *alanine-glyoxylate aminotransferase* (AGT) is involved in the breakdown of oxalates, and it is dependent on vitamin B$_6$. So if someone has a vitamin B$_6$ deficiency, they will have problems breaking down oxalates, and taking larger doses of vitamin B$_6$ may reduce the risk of kidney stone formation.[4]

4. **Supplement with calcium and magnesium citrate, and consider drinking lemon juice.** These all can help to neutralize oxalates in the urine. Citrate helps to prevent the formation of kidney stones by binding to calcium oxalate crystals and can prevent crystal growth.[5] If someone has high oxalate levels and/or low citric acid (both of these are measured on an organic acids test) and they want to continue eating some high-oxalate foods, then they definitely should consider taking calcium and/or magnesium citrate, or they can drink some lemon juice.

   However, if you take this approach, you would want to take these right before you eat the high-oxalate foods. For example, if you have a smoothie with spinach, raspberries, and other foods high in oxalates, then you might want to add some calcium and/or magnesium citrate powder to the smoothie as well. Or you can drink four ounces of lemon juice. But if you test high for oxalates, it is also a good idea to minimize your consumption of higher-oxalate foods.

5. **Supplement with arginine and omega-3 fatty acids.** Both L-arginine and fish oils can help reduce the deposition of oxalate crystals while reducing oxidative damage.[6,7,8]

6. **Stay well hydrated.** Regardless of whether you have high oxalates, you want to stay well hydrated, and drinking plenty of water will help with the excretion of oxalates from the body.

In summary, oxalates can be a problem, but I would try not to stress about completely avoiding oxalates. There are plenty of very low- to moderately low–oxalate foods you can eat. As for higher-oxalate foods that are commonly consumed on a more restrictive diet (i.e., Level 3 Hyperthyroid Healing Diet), such as sweet potatoes, ultimately it's your decision as to whether or not you should avoid these, but over the years I've had a lot of people eat sweet potatoes without it affecting their recovery. For more information on high- and low-oxalate foods, remember to read the book *Toxic Superfoods* by Sally K. Norton, and if you're on Facebook, then you might also want to join the group Trying Low Oxalates.

Chapter 16 Highlights

- Oxalates are small molecules that have the ability to form crystals, which in turn can deposit in different areas of the body, including the thyroid gland.
- Some foods high in oxalates (i.e., sweet potatoes) are allowed on all three levels of the Hyperthyroid Healing Diet.
- Three causes of high oxalates include (1) eating foods high in oxalates, (2) overgrowth of yeast/fungi, and (3) having problems with oxalate metabolism.
- Some potential symptoms of high oxalates include sandy stools, bladder irritability, pain on urination, urethral irritation, eye pain, body aches, tendon pain, moodiness, and irritability.
- Some of the foods higher in oxalates include spinach, Swiss chard, nuts, soy, peanuts, raspberries and blackberries, beets, sweet potatoes, chia seeds, and collagen.
- Foods that are lower in oxalates include meat and poultry, seafood, eggs, flaxseeds, arugula, collard greens, cauliflower, lettuces, mushrooms, apples, blueberries, cranberries, and coconut.
- Oxalate dumping is the excretion of stored oxalates from the tissues of the body into the bloodstream.
- Here are some things you can do to lower oxalates: reduce your intake of high-oxalate foods, address yeast/fungi overgrowth, supplement with vitamin B6, supplement with calcium and magnesium citrate, supplement with arginine and omega-3 fatty acids, and stay well hydrated.

To access the book references and resources, visit
SaveMyThyroid.com/HHDNotes.

CHAPTER
17

Mold in Food

Mold in food is something that is commonly overlooked, yet in some situations it can have a profound effect on one's health. Obviously, mold from other sources, especially water-damaged buildings, is also a big issue for many people. But I'm not going to get into great detail about mold from other sources, as since this is a diet-related book, it makes sense to focus on mold in food.

Mycotoxins are defined as secondary metabolites produced by microfungi that are capable of causing disease and death in humans and other animals.[1] They are frequently classified by the organ they affect. They can be hepatotoxins (affecting the liver), nephrotoxins (affecting the kidneys), neurotoxins (affecting the nervous system), immunotoxins (affecting the immune system), etc. Some mycotoxins affect multiple organs.

Over three hundred types of mycotoxins are produced by molds.[2] The concern isn't just with humans, as mold can affect livestock as well, which can indirectly affect humans. Aflatoxins are one of the most significant mycotoxins affecting livestock, although others include trichothecenes, zearalenone, fumonisins, ochratoxins, and patulin. Grains, such as corn, wheat, and barley, may be easily contaminated with mold, which is how the livestock get these mycotoxins.

How Is Mold Toxic to Your Health?

I want you to understand that not everyone has the same reaction to mold. Genetics plays an important role in how people will react to mold. HLA is part of the immune system and is involved in antigen presentation. Certain HLA genotypes make people more susceptible to mycotoxins and cause many different symptoms. The reason people with these genes are more likely to react to mold is because having one of these HLA genotypes will reduce the person's ability to clear the mycotoxins produced by the mold, which, in turn, is responsible for the symptoms people will experience.

Exposure to mold is well known to trigger inflammation, allergies, and asthma; oxidative stress; and immune dysfunction in both human and animal studies. Mold spores, mycotoxins, and fungal fragments can be measured in buildings and in people who are exposed to these environments. Arguably, mold from sources other than food (i.e., water-damaged buildings) usually have a greater impact on one's health than mold in food, but it still can be a problem in genetically susceptible people. Plus, I don't know about you, but even though I don't think I'm genetically susceptible to the effects of mold, I still want to try my best to avoid "moldy" food.

Mold in Food Can Cause More Than Just Symptoms

It's scary to read some of the journal articles discussing the potential side effects of toxic mold. For example, certain aflatoxins are potent human liver carcinogens and have been estimated to contribute to 25,000 to 155,000 cases of hepatocellular carcinoma each year.[3] The same study mentioned that aflatoxin contamination could cause losses to the corn industry ranging from $52.1 million to $1.68 billion annually in the United States. Getting back to hepatocellular carcinoma, a different study showed that of the 550,000 to 600,000 new hepatocellular carcinoma cases worldwide each year, up to 155,000 may be attributable to aflatoxin exposure.[4]

Ochratoxin A is another abundant mycotoxin contaminant in food and has been shown to possess carcinogenic, nephrotoxic, teratogenic, and immunotoxic properties.[5] It's especially associated with nephrotoxicity, which is rapid deterioration in kidney function. If you see a low eGFR and/or high creatinine on a comprehensive metabolic panel, this doesn't always mean that it's related to mycotoxins from mold, but the problem is that most medical doctors, including nephrologists, wouldn't even consider mycotoxins to be a factor. On a side note, it's very common for people with hyperthyroidism to have a low creatinine, which is usually associated with decreased muscle mass.

One more mycotoxin I'd like to briefly discuss here is zearalenone, which is an estrogenic mycotoxin commonly found on plants such as corn or small grains. It is mainly produced by *Fusarium* fungi and has been proven to affect the reproductive capacity of animals by binding to the estrogen receptors.[6] Another study looked at the effect of zearalenone metabolites on human health, and the authors mentioned how exposure to this mycotoxin may lead to numerous diseases of the reproductive system such as prostate, ovarian, cervical, or breast cancers.[7]

How Does Food Become Moldy?

Mold spoilage results from having a product contaminated with fungal spores that germinate and form a visible mycelium (the growing body of a fungus) before the end of the shelf life.[8] Mycotoxin contamination can occur pre-harvest when the crop plant is growing or post-harvest during processing, packaging, distribution, and storage of food products.[9] Mold growth and contamination with mycotoxins can occur with all crops and cereals that are stored under higher temperatures and humidity for a prolonged time.[10] Corn is considered to be the crop most susceptible to mycotoxin contamination, while rice is the least.[11]

To avoid fungal spoilage in the food industry, a great amount of effort is used to prevent contamination and inhibit fungal growth during the manufacturing process. Chemical preservatives have been used in the food industry to protect food from undesirable growth and thus extend product shelf-life,[12] but there is an increased public concern about the extensive use of chemical preservatives being used in our food.[13] In addition, an increasing number of molds are becoming resistant to certain food preservatives, such as sorbic acid and benzoic acids.[14]

While purchasing food that is already moldy is a big concern, of course sometimes mold spoilage occurs in the consumer's home. It can occur in your cupboard, or even in the refrigerator. And since mycotoxins aren't destroyed by heat, cooking moldy food isn't the answer.

What Are the Symptoms of Toxic Mold?

There can be many symptoms associated with a mold toxicity, but the following are some of the most common ones:

- Severe fatigue
- Anxiety
- Insomnia
- Memory loss
- Migraines
- Skin rashes
- Respiratory distress
- Sinus problems
- Excessive thirst
- Neurological symptoms
- Frequent static shocks

Now, to be fair, most people won't develop these symptoms just by eating moldy food. In most cases people will experience moderate to severe symptoms upon inhalation of mycotoxins, which usually takes placed in a water-damaged building. This can be your home, place of work, school, etc. If you are experiencing severe fatigue, sinus problems, and/or neurological symptoms related to mold, it very well may be due to a combination of inhaling mycotoxins and eating contaminated food, but it usually isn't related to food alone.

What Foods Are Commonly Contaminated with Mold?

Here are some of the foods more commonly contaminated with mold:[15]

- Peanuts
- Brazil nuts
- Pecans
- Walnuts
- Almonds
- Filberts
- Pistachio nuts
- Cottonseed
- Corn
- Sorghum
- Millet
- Figs
- Soybeans

Yet Another Reason to Avoid Corn

Although I just listed over one dozen different foods that can be contaminated with mold, corn is one of the biggest culprits. Many people avoid non-organic corn because most corn is genetically modified, but even if it's organic, it can be contaminated with mold. The problem is that many packaged foods contain corn, and this is especially true for many gluten-free products.

Does this mean you can never have organic corn on the cob or that corn-based taco that you crave? While in many cases it can benefit your health to give up corn completely, I realize that not everyone will choose to do this. Just make sure you check out the end of this chapter when I discuss how to reduce your mold exposure from foods.

Another concern is eating livestock that has been given feed contaminated with mycotoxins. We need to consider the negative effect they have on the animal's health, as exposure to mycotoxins can cause immunotoxicity and impair reproductive function in farm animals.[16] Then, of course, we eat the contaminated dairy, eggs, or meat. It truly seems like a no-win situation, as you can eat organic chicken, and while this is a healthier option than conventional chicken, it's very possible that the chicken was fed organic corn that was contaminated with mycotoxins.

Other Foods That Can Be Contaminated with Mold

Unfortunately, the foods I just listed aren't the only foods that can be contaminated with mold. Milk can be contaminated with aflatoxins,[17] and dark chocolate can be a source of mold, as mycotoxins can form during the various steps in cocoa processing.[18] Even some spices are more suitable substrates for mold growth and mycotoxin development.[19] One study showed that among Indian herbal samples, black pepper and long pepper are the most highly contaminated with aflatoxin B1.[20] Wine can also be a source of mycotoxins, especially ochratoxins.[21]

Doesn't the Government Regulate Mold Contamination in Food?

Currently, about one hundred countries have established limits on the presence of major mycotoxins in food and feed.[22,23] Due to the extreme concerns about aflatoxin contamination in food and feed and their negative public health and economic impacts, aflatoxins have been closely controlled by the FDA since 1969.[24] Among all mycotoxins, aflatoxins are the only ones regulated by established FDA action levels.[24]

The FDA has set the recommended maximum levels at 2–4 ppm for fumonisins in human foods such as corn and processed corn-based products and at 5–100 ppm in different animal feeds, which it considers achievable with the use of good agricultural and manufacturing practices.

How to Reduce Your Exposure to Mold in Foods

Probably the best way to reduce your exposure to mold in food is to limit your consumption of the foods that are most likely to be contaminated. For example, corn is commonly contaminated with mold, and since there are other reasons to avoid corn (i.e., it's a common allergen, is commonly genetically modified), you might want to make an effort to eliminate it from your diet not only while trying to heal from your hyperthyroid condition, but even after you have regained your health.

If you eat nuts and seeds, you need to be careful about how they are stored. I would recommend storing them in the refrigerator or freezer. I would also recommend inspecting nuts before eating them to make sure they're not moldy. I would do this with other foods as well (i.e., certain fruits such as strawberries, raspberries, and apples). If there are any small spots of mold, you might be tempted to cut them out, but I would throw out the entire nut, piece of fruit, or whatever food is contaminated with mold.

If you eat meat, eat 100 percent grass-fed beef and pasture-raised poultry. Remember that even if it's organic, the animals might be fed grains that are contaminated with mycotoxins. If you choose to drink coffee, purchase a brand such as Purity or Bulletproof that tests for mycotoxins.

Organic, pasture-raised chickens and eggs are also preferred. Otherwise you might be eating chicken and/or the eggs of chickens that were fed corn. I realize that all of this might sound overwhelming, and I understand that you might not be able to completely avoid all potential food sources of mold, but just try your best. For example, while I always buy organic chicken and eggs, I can't say that I always buy pasture-raised chicken, and the same thing applies to eggs.

In summary, mold in food can sometimes have a profound impact on one's health. This doesn't mean that you need to completely avoid all of the foods that are more commonly contaminated with mold, although many of these foods are excluded from a Level 3 Hyperthyroid Healing Diet, while others, such as grains and certain nuts (i.e., almonds), are excluded from a Level 2 Diet. Be careful how certain foods are stored, and while organic meat and poultry are preferred, remember that the animals still might be fed grains that are contaminated with mycotoxins.

Chapter 17 Highlights

- Mold in food is something that is commonly overlooked, yet in some situations it can have a profound effect on one's health.
- Grains, such as corn, wheat, and barley may be easily contaminated with mold, which is how the livestock get these mycotoxins.
- Genetics plays an important role in how people react to mold.
- Exposure to mold is well known to trigger inflammation, allergies and asthma, oxidative stress, and immune dysfunction in both human and animal studies.
- Some of the more common symptoms associated with a mold toxicity include severe fatigue, anxiety, insomnia, memory loss, migraines, skin rashes, respiratory distress, sinus problems, neurological symptoms, and frequent static shocks.
- Foods commonly contaminated with mold include peanuts, Brazil nuts, pecans, walnuts, almonds, filberts, pistachio nuts, corn, sorghum, millet, figs, soybeans.
- Milk, dark chocolate, some spices, and wine can also be contaminated with mold.
- The best way to reduce your exposure to mold in food is to limit your consumption of the foods that are most likely to be contaminated.

To access the book references and resources, visit SaveMyThyroid.com/HHDNotes.

CHAPTER
18

When Is a Low FODMAP Diet Necessary?

ODMAP stands for *fermentable oligosaccharides, disaccharides, monosaccharides, and polyols*. This is yet another category of food some people can have problems with. This is especially true with those who have small intestinal bacterial overgrowth, also known as SIBO.

Although I don't have a practice that focuses on SIBO, since 2016 I've been fascinated with this condition. I've attended SIBO conferences and online SIBO summits, have gone through online training programs, etc. I've even interviewed some SIBO experts on my podcast. And the reason for all of this is because SIBO is quite common, and in some cases it can be very difficult to treat.

What Is SIBO?

Normally there should be a smaller amount of bacteria in the upper small intestine when compared to other parts of the gastrointestinal tract. But it's not only the increase in the number of organisms which characterize SIBO, but the type of organisms as well. For example, under normal circumstances, most of the bacteria in the upper small intestine should be gram-positive. But with SIBO it's common to have a greater amount of gram-negative organisms, such as *E. Coli* and *Klebsiella pneumoniae*, although gram-positive organisms such as *Enterococcus* can also be present in greater numbers.[1]

SIBO vs. Irritable Bowel Syndrome

Small intestinal bacterial overgrowth (SIBO) is one manifestation of gut microbiome dysbiosis and is highly prevalent in IBS (irritable bowel syndrome).[2] While not all cases of IBS involve SIBO, a lot of them do. For years many people with IBS were told by gastroenterologists that there was nothing they could do other than try to avoid foods that caused digestive symptoms. But when SIBO is the cause, this can be addressed, although it admittedly can be challenging at times.

When I went through my SIBO training, I discovered that food poisoning is the most common cause of irritable bowel syndrome with diarrhea (IBS-D). This in turn has a negative effect on gut motility, and this is what leads to small intestinal bacterial overgrowth. This doesn't mean that every case of SIBO is caused by food poisoning, but if you had an episode of food poisoning in the past and shortly thereafter developed SIBO, then there is a good chance it's related.

I won't get into great detail about the mechanism behind this, but I will say that the way food poisoning can result in SIBO is through an autoimmune process that damages nerves critical to gut function. Unfortunately, at the time of writing this book, there is no known way to reverse this autoimmune process. The good news is that when SIBO is caused by food poisoning, it still can be treated, although the person might need to take a prokinetic continuously to prevent it from coming back. Prokinetics can help with gut motility, and I'll discuss them later in this chapter.

Should Everyone with SIBO Follow a Low FODMAP Diet?

Getting back to the low-FODMAP diet, it is commonly recommended for those with SIBO. But there are a few things you need to know about this diet. First of all, it isn't a permanent solution for SIBO. If someone follows a low-FODMAP diet, the overall goal should be to address the bacterial overgrowth. I'll discuss this later in this chapter. Second, not everyone with SIBO needs to follow the exact same diet, and there are modifications of the low-FODMAP diet, including Dr. Allison Siebecker's SIBO-Specific Diet, and Dr. Nirala Jacobi's SIBO Biphasic Diet, just to name a few.

What Are the Richest Food Sources of FODMAP Carbohydrates?

I came across a table from a well-researched journal article that lists the richest food sources of FODMAP carbohydrates.[3] According to the table there are six categories of FODMAPs. These include fructo-oligosaccharides (fructans), galacto-oligosaccharides (GOS), lactose, fructose, sorbitol, and mannitol. Some of the foods that fall under the different categories include wheat, rye, onions, garlic, legumes, milk, honey, apples, watermelon, mushrooms, and cauliflower.

I just want to remind you that those who follow a low-FODMAP diet might not necessarily need to avoid foods in all of the categories listed in the table. That being said, foods that fall into the fructans and GOS category should be excluded by anyone trying to follow a low-FODMAP diet, as these foods are always malabsorbed and fermented by intestinal microflora.[4] On the other hand, some people will be able to tolerate foods such as honey, apples, pears, and watermelon. For a more comprehensive list, check out the resources at **savemythyroid.com/HHDNotes**.

Which FODMAP Foods Should Be Avoided?

So how does someone who needs to follow a low-FODMAP diet know which foods they can and can't eat? As I just mentioned, everyone who needs to follow a low-FODMAP diet will probably need to avoid eating foods in the fructans and GOS category. As for whether they are able to eat foods in the other categories, there are a few different ways to find this out. One way is through a breath test. For example, if someone wants to find out if they have problems absorbing fructose, then they can do a breath test to determine this. They can also choose to do a breath test for lactose and sorbitol.

Another way to determine if you can tolerate these other foods is simply to eat them and see how you feel. If someone has SIBO, they might be concerned that eating these foods will worsen their condition, but the worsening of symptoms upon eating certain foods doesn't mean that the overgrowth itself is worsening. I'm not suggesting that you continue eating any foods that cause symptoms such as gas, bloating, etc. But there's nothing wrong with trying to find out which foods you can and can't tolerate while addressing the cause of the problem.

The reason for this is that some people with SIBO can tolerate certain foods that others can't. So for example, some with SIBO can't eat cruciferous vegetables without experiencing gas and/or bloating, while others do perfectly fine. Another thing to keep in mind is that some people are able to eat smaller quantities of certain higher FODMAP foods without experiencing any symptoms, but they experience digestive symptoms when they eat larger servings. For example, they might not experience bloating or gas when eating half a cup of broccoli, but if they exceed this, they experience these symptoms.

Should You Combine a Low FODMAP Diet with a Hyperthyroid Healing Diet?

Although one can certainly try to follow a low-FODMAP diet and at the same time follow one of the Hyperthyroid Healing Diets discussed in this book, the problem is that combining these diets might be too restrictive. This is especially true with a Level 3 Hyperthyroid Healing Diet. If someone has

SIBO, I would not combine a Level 3 Hyperthyroid Healing Diet with a low-FODMAP diet, or any other SIBO-related diet.

In other words, if you have SIBO, I would follow a low-FODMAP diet or some variation of it, and while doing this I would focus on addressing the SIBO (i.e., through antimicrobial herbs). While you probably would be okay combining this with a Level 1 or Level 2 Hyperthyroid Healing Diet, I would not follow a Level 3 Hyperthyroid Healing Diet until you have addressed the SIBO. Once this has been done you can follow a Level 3 Hyperthyroid Healing Diet if you'd like.

This is especially important for those with Graves' disease, as most of the immune system cells are located in the gut. Therefore, you need a healthy gut in order to have a healthy immune system. If you have SIBO, you probably need to address it in order to regain your health.

This doesn't mean that you can't address other triggers and underlying imbalances related to your Graves' disease condition at the same time, and from a food perspective, you still want to avoid common allergens, and perhaps even certain foods such as nightshades. But if you try to follow a low-FODMAP diet while avoiding other nutrient-dense foods (eggs, nuts, etc.), then it is possible to develop nutrient deficiencies.

More about Addressing SIBO

My goal here isn't to give you everything you need to know about SIBO, as that's very difficult to accomplish in a single chapter. If you want to learn more about SIBO, there are some great resources out there, including Shivan Sarna's *Healing SIBO* book and Dr. Nirala Jacobi's *The SIBO Doctor* podcast. However, I will share some of the basics here so you can at least figure out if you have SIBO and, if so, what steps you can initially take to address it.

How to Find Out If You Have SIBO

Although symptoms can provide a lot of valuable information, if SIBO is suspected, it is a good idea to test. Some of the more common symptoms of SIBO include abdominal bloating, pain, or gas, especially when eating higher FODMAP foods. Constipation and/or diarrhea are also common symptoms. Some people will experience weight loss, while others might experience skin issues, including rashes or eczema.

The gold standard of testing SIBO is through a breath test. With the breath test the patient fasts overnight, and then in the morning they will start with a baseline breath test, followed by the consumption of a substrate (i.e., lactulose or glucose). After the baseline breath test, the lab will measure a breath sample approximately every twenty minutes. What the lab is looking for is bacterial fermentation, and it measures this fermentation by measuring the levels of hydrogen and methane. In other words, if someone has SIBO, there will be more fermentation, which will lead to higher levels of hydrogen, methane, or both gases. More recently, hydrogen sulfide has been able to be tested through some labs as well.

Let's take a look at the main breath tests used:

Lactulose breath test. Lactulose can't be absorbed by humans but can be broken down by bacteria. As bacteria consume lactulose, they produce hydrogen and/or methane gases, which are measured with the breath test. This is most commonly used because it can diagnose SIBO in the distal end of the small intestine.

Glucose breath test. The glucose breath test seems to be more accurate, but the reason this test isn't as commonly used is that glucose is absorbed in the beginning of the small intestine. As a result, if someone has SIBO that is occurring in the distal small intestine, then it is less likely to be detected.

However, some bacteria don't ferment lactulose, and as a result, if SIBO is suspected yet the lactulose test comes back negative, then you should consider doing a glucose breath test. Another option is to do both the lactulose and glucose tests initially, although many labs don't offer both types of testing.

Hydrogen sulfide breath test. Up until recently hydrogen sulfide couldn't be tested, and I can't say that everyone who is suspected to have SIBO needs to do this test. Elevated levels of hydrogen sulfide are usually associated with diarrhea. As a result, if someone is experiencing constipation, then they probably don't need to test for hydrogen sulfide, although it's worth mentioning that as of writing this book, there is a test called the Trio-Smart breath test that tests for methane, hydrogen, and hydrogen sulfide.

Can a Stool Panel Detect SIBO?

Hydrogen and methane are produced by microorganisms (bacteria and archaea), and this is what's being measured on the breath tests. *Methanobrevibacter smithii* is an archaea that accounts for most of the methane production in the body. Some comprehensive stool panels test for this "methanogenic" archaea, and if this is high, then it suggests that someone may have SIBO. However, this isn't conclusive, since stool testing evaluates the large intestine, and the breath test remains the gold standard for determining if someone has SIBO. In short, you can't use stool testing to confirm or rule out SIBO.

Three Ways to Treat SIBO

1. **Prescription antibiotics.** Rifaximin (brand name Xifaxan) is the antibiotic most commonly recommended for SIBO. While I'm not a big fan of antibiotics, Rifaximin is different than most other antibiotics. First of all, according to the research, it doesn't harm the beneficial bacteria in the large intestine like most other antibiotics do, and has actually been shown to increase *bifidobacterium*, *Faecalibacterium prausnitzii* and *lactobacillus*.[5]

In addition, bacterial resistance isn't too common when using Rifaximin. That being said, not everyone with SIBO will respond to Rifaximin, and it's usually not my first choice of treatment for patients with SIBO.

2. **Herbal antimicrobials.** I personally prefer to use herbal antimicrobials when dealing with SIBO. Some of the natural agents that can help eradicate SIBO include berberine, oregano oil, neem, and allicin. Keep in mind that while garlic is a high FODMAP food, most people with SIBO can tolerate an allicin supplement, although not everyone. As for whether the herbs are as effective as Rifaximin, there actually was a study that showed that herbal therapy is equivalent to Rifaximin for treating SIBO.[6] However, just as is the case with Rifaximin, not everyone with SIBO will respond to the herbal antimicrobials.

3. **Elemental diet.** Unlike the low-FODMAP diet, the elemental diet is actually considered to be a treatment for SIBO. In fact, the elemental diet can be the most effective treatment when it comes to alleviating the symptoms of SIBO. However, it is arguably the most challenging diet to follow. It's considered to be an antimicrobial approach because the goal is to starve the bacteria but at the same time supply the person with sufficient nutrients in an easily absorbed form.

The elemental diet consists of protein, fat, carbohydrates, amino acids, vitamins, minerals, and either glucose or maltodextrin. You can get a premade formula from a company such as Integrative Therapeutics, or if you visit **www.siboinfo.com** and visit the resources page, you can get a recipe to make your own. The elemental diet can help to lower both methane and hydrogen levels, as well as hydrogen sulfide, and typically you want to follow it for two or three weeks, and then do another breath test immediately upon completion of it.

The Role of Prokinetics in Preventing a Relapse

Prokinetics help to stimulate the migrating motor complex (MMC), and since many cases of SIBO are caused by a dysfunctional MMC, taking prokinetics can be important in preventing a relapse after receiving treatment for SIBO. It's also important to understand that the MMC works in a fasting state, so while some practitioners recommend that patients eat regularly throughout the day to help stabilize their blood sugar levels, those with SIBO probably shouldn't snack in between meals and should go at least twelve hours overnight without eating.

As for what prokinetics you should take, I like an herbal formulation called Iberogast. Ginger can also be a good prokinetic, and 5-HTP can also be beneficial. Low-dose naltrexone (LDN) is commonly used to modulate the immune system in those with autoimmune conditions such as Graves' disease, but it can also act as a prokinetic. Erythromycin is commonly used as an antibiotic, but in very low doses it can also help to stimulate the MMC.[7] Prucalopride (brand name Motegrity) might be the most effective prokinetic out there.

How long after SIBO has been eradicated should someone take a prokinetic? It depends on the person, as most will need to take them for at least two to three months. If someone has SIBO due to an autoimmune process involving the migrating motor complex, they might need to take prokinetics on a permanent basis.

If you suspect you have SIBO, it probably would be a good idea to work with a healthcare practitioner who has experience treating it. Unfortunately, not all gastroenterologists are familiar with treating SIBO, and if they do treat it they'll most likely recommend antibiotics. Not all natural healthcare practitioners are familiar with treating SIBO either, and at times SIBO can be complex to treat, which is why there are conferences and summits dedicated to SIBO.

SIBO vs. SIFO

Whereas SIBO is *small intestinal bacterial overgrowth*, SIFO stands for *small intestinal fungal overgrowth*. SIFO is characterized by the presence of an excessive number of fungal organisms in the small intestine associated with gastrointestinal symptoms.[8] The symptoms of SIFO are similar to SIBO, with the most common symptoms including belching, bloating, indigestion, nausea, diarrhea, and gas.[8] Just as is the case with SIBO, it's also possible for someone with SIFO to experience extra-intestinal symptoms such as fatigue, joint pain, brain fog, headaches, and other symptoms that can improve with treatment.

How can one differentiate SIBO from SIFO? The gold standard is aspiration and culture from the duodenum or jejunum of the small intestine. This can be done by a gastroenterologist, but it might be challenging to find a GI doctor who is willing to do this procedure.

What are some other options if someone can't get this done? If someone has symptoms similar to SIBO but has a negative breath test, then this can be suggestive of SIFO, although it's not conclusive. Or if someone with a confirmed or suspected case of SIBO doesn't respond to treatment, then SIFO might be the culprit. This is especially true if the person took Rifaximin and didn't respond.

One can also do some testing to see if there is a yeast overgrowth, such as testing the candida antibodies through the blood, or they can do an organic acids test. The problem is that a positive finding doesn't confirm yeast overgrowth in the small intestine. That being said, if the person has symptoms suggested of SIBO or SIFO, and they test positive for a yeast overgrowth, then it probably would be a good idea to put that person on a low sugar diet along with giving them some antifungal herbs or medication (i.e., Nystatin). In my opinion, I think it's worth starting with antifungal herbs, and if this doesn't help, then perhaps consider antifungal medication.

In summary, some people with hyperthyroidism have problems with high FODMAP foods. This is especially true for many who have SIBO, although it's possible to have problems even without this condition. In this chapter I mentioned six categories of FODMAPs, and foods which fall into the fructans and GOS category should be excluded by anyone trying to follow a low-FODMAP diet. If you have Graves' disease and SIBO, I wouldn't recommend combining a low-FODMAP diet with a Level 3 Hyperthyroid Healing Diet, as it can be too restrictive. If you have SIBO, in addition to following a low-FODMAP diet, you want to try to eradicate it either through prescription antibiotics, herbal antimicrobials, or an elemental diet.

Chapter 18 Highlights

- FODMAP stands for fermentable oligosaccharides, disaccharides, monosaccharides and polyols.
- Small intestinal bacterial overgrowth (SIBO) involves having too much bacteria in the small intestine.
- A low-FODMAP diet is commonly recommended for those who have SIBO.
- The six categories of FODMAPs include (1) fructo-oligosaccharides (fructans), (2) Galacto-oligosaccharides (GOS), (3) lactose, (4) fructose, (5) sorbitol, and (6) mannitol.
- Some of the foods that fall under the different FODMAP categories include wheat, rye, onions, garlic, legumes, milk, honey, apples, watermelon, mushrooms, and cauliflower.
- Everyone who needs to follow a low-FODMAP diet will probably need to avoid eating foods in the fructans and GOS categories.
- Combining a low-FODMAP diet with a Level 3 Hyperthyroid Healing Diet probably will be too restrictive.
- Some of the more common symptoms of SIBO include abdominal bloating, pain, or gas, especially when eating higher FODMAP foods. Constipation and/or diarrhea are also common symptoms.
- The gold standard of testing SIBO is through a breath test.
- Three ways to treat SIBO include (1) prescription antibiotics, (2) herbal antimicrobials, and (3) an elemental diet.
- Since many cases of SIBO are caused by a dysfunctional MMC, taking prokinetics can be important to prevent a relapse after receiving treatment for SIBO.
- Small intestinal fungal overgrowth (SIFO) is characterized by the presence of an excessive number of fungal organisms in the small intestine associated with gastrointestinal symptoms

To access the book references and resources, visit
SaveMyThyroid.com/HHDNotes.

Eating Out and Snacking

lthough you should try to eat at home as much as possible, I understand that there are times when you might want to go out to eat. Sometimes it's just for a single meal, while at other times it will be for multiple meals as part of a vacation. Without question it can be more challenging to stick with one of the Hyperthyroid Healing Diets when eating out, but it doesn't mean that it's impossible.

It really all comes down to proper planning, and of course some willpower. I can't help you much with the willpower part, but I can give you tips to plan. If you just randomly go to a restaurant or a party without being prepared, then you are more likely to consume foods you are trying to avoid. So the goal of this chapter is to give you some tips so you can properly prepare for single meals out, parties, vacations, and even air travel.

Mentally Prepare Before You Go Out

As I said, I can't do much when it comes to giving you willpower, but this doesn't mean I can't give you some tips in this area. When I was in chiropractic school I saw a practitioner who did food sensitivity testing, so I did a test, and after receiving the results, the practitioner put me on my very first elimination diet. Just a reminder that I ate horribly growing up, so the diet wasn't easy to stick to at the time. To make it even more challenging, while I was on this diet, there was an out-of-town seminar that a friend and I decided to attend.

I went to chiropractic college in Marietta, Georgia, and the seminar was taking place in Orlando. My friend's parents lived in Daytona, so in order to save money on a hotel, we stayed at his parents' house. When we arrived, they wanted to eat pizza for dinner! A lot of people love pizza, and that definitely includes me, so I wasn't sure if I would be able to resist having pizza in this situation.

However, I ordered a salad without dressing while everyone else ordered delicious New York–style pizza. I definitely thought about cheating, but before going to the restaurant I had made up my mind that I wasn't going to cheat. I actually had made up my mind before we left for Orlando, although I honestly didn't expect myself to be sitting in a restaurant with everyone around me stuffing their faces with pizza. I was able to avoid the temptation, and ever since then I have used this as motivation whenever following a certain diet.

The point of this story is that before you go out to eat, you need to make up your mind that you won't cheat under any circumstances. Of course, there's also the concern of cross contamination, which I'll discuss shortly, but you need to tell yourself that you won't eat any bread or pasta, anything with refined sugars or oils, etc. Before heading out to eat, I suggest envisioning yourself eating whole, healthy foods while at the restaurant.

Concerns with Eating Non-Organic

When eating out, not only is there a risk of being exposed to a common food allergen, but also it is more difficult to eat organic. For example, if you go to a restaurant and have a salad with grilled chicken, even if there is no cross contamination, chances are the food won't be organic, which means that you'll be exposed to the chemicals used on the vegetables in the salad, and the chicken also won't be of the highest quality. While this isn't ideal, in most cases, doing this on an occasional basis isn't a big deal.

On the other hand, if you eat out on a frequent basis and eat a lot of foods containing pesticides, herbicides, hormones, antibiotics, etc., then this very well might affect your recovery. And of course the same thing applies if you eat at home but purchase mostly non-organic foods. Don't get me wrong, I'd rather you eat non-organic vegetables than pull out a box of cookies, but the quality can have an impact on your health.

I would try your very best to buy all fruits, vegetables, meat, and poultry organic. And beef should be 100 percent grass fed, and ideally poultry should be pasture raised, although you're still doing a great job if you eat organic poultry that's not pasture-raised. Getting back to the produce, if for any reason you're unable to purchase organic fruits and vegetables, I suggest checking out the Dirty Dozen and Clean Fifteen lists by the Environmental Working Group (www.ewg.org), trying your best to avoid all fruits and vegetables on the Dirty Dozen list, and choosing produce off of the Clean Fifteen list. Just keep in mind that not everything on the Clean Fifteen list is permitted when following one of the Hyperthyroid Healing Diets.

Preparing for a Single Meal Out

This is the easiest to prepare for, although it still can be challenging. This is especially true when it's your very first time eating out upon following a Hyperthyroid Healing Diet. First of all, you want to choose your restaurant wisely, and hopefully you're in a position where you will have a say as to where you go out to eat. If a friend or family member invites you to go to a specific restaurant, it might be more challenging, but this doesn't mean you still can't eat healthily.

In either situation, you want to first view the menu, which you most likely can do online. Most places will have healthier options, such as meat with a side of vegetables, or a salad with grilled chicken. And if there isn't anything on the menu you can eat, you can always call the restaurant and see if they would be willing to prepare something for you. In most cases, doing this won't be necessary.

A big concern when eating out is cross contamination, and the truth is that it can be difficult to completely avoid cross contamination when eating out. I would definitely recommend calling the restaurant ahead of time, or if it's nearby you might even want to visit it before going out to eat there. It's also nice to see the restaurant rating if you can, and just get a feel for the overall atmosphere. But just calling is also fine, and you should ask if you can speak with a manager about your upcoming visit, and discuss your concerns about cross contamination. For example, if they don't have a dedicated gluten-free oven or grill, then perhaps they can use a separate skillet to cook your food.

The Gluten Avoidance Question: Preference or Sensitivity?

When you go to a restaurant and ask to order something gluten-free, many times they will ask you if this is related to a preference or sensitivity. Even if you don't have celiac disease and you don't think you have a gluten sensitivity, I still would tell the server that it's due to a sensitivity. If you tell them that it's a preference, then there is a chance that the people who prepare the food won't change their gloves, which of course can be a big deal when trying to avoid cross contamination.

Preparing for a Special Occasion

Attending a party, wedding, bar mitzvah, or other special event can also be challenging from a diet perspective. Not only do you have to resist the temptations, but if it's a smaller gathering you might be embarrassed to not eat anything there, as you probably wouldn't want to offend the host. As for resisting the temptations, I would suggest trying to find out what's being served at the party, wedding, etc.

One thing you can do is contact the host and let them know that you have a health condition that requires a special diet. Not that you would expect the host to cater to you, but this will accomplish two things. First, you will find out if there will be food you can eat at the special event. If not, you can either eat before the special event and/or bring your own snacks. The second thing this will accomplish is to let the host know that you are following a diet for a certain health condition, so they will know ahead of time that you won't be eating everything they prepare.

Will some people still get offended that you won't eat the dessert they worked so hard to prepare? Sure, this may happen, but if someone truly doesn't understand your situation and/or gives you a hard time about this, then you might not want to go in the first place. Another thing you can do is not only let the host know about the special diet you're on but also offer to bring your own dish that others attending can enjoy.

Even if you find out that there is food you will be able to eat, you still might want to eat something before the special event takes place. There are a few reasons for this. First of all, it might take awhile for the food you can eat to be served, and in the meantime you might be surrounded by unhealthy foods. A second reason is that even if the host tells you there are healthier foods you can eat, there is always the chance that they misunderstood what you could and couldn't eat.

Obviously you can use your own judgment, as perhaps you're attending a party held by a good friend who understands the types of food you're trying to avoid, and if she happens to be a health nut who only prepares healthy food, then you probably can take her word for it. While this is an ideal scenario, most of the time this won't be the case when attending a special event, so you just want to prepare ahead of time.

Preparing for a Vacation

Going on a vacation can be an even greater challenge when trying to follow one of the Hyperthyroid Healing Diets. But once again, planning ahead is the key. First of all, I highly recommend staying somewhere with a refrigerator and kitchen or kitchenette. Thankfully, Airbnb and Vrbo have made this a lot easier to do, although there are also some hotels that offer a kitchen. I recently visited my dad in upstate New York and stayed in an Airbnb, and even though it was a smaller town, the local grocery store had some good organic selections, so it wasn't too challenging to eat healthily while I was out of town.

Even if you have a kitchen or kitchenette where you stay, you might still decide to go out to eat at times while on vacation. I would try to limit it to once or twice, and just as I mentioned earlier, make sure you do some research ahead of time. This will allow you to find restaurants with healthier options on their menus. Once again, if necessary, feel free to call the restaurant to speak with a manager.

You also might want to download the app Find Me Gluten Free or visit the website **www.findmeglutenfree.com**. This lists restaurants that have gluten-free options, although not all of the restaurants listed are healthy options. Some of the value lies in the comments, as they might be able to give you an idea as to whether cross contamination is common.

In the comments it's common to find people with celiac disease who visited the specific restaurant you're researching, and they will tell you if they got sick or not after eating there. Of course, this isn't the case with every restaurant, but if a restaurant has been on the app for awhile, there's a good chance there are reviews from customers who ate there who are gluten sensitive.

When on vacation, make sure you bring some healthy snacks. It would also be nice if there was a grocery store nearby that had healthier snack options. The good news is that many conventional grocery stores have some healthier food options, although if there is a health food store nearby, that would be even better.

If you are planning to go on vacation with friends or family members, it probably will be even more difficult to eat healthily. Don't be surprised if one or more of the people from your party encourage you to stray from the diet. After all, "You're on vacation!" All I can say is that you need to be strong and try your best not let them influence you. If you decide to stray from the diet on your own, that's one thing, but you don't want to end up cheating because a friend or family member encouraged you to do so.

How to Eat Healthy When Cruising

My family and I have been on a few cruises, and all I can say is this: if I was on a cruise while I was dealing with Graves' disease, I'm pretty sure that I would have cheated multiple times. Perhaps you have more willpower than I do, but I can't imagine being on a cruise ship with all of the temptations that are included in what you paid for and not straying from the diet at least a couple of times. This doesn't mean that there aren't healthier options on some cruise ships, and the ones I have been on did offer gluten- and dairy-free options on the menu and even at the buffet. But I just think you're putting yourself in a very difficult position.

If you already paid for a cruise and can't cancel (or don't want to), then I would just try to do your best to eat well. On the reservation, make sure you let them know about the foods you want to avoid. I would also highly recommend bringing your own snacks on the cruise ship. While it's certainly not impossible to follow a Level 3 Hyperthyroid Healing Diet on a cruise, it might be best to try following a Level 1 or 2 Hyperthyroid Healing Diet.

Considering Postponing Your Vacation

In many cases it won't be necessary to do this, but I feel the need to bring this up as an option. While the main goal of going on a vacation shouldn't be to eat crap all day, the truth is that this is what many people do. I'll be the first one to admit that I've fallen off the wagon (from a diet perspective) when going on vacation. One of the main goals of going on a vacation should be to rest and relax. If you are used to going on vacation and eating horribly, I would change your perspective and think about vacationing as a way to enhance your health even further.

I'm not suggesting that every future vacation needs to be like this, but at least while regaining your health, you should look at your vacation as an opportunity to get some much-needed rest and relaxation, and while doing this you should look to nourish your body. This admittedly isn't easy to do if you plan on going to Disney World, Universal Studios, or somewhere similar. This is coming from someone who absolutely loves amusement parks, as these vacations can be a lot of fun, but they're usually not "relaxing" vacations.

Not only are they not relaxing, but it is very difficult to eat healthily at an amusement park. While many of them have gluten- and dairy-free options these days, this doesn't mean that they are "healthy" gluten- and dairy-free options. For example, one of our favorite amusement parks to visit is a place called Holiday World, which believe it or not is in Santa Clause, Indiana! I bring this up because it's the only place I've ever seen that has gluten-free funnel cake! Of course, many amusement parks offer gluten-free pizza and chicken nuggets, as well as burgers with gluten-free buns, etc. But once again, just because something is gluten-free doesn't mean that it's healthy.

If you find yourself in an amusement park and want to stick with one of the diets the best that you can, besides bringing your own healthy snacks, I would just try to eat whole foods. For example, you can order a salad with grilled chicken but pass on any croutons and cheeses and see if you can get olive oil to use as your dressing. Or just have a piece of grilled chicken alone, as while many offer grilled chicken sandwiches, you can simply order it without the bun.

Some amusement parks offer rotisserie chicken with vegetables on the side, which is great. In most cases it won't be organic, but if you're looking for organic food to be served at an amusement park, you'll just have to wait until I build my future amusement park called Save My Thyroid Land.

Preparing for Air Travel

Air travel is yet another situation that is not ideal when trying to eat healthily. This is especially true if you have a very long flight. That being said, you can also do some planning so that you avoid the junk food in the airport terminal and on the plane.

The best thing you can do is bring your own food. Bring plenty of healthy snacks, and you can even bring a meal or two to eat in the terminal or on the plane. You can also eat a healthy meal right before heading to the airport, although you might not choose to do this if you have an early morning flight.

Depending on the airport, there might be restaurants in the terminal with healthier options. Once again, cross contamination can be a big concern, so unless there is a restaurant in the airport terminal that serves organic food and/or has a dedicated allergen-free kitchen, then I would encourage you to bring your own food. As I'm sure you know, once you're on the plane, the menu options are extremely limited, so I definitely would make sure you bring your own food on the plane, especially if you have a long flight. If it's a short flight, you might be fine without eating on the plane, but I still would bring a healthy snack or two along, just to play it safe.

Skipping a Meal Is Better Than Eating Unhealthy

One of the challenges with hyperthyroidism is that many people have a voracious appetite. This definitely described me when I was dealing with Graves' disease. I'm sure at the time I would have cringed at the thought of skipping a meal. This is why it's a good idea to bring a healthy snack or two wherever you go. After all, even with proper planning you might end up in a situation where you are very hungry and have no healthy food options around you.

For example, if you are flying, there is always a chance that your flight will get delayed by a few hours. And if you haven't brought extra snacks, your voracious appetite might get the best of you, and you might end up eating at the closest restaurant to you. If you don't end up needing your snacks, you of course can eat them later or on another day.

Another tip I'd like to share with you is to bring your own extra virgin olive oil to put on salads. First of all, olive oil is very healthy and is allowed on all of the Hyperthyroid Healing Diets. Second, while many restaurants will have their own olive oil, you can't trust the quality of it, as olive oil adulteration is a big concern. For more information on this, I would recommend reading the book *Extra Virginity: The Sublime and Scandalous World of Olive Oil* by Tom Mueller.

Healthy Snack Options

I've mentioned healthy snacks a few times in this chapter, but you might be wondering what some healthy snack options are. If you're following a Level 3 Hyperthyroid Healing Diet, then some healthy snacks to consider include fruit, AIP-friendly beef jerky, unsweetened coconut yogurt, tiger nuts, coconut chips, kale chips, and sweet potato chips. These are also allowed on a Level 1 or Level 2 Diet, but if you are on one of those diets you can also eat the nuts and seeds listed in chapters 6 and 7.

Here are some snacks that you can consider eating:

- Fruit (all three diets)
- Baby carrots (all three diets)
- AIP-friendly beef jerky (all three diets)
- Unsweetened coconut yogurt (all three diets)
- Tiger nuts (all three diets)
- Coconut chips (all three diets)
- Kale chips (all three diets)
- Plantain chips (all three diets)
- Sweet potato chips (all three diets)
- Certain nuts and seeds (Level 1 and Level 2 Diets)

In summary, it is challenging to eat well when you eat away from home. However, it's not impossible, as it comes down to proper planning, as well as having the willpower to avoid certain temptations. While preparing for a single meal out isn't too difficult, it can be more challenging to prepare for a special occasion or go on a vacation.

Of course, I would recommend following the advice I gave in this chapter, and just remember that it's better to skip a meal every now and then than to wreck your diet by eating an unhealthy meal. It's probably a good idea to carry some healthy snacks with you just in case a situation arises where you're out and about and there are no healthy options available.

Chapter 19 Highlights

- Without question it can be more challenging to stick with one of the Hyperthyroid Healing Diets when eating out, but it doesn't mean that it's impossible.
- When eating out, there is not only a risk of being exposed to a common food allergen, but it is also more difficult to eat organic.
- If for any reason you're unable to purchase organic fruits and vegetables, I would check out the Dirty Dozen and Clean Fifteen lists by the Environmental Working Group (www.ewg.org).
- If eating out, you want to choose your restaurant wisely, view the menu online before visiting it, and if necessary call the restaurant ahead of time to see if they can prepare something for you.
- Planning is also important when attending a party or wedding or going on vacation.
- When going on vacation, I highly recommend staying somewhere with a refrigerator and kitchen or kitchenette.
- Air travel is yet another challenging situation when trying to eat healthily. You want to bring plenty of healthy snacks and eat a healthy meal before heading to the airport.
- Skipping a meal is better than eating unhealthily.
- Healthy snack options include fruit, baby carrots, AIP-friendly beef jerky, unsweetened coconut yogurt, tiger nuts, coconut chips, kale chips, and sweet potato chips.

To access the book references and resources, visit
SaveMyThyroid.com/HHDNotes.

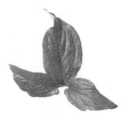

Beyond The Hyperthyroid Healing Diet

CHAPTER
20

Optimize Your Adrenals

I'm confident that stress was a big factor in the development of my Graves'
disease condition, and I find that it's also a major factor with most of my
patients. As a result, improving one's stress-handling skills is extremely
important to the recovery process. Unfortunately, this is one of the most
overlooked steps people take when trying to improve their health.

This of course isn't the case with everyone, but I know that when I was
diagnosed with Graves' disease I was in denial that poor stress-handling skills
was a factor. While I admitted that I dealt with a lot of stress at the time, I
thought I handled my stress pretty well . . . even though I didn't actively do
anything to improve my stress-handling skills. But reality set in when I got
the results of my adrenal saliva test, which revealed that my adrenals were
in the tank.

The Truth about Stress Management and Hyperthyroidism

I've mentioned numerous times in this book that most of the time improving
your diet alone won't restore your health, but it's an important piece of the

puzzle. If someone eats a 100 percent clean diet consisting of whole, healthy foods and avoids the foods they shouldn't be eating, this might not be enough to help them regain their health. But if they eat inflammatory foods, especially on a consistent basis, then there is almost no chance for the person to restore their health.

Similarly, stress management should be part of your hyperthyroid healing journey if you want to receive optimal results. Like diet, improving one's stress handling skills alone probably won't be enough to restore your health, but not blocking out time for stress management on a regular basis can be a reason why you don't recover. Even if you don't think stress is a factor, I recommend blocking out time daily for stress management.

A Common Scenario I See in Practice

Just as is the case with most healthcare practitioners, before I see a patient, I have them complete some forms, including a health history questionnaire. On this questionnaire I ask them to rate their stress levels and stress handling. While some people rate their stress levels as being high and/or their stress handling as low, it's not uncommon to see the opposite pattern (stress levels rated low and stress handling rated high).

Or they might list their stress levels as being low, but also list their stress handling as low or average. And while their *current* stress levels very well might be low, some people don't take into account their past stress levels. For example, I recently had a patient who rated her stress levels as 3 on a scale of 1–10, with 1 meaning the person has low stress levels, and 10 meaning their stress levels are extreme. This represented her current stress levels, but during our initial consultation she admitted that not too long ago she retired from a very stressful job that she worked at for thirty-five years, which in turn might have been a key factor in the development of her hyperthyroid condition.

While there is no question that eliminating this stressor will have a positive impact on her health, this alone probably won't be enough to reverse her hyperthyroid condition. Not only should she still incorporate DAILY stress-management techniques into her life, but depending on the results of her adrenal testing, she most likely will also need to do things to restore the health of her adrenals. I'll talk more about this later in this chapter.

Don't Have Time for Stress Management?

When I tell my hyperthyroid patients that they need to block out time for stress management on a daily basis, one of the most common objections is that they don't have any time for this. As I learned the hard way, those who don't have time for stress management usually need it the most. The good news is that you don't have to start with an hour of stress management daily, or even thirty minutes.

I recommend initially blocking out five minutes per day for stress management, which just about everyone can do. I want you to get into the routine of managing your stress, and once you accomplish this, you can gradually increase the duration so that eventually you're blocking out at least fifteen to twenty minutes per day, which can make a big difference not only in regaining your health but also in preventing other health issues from developing in the future (especially when combined with eating a healthy diet).

Wait, you don't have five minutes per day to spend on stress management? Once again, if this describes you, then remember what I said about those not having the time to incorporate stress management usually needing it the most. This is especially true if you can't even find the time to block out five minutes per day.

What Are the Adrenals?

Before I talk about acute vs. chronic stress, I want to briefly discuss the function of the adrenals. The adrenal gland is made up of two parts, the cortex and the medulla. The adrenal cortex is responsible for producing glucocorticoids, mineralocorticoids, and androgens. The adrenal medulla produces catecholamines, epinephrine, and norepinephrine.

When it comes to the adrenals, one also can't ignore the importance of both the pituitary gland and hypothalamus. For example, in response to circadian rhythms or stressors, paraventricular neurons (PVN) in the hypothalamus make and secrete corticotropin-releasing hormone.[1] This hormone binds to receptors on the anterior pituitary gland, which leads to the synthesis of ACTH (or corticotrophin), which signals to the adrenals to produce cortisol.

While someone can certainly have problems directly related to the adrenals, many times the main problem is with the hypothalamic-pituitary-adrenal (HPA) axis. In fact, cortisol is the major glucocorticoid, and it increases in response to stress, which in turn activates the HPA axis. When the stress is chronic, it can lead to dysregulation of the HPA axis, which can be a factor in the development of conditions such as Graves' disease.

Acute vs. Chronic Stress

It's important to understand that not all stress is bad. For example, exercise puts stress on the body, but this type of stress is beneficial, assuming you don't overtrain, which I did prior to being diagnosed with Graves' disease, and I further discuss this in chapter 23. Stress is essential to survive, as it helps us to adapt to our environment.

The problem is when stress becomes chronic. Our bodies were designed to handle acute stress situations. While extreme acute stress situations can sometimes cause problems, chronic stress is usually what gets us into trouble from a health perspective.

How Stress Affects the Sex Hormones

I want to briefly discuss something called the *pregnenolone steal*, also known as the *cortisol steal*. All of the steroid and sex hormones are derived from cholesterol. As a result, if you have low cholesterol levels, which is common with hyperthyroidism, then this can result in low levels of estrogen, progesterone, testosterone, etc.

I felt the need to bring this up not only because many people with hyperthyroidism have lower cholesterol levels, but for those who have high cholesterol, it's common for medical doctors to prescribe statins to their patients, which in turn can result in low cholesterol levels. As a result, this can have a negative effect on the sex hormones, as well as cortisol, which is also derived from cholesterol.

Anyway, the hormone pathway starts with cholesterol, and pregnenolone is a hormone that is synthesized from cholesterol. This takes place in the mitochondria, and if someone has dysfunction of the mitochondria, then this in turn can affect the production of pregnenolone. But under normal circumstances, pregnenolone converts into either progesterone or DHEA, and these in turn will convert into other hormones.

As an example, DHEA can convert into androstenedione, which is a precursor of testosterone, and testosterone can convert into estradiol, and it does this with the assistance of an enzyme called *aromatase*. Testosterone converts into dihydrotestosterone (DHT) thanks to the enzyme *5α-reductase*. Pregnenolone can also convert into progesterone, which in turn converts into 17-hydroxy progesterone, which converts into cortisol.

Cortisol Is a Priority Over the Sex Hormones

Although it's awesome to have healthy sex hormones, the body will always prioritize the production of cortisol. As a result, if someone is dealing with chronic stress, cortisol will be produced at the expense of DHEA. Remember that pregnenolone can be converted into both progesterone and DHEA, and DHEA will convert into the other hormones I mentioned. When chronic stress is a factor, it inhibits an enzyme called *17,20 lyase*. This enzyme helps to convert 17-OH pregnenolone into DHEA, and 17-OH progesterone into the hormone androstenedione.

Consequently, if these enzymes are inhibited, there will be a decrease in both DHEA and androstenedione. These hormones are precursors to testosterone, and testosterone converts into estradiol and DHT. So when looking at the big picture, the pregnenolone steal can result in decreased levels of DHEA, androstenedione, testosterone, estradiol, and DHT. It's important to understand that not all of these hormones will become low simultaneously. A common scenario is that initially you might see some of these hormones very low, while other hormones will look fine. Or perhaps they will be in the lab reference range, but not within the optimal range.

Either way, the pathway that converts pregnenolone into progesterone will predominate. However, remember that cortisol is a priority over progesterone. Because of this, progesterone will also decrease as cortisol production increases. Now you can understand why this is also called the *cortisol steal*. There are two main ways to stop and reverse this process: by (1) decreasing the stressors in your life and (2) improving your stress-handling skills.

I don't want you to think that all sex hormone imbalances are caused by the pregnenolone steal. Obviously we live in a toxic world where endocrine-disrupting chemicals can play a role, and there can be other factors. And while it's important to decrease your toxic load, which I'll discuss in chapter

24, improving your adrenal health is a good starting point, which is what this chapter is about.

How to Optimize Your Adrenal Health

If you currently have compromised adrenals, then it will take time to restore them back to normal. While I do recommend nutritional supplements to my patients in order to support the adrenals, if this is all you do, then you will never achieve optimal adrenal health. You need to focus on diet and lifestyle, which is of course what this book is all about. Let's take a look at some things you can do to regain the health of your adrenals.

Eat well. The main purpose of this book is to show you what foods to eat and which to avoid, so you can reverse your hyperthyroidism. I've already mentioned multiple times in this book that food alone usually won't accomplish this, but it is a huge piece of the puzzle. Anyway, I won't discuss this any further, as you can always refer back to section 2 as a reminder of which foods you should and shouldn't eat, which depends on which Hyperthyroid Healing Diet you choose to follow.

Block out regular time for stress management. I already mentioned this earlier in this chapter, and I recommended to start with five minutes per day and to do this *every* day. Remember that if you don't feel like you have the time to dedicate five minutes per day, then you *really* need to do this. Also, you might wonder what you should do if you're already blocking out some time for stress management but not on a daily basis.

For example, someone might be practicing meditation or yoga three days per week, and perhaps even spending thirty to sixty minutes doing this. In this situation, I would suggest to block out at least five minutes for stress management on the other four days of the week. If you're already in the routine of practicing stress management, it's fine to have days when you're doing it for thirty minutes or longer and other days when you're only dedicating five minutes to it.

Get sufficient sleep. I can easily dedicate an entire chapter to getting quality sleep. And guess what? I did write an entire chapter on this topic, which is chapter 22.

Nutritional Supplements and Herbs That Can Support Adrenals

Once again, I commonly recommend adrenal support in the form of nutritional supplements and herbs, but in many cases it's perfectly fine to initially focus on eating well, daily stress management, and getting sufficient sleep. That being said, some of the nutritional supplements and herbs that can support the adrenals include licorice root, rhodiola, holy basil, eleuthero, phosphatidylserine, adrenal glandulars, the B vitamins, and vitamin C. Remember that I have a bonus chapter where I discuss nutritional supplements and herbs that can support different areas of the body, including the adrenals. So for more information on these, including suggested doses, visit **savemythyroid.com/HHDNotes**.

Which Stress-Management Techniques Should You Incorporate?

There are many different stress-management techniques you can choose from. And while you don't need to stick with a single one, if you're not already incorporating any stress-management techniques then it's a good idea to start with one. Choose one you think you'd be willing to do on a regular basis, and if for any reason it's not a good fit for you, then you can always switch to a different one. I'll list a few in this book, but just keep in mind that there are many others to choose from.

1. **Deep breathing.** This will be the easiest place to start for many people, as simply incorporating deep breathing techniques can do wonders from a

stress-handling perspective. Research shows that deep breathing can result in an improvement in both mood and stress.[2] I like something called the *4-7-8 breathing technique*, which involves breathing in for a count of four seconds, holding that breath for seven counts, and taking eight seconds to exhale. A few studies actually show that this specific breathing technique offers some health benefits.[3,4]

2. **Meditation.** I think it's safe to say that this is the most well-known type of stress-management technique. A number of different types of meditation are practiced, and most of them involve four elements.[5] This includes a quiet location, a specific position, a focus of attention, and an open attitude. While meditation is great to practice for stress-management purposes, there are other health benefits as well, such as pain management.

I want to briefly mention something called *mindfulness meditation*. Mindfulness simply means being aware of the present moment, and mindfulness meditation is a type of meditation that allows us to focus more on our inner and outer experiences. So essentially it makes us more aware of all of the surrounding physical and mental activities.

I'd like to reveal some of the studies that show some of the benefits of meditation. One randomized controlled trial I came across demonstrated that meditation may change brain and immune function in positive ways.[6] Another randomized controlled trial examined the effects of a one-month mindfulness meditation versus somatic relaxation training reporting distress.[7] The study showed that brief training in mindfulness meditation or somatic relaxation reduces distress and improves mood states. Another study showed that the practice of meditation reduced psychological stress responses and improved cognitive functions.[8]

If you've never meditated before, you might be wondering how you can learn to do so. There are many different ways, including reading books, watching YouTube videos, and even attending online classes. There are a few phone apps to consider as well, including Calm, Headspace, and the Mindfulness App. And if you prefer working in person with someone, you can do an online search to see if there are some local groups or classes.

3. **Yoga.** Yoga is another type of stress-management technique, and there are many different yoga techniques to choose from. I'm definitely not an expert when it comes to the different techniques, although I'll mention here that hatha yoga is the most commonly practiced type in the United States and Europe. Some of the major styles of hatha yoga include Iyengar, Ashtanga, Vini, Kundalini, and Bikram yoga.[9] There are even certain yoga postures that are known to improve thyroid health, including a shoulder stand position known as *sarvangasana*.

While you might be able to learn how to do yoga by watching online videos, it probably is best to learn this from a certified yoga instructor. This doesn't have to be in person, although it certainly can be, as you can join a local yoga studio. But there are also online yoga classes to consider joining.

The best of both worlds would be to find a local yoga studio that also offers an option to do online classes. This way you can attend in person a few times per week but also have the option to do it from home. Even if you have to choose one or the other, that's perfectly fine. It's just important that you get into the routine of practicing it while being taught the correct way.

As for the research, there is no shortage of studies that demonstrate how yoga can help with stress. A systematic review of the literature examined the mechanisms through which yoga reduces stress.[10] This review showed seven mechanisms. Three of these are psychological mechanisms and include positive effect, mindfulness, and self-compassion.[10] Four of these mechanisms are biological and include the posterior hypothalamus, interleukin-6, C-reactive protein, and cortisol.[10]

4. Biofeedback. Biofeedback is a stress-management technique that can modify physiology to improve physical, mental, emotional, and spiritual health.[11] This involves measuring a person's quantifiable bodily functions (e.g., blood pressure, heart rate, muscle tension) and, by using this information, providing guidance and reinforcement for the successful management of the physiological response to stress.[12] Some smaller studies have shown the effectiveness of biofeedback.

One study assessed whether a self-directed, computer-guided meditation training program is useful for stress reduction in hospital nurses.[13] The study showed that this program helped hospital nurses reduce their stress and anxiety. Another study showed that heart rate variability biofeedback decreases blood pressure in prehypertensive subjects.[14]

Although many types of biofeedback devices are utilized at clinician's offices, you can also purchase a device to use at home. Heart Math is a company that has some amazing technology. I own their emwave2 and the Inner Balance. The emwave2 and Inner Balance programs measure heart rate variability (HRV), which involves a variation in the interval between heartbeats.

HRV is a measure of the autonomic nervous system's function and reflects an individual's ability to adaptively cope with stress.[15] Having a higher HRV is a sign of good adaptation and characterizes a person with efficient autonomic mechanisms, while having a lower HRV is usually an indicator of abnormal and insufficient adaptation of the autonomic nervous system.[16]

Even under resting conditions, there is supposed to be some degree of heart rate variability. HRV can be an important indicator of health and fitness. Having low HRV usually means that there is an imbalance of the autonomic nervous system, which in turn can increase the risk of developing certain health conditions. I personally use the Inner Balance from Heart Math as my main form of stress management. For more information, visit **www. heartmath.com**, as they have some videos and articles that discuss HRV in greater detail and how their programs can help.

Some of the factors that influence HRV include exercise, one's breathing patterns, and even your feelings and emotions. Having a negative attitude or being stressed out will most likely lead to a decrease in HRV. However, having a positive attitude and doing a good job of managing your stress can lead to increased HRV.

5. **Hypnotherapy.** Hypnotherapy is also considered to be a type of MBM. Hypnosis is a state of deep concentration and can be used to help people with many different conditions. The research shows that hypnosis can not only be used for stress and anxiety,[17,18] but also might help with depression,[19] sleep disorders,[20] and irritable bowel syndrome.[21,22]

6. **Other stress-management techniques.** Some other stress-management techniques include music therapy, visualization, tai chi, and qigong. While I recommend that someone should choose one or more stress-management techniques to focus on, any of these can be of tremendous benefit. Although these techniques can help greatly to manage your stress levels, remember that they can also help with other conditions, such as pain, high blood pressure, and depression.

Should You Do Adrenal Testing?

In the beginning of this chapter I mentioned how I was in denial about stress being a factor in the development of my Graves' disease condition. It took an adrenal saliva test to convince me that stress not only was a factor, but was a very big factor. It taught me that you can't always go by symptoms when evaluating the adrenals, and the same is true with other areas of the body, as you can't always rely on symptoms to determine whether someone has an adrenal problem, dysbiosis of the gut microbiome, etc. Because of my experience, I recommend adrenal testing to most of my patients.

While some people reading this book are in denial like I was, others don't need any convincing that stress is a big problem in their lives. And if this describes you, then you might wonder why you can't just assume that your adrenals are compromised, and then take action to improve your adrenal health. After all, I did say that diet and lifestyle changes are the most important factors when restoring one's adrenal health, right?

While you certainly can and should eat a healthy diet, do things to improve stress handling, and try to get more sleep, many times additional support in the form of nutritional supplements and herbs can be a valuable part of the healing process. For example, in 2008 my adrenal saliva test revealed low cortisol levels, so the supplement protocol I followed was tailored to my results. On the other hand, if someone has elevated cortisol, then different supplements are required, which you can learn more about by checking out my bonus chapter on nutritional supplements.

How Can You Test the Adrenals?

As I mentioned already, I tested my adrenals through the saliva when I dealt with Graves' disease, and I've recommended saliva testing to many of my patients over the years. But more recently I've also incorporated dried urine testing. Although I discuss some of the different types of testing in chapter 27, let's briefly take a look at the three main options to test the adrenals:

Blood testing. While blood testing has some advantages over saliva and urine testing, it also has some disadvantages. The benefits are that it can test for adrenocorticotropic hormone (ACTH), and you can also test for adrenal auto-antibodies, which are usually present in Addison's disease. However, with blood testing, you can't look at the circadian rhythm of cortisol. This is important because cortisol should be at its highest levels in the morning and should gradually decrease throughout the day. Another disadvantage is that in most cases you have to visit a lab or doctor's office, and some people get stressed out when getting blood drawn, which can lead to a false elevation of cortisol.

Saliva testing. I'm a big fan of saliva testing, and the main benefits of saliva testing are that you can look at the circadian rhythm of cortisol and collect the samples from the comfort of your home. The downside is that some people find it difficult to generate enough saliva for the samples. Most conventional medical doctors who test for cortisol will do so in the blood, but the research shows that you can measure salivary hormones with a high level of sensitivity and specificity.[23] In states of altered cortisol binding, salivary biomarkers are more accurate measures of adrenal reserve than serum cortisol.[23]

Urinary testing. Over the last few years I've done more and more dried urine testing. If focusing solely on the adrenals, saliva is still the main test I recommend, but if I also want to look at the sex hormones and the hormone metabolites, then I may recommend dried urine testing. I'll discuss dried urine testing in greater detail in chapter 27.

It's also worth mentioning that there are other types of urine tests related to the adrenals, but these don't take into account the circadian rhythm of cortisol. For example, some labs offer a twenty-four-hour urinary cortisol test, where you collect all of your urine over a twenty-four-hour period. This can determine the total cortisol, which can be helpful in diagnosing a condition such as Cushing syndrome but otherwise doesn't have much value.

In summary, stress is a big factor in many people with hyperthyroidism, especially those with Graves' disease. It shouldn't be surprising that most people with hyperthyroidism have adrenal imbalances. I usually recommend saliva or dried urine testing to evaluate the adrenals, and while nutritional supplements and herbs can be helpful, they're not a replacement for eating well, getting sufficient sleep, and blocking out time for stress management.

Chapter 20 Highlights

- I'm confident that stress was a big factor in the development of my Graves' disease condition, and I find that it's also a major factor with most of my patients.
- Those who don't have time for stress management usually need it the most.
- Stress management should be part of your hyperthyroid healing journey if you want to receive optimal results.
- I recommend initially blocking out five minutes per day for stress management and then gradually increasing the duration.
- While someone can certainly have problems directly related to the adrenals, many times the main problem is with the hypothalamic-pituitary-adrenal (HPA) axis.
- Our bodies were designed to handle acute stress situations, not chronic stress.
- Although it's awesome to have healthy sex hormones, the body will always prioritize the production of cortisol.
- There are several things you can do to optimize your adrenal health: eat well, block out regular time for stress management, get sufficient sleep, consider certain nutritional supplements and herbs
- Here are some stress-management techniques to consider: deep breathing, meditation, yoga, biofeedback, hypnotherapy.
- The two primary ways I test the adrenals in my practice are (1) saliva testing and (2) dried urine testing.

To access the book references and resources, visit
SaveMyThyroid.com/HHDNotes.

CHAPTER
21

Gut Healing and the 5-R Protocol

Having a healthy gut is important with any health condition, including hyperthyroidism. It is estimated that 70 to 80 percent of immune system cells are located in the gastrointestinal tract, so it should be obvious why anyone with any autoimmune condition would want to have a healthy gut, and this of course includes those with Graves' disease. As for toxic multinodular goiter, a common cause is problems with estrogen metabolism, and having a healthy gut plays a role in this. Even with subacute thyroiditis, since most cases are related to a virus, a healthy gut is obviously important, as having a healthy immune system is important to keep viruses in check.

What is the difference between the gut microbiota and the gut microbiome? The assemblage of microorganisms (bacteria, archaea, lower and higher eukaryotes, and viruses) present in a defined environment defines the term *microbiota*.[1] *Microbiome*, on the other hand, refers to the entire habitat and surrounding environmental conditions of a given microbiota and their collective genomes.[1]

Reminder: The Triad of Autoimmunity

In chapter 2 I mentioned the triad of autoimmunity, which relates to three components necessary for autoimmune conditions such as Graves' disease to develop. These include (1) a genetic predisposition, (2) exposure to one or more environmental triggers, and (3) an increase in intestinal permeability. This chapter essentially focuses on the third component of this triad.

And once again, the "leaky gut" component isn't just important when it comes to Graves' disease. So regardless of what type of hyperthyroid condition you have, it is essential to optimize your gut health. This goes back to Hippocrates, who said that "all disease begins in the gut."

What Is a "Leaky" Gut?

A leaky gut is also known as "an increase in intestinal permeability," and this involves damage to the enterocytes (cells of the small intestine). What happens is that one or more factors will either cause damage to the tight junctions connecting the enterocytes (referred to as *paracellular permeability*) and/or will actually penetrate these cells (referred to as *transcellular permeability*). Either way, this increase in intestinal permeability allows proteins and other larger molecules to pass into the bloodstream, which can in turn can trigger an immune system response.

Dr. Alessio Fasano is a pediatric gastroenterologist and researcher, and he has done a lot of research on intestinal permeability and autoimmunity. In a journal article entitled "Tight Junctions, Intestinal Permeability, and Autoimmunity Celiac Disease and Type 1 Diabetes Paradigms," Dr. Fasano concluded, "Genetic predisposition, miscommunication between innate and adaptive immunity, exposure to environmental triggers, and loss of intestinal barrier function secondary to dysfunction of intercellular tight junctions all seem to be key components in the pathogenesis of autoimmune diseases."[2]

This is just confirmation that in order to reverse the autoimmune process, you need to heal the gut.

The Importance of the Mucosal Barrier

The mucosal epithelium is an important barrier that protects us against pathogenic viruses and bacteria. The first component of this barrier is mucus, which is not only found in the GI tract but also other parts of the body. In the large intestine there are two layers of mucus, while in the small intestine there's only one.

Even though nobody would want to chat about mucus at a cocktail party, it really is amazing how important mucus is to our health. Mucus is produced continuously by intestinal cells, and each region of the gastrointestinal tract produces its own unique form of mucus. I mentioned how mucus protects us against microorganisms such as viruses and bacteria, along with digestive enzymes and acids, digested food particles, microbial by-products, and food-associated toxins.[3] The mucus layer adjacent to the epithelial barrier of the GI tract is also essential in the maintenance of intestinal homeostasis and contains a thriving biofilm including beneficial and pathogenic microbial populations.[3]

What Can You Do to Fortify Your Mucosal Barrier?

It wasn't until I started doing research for this book that I discovered how important *Akkermansia muciniphila* is to the mucosal barrier. This microbe is measured in some comprehensive stool panels, but I didn't realize the potential negative consequences of it being too low. *Akkermansia muciniphila* can convert mucin into beneficial by-products, regulate intestinal homeostasis, and maintain gut barrier integrity.[4] It is also known to competitively inhibit other mucin-degrading bacteria and improve metabolic functions and immunity responses in the host.[4]

There are many more benefits of this microbe. But the million-dollar question is "how can we increase this microbe when it's deficient on a stool test?" Prebiotics may help, along with polyphenol-rich foods. And there is also a company that has an *Akkermansia muciniphila* supplement.

In his excellent book *Super Gut*, Dr. William Davis discusses how you don't want too much or too little *Akkermansia muciniphila*. His research shows that oleic acid (found in extra-virgin olive oil) can stimulate the proliferation of *Akkermansia*. However, he also mentions that approximately 5 percent of the population doesn't have any *Akkermansia* and thus might need to rely on supplementation. I will say that I have seen a decent number of patients have less than detectable levels of *Akkermansia muciniphila* on a comprehensive stool panel. And while taking an *Akkermansia muciniphila* probiotic supplement is something to consider in this situation, I'm not sure if this is something everyone with low levels of this microbe needs to do.

The 5-R Protocol and Hyperthyroidism

When it comes to having a healthy gut, you want to focus on the components of the 5-R protocol:

1. Remove
2. Replace
3. Reinoculate
4. Repair
5. Rebalance

Let's go ahead and take a look at each one of these components:

1) REMOVE

This is perhaps the most important component of the 5-R protocol, as it involves removing anything that will disrupt the gut. The main focus of this book is on food, and you've learned that food can have a negative impact on the gut and that certain foods can even cause an increase in intestinal permeability (a leaky gut). In fact, one of the main focuses of all three Hyperthyroid Healing Diets is to remove common allergens and reduce lectins and other compounds that can have a negative effect on gut healing.

But there are factors other than food that can cause a leaky gut and/or intestinal dysbiosis. Remember that *intestinal dysbiosis* refers to an imbalance of the gut flora. Certain medications can disrupt the gut microbiome. Even though antibiotics are sometimes necessary to take, you probably know that they can have a negative impact on the gut microbiome, as can acid blockers and NSAIDs. And the research shows that antithyroid medication (methimazole and PTU) can also disrupt the gut microbiome and affect the intestinal barrier.[5]

This doesn't mean that there isn't a time and place for taking antithyroid medication. Everything comes down to risks versus benefits, and while I personally chose to take an herbal approach for symptom management when I dealt with hyperthyroidism, this isn't always effective. You just need to keep in mind that if you are taking antithyroid medication, then healing the gut may be a little more challenging, but over the years I've had many people with hyperthyroidism take antithyroid medication and restore their health.

The Impact of Other Chemicals on the Gut Microbiome

There are many other chemicals that can have a negative effect on the gut microbiome. In chapter 26 I discuss the negative impact of glyphosate on our health, and one of the main problems with glyphosate is that it can disrupt the gut microbiota.[6] Certain xenoestrogens, including bisphenol A (BPA) and phthalates can also have a negative effect on the gut microbiome.[7] Trichloroethene (TCE) is a widely used industrial solvent, and it's associated with the development of certain autoimmune conditions by affecting the microbiome.[8] Even heavy metals can have a negative impact on the gut.[9]

So hopefully you understand that even if you eat a healthy diet, exposure to certain environmental toxicants can disrupt the gut. Obviously it's impossible to completely avoid environmental toxicants, but this doesn't mean that there is nothing you can do. In chapter 24 I go into greater detail about how to reduce your exposure to these environmental toxicants.

Lions and Tigers and Gut Infections . . . Oh My!

This is yet another topic I could easily dedicate a few chapters to. But since this isn't a book that focuses on gut infections, I'm not going to spend too much time on this. It's important to mention that even though I just used the term "infections," just because you have certain microorganisms present doesn't mean you have an actual infection.

Also keep in mind that a yeast overgrowth or small intestinal bacterial overgrowth (SIBO) aren't infections, as it's normal to have yeast in our gastrointestinal tract, but you just don't want an overabundance of it. And with SIBO, you have too much bacteria in the small intestine, which can cause symptoms such as bloating, gas, and changes in bowel habits.

What I'd like to do is separate this into three different categories: bacterial gut infections, viral gut infections, and parasitic gut infections:

Viral infections. When thinking of viruses, many people tend to think of the more common ones, including influenza, Epstein-Barr, cytomegalovirus, etc. But there are at least 320,000 mammalian viruses.[10] Although viruses commonly infect the upper respiratory tract and lungs, they also can affect the colon, liver, spinal cord, and even white blood cells.

While many viruses can without question cause harm, there is evidence that some may be protective. That being said, certain viruses that invade the colon can become problematic, including adenovirus and norovirus. Having a healthy gut microbiome and mucosal barrier are important factors to prevent viruses from having a negative effect on your gastrointestinal tract.

Bacterial infections. There are a lot of different bacteria that can cause problems, including *Clostridium difficile, Yersinia enterocolitica, Klebsiella pneumonia*, and *Citrobacter freundii*. Some of these are completely normal to have in the gut, but they can become "opportunistic" under certain circumstances. In other words, in some situations certain bacteria that normally inhabit the gut can become harmful.

Helicobacter pylori (*H. pylori*) is yet another well-known bacteria that can cause problems. This is a gram-negative bacteria that can infect the stomachs of humans, and it is associated with peptic ulcer disease, gastric carcinoma, and gastric lymphoma.[11] Keep in mind that while some people will experience symptoms such as heartburn, indigestion, and nausea, the absence of symptoms doesn't rule out *H. pylori*.

As for how *H. pylori* is transmitted, the most common method is the oral-oral route (i.e., kissing), and the fecal-oral route (i.e., contaminated water).[12] It's also worth mentioning that a few studies show a correlation between *H. pylori* and Graves' disease.[13,14] However, this doesn't mean that *H. pylori* is always a trigger. Some practitioners even feel like you shouldn't address it unless you experience common symptoms associated with this bacteria, such as heartburn and acid reflux.

Parasites. There are two main classes of intestinal parasites, which include helminths and protozoa. Helminths are worms with many cells, and include tapeworms, pinworms, and roundworms. Adult helminths are unable to multiply in the human body. On the other hand, protozoa can multiply inside the human body, and the most common protozoa in the United States are giardia and cryptosporidium. Next I'm going to discuss some of the more common intestinal parasites, as well as a few other types of parasites.

Giardia lamblia. This is a parasite of the small intestine that causes extensive morbidity worldwide.[15] It lives in soil, food, and water and can cause giardiasis, which is an infection of the small intestine. You can become infected by coming into direct contact with someone who has giardiasis, or by drinking water from contaminated lakes or streams, or contaminated foods. The main symptom someone presents with is diarrhea, although other symptoms can include gas, bloating, headache, loss of appetite, low-grade fever, and weight loss.[16]

Cryptosporidium. This is another type of protozoan parasite that can lead to gastroenteritis. Infection of this parasite leads to cryptosporidium enteritis, which is an infection of the small intestine and usually causes watery diarrhea, although other symptoms can include fever, nausea, and vomiting.[17] Two common causes of this infection include drinking from contaminated public water supplies and swimming in contaminated pools and lakes.[17]

Blastocystis hominis. *Blastocystis hominis* was once considered to be a member of the normal intestinal flora, but in recent years it has been labeled as a very controversial pathogenic protozoan.[18] One study showed that the frequency rate of intestinal symptoms was 88.4 percent, with abdominal pain being the most frequent symptom (76.9 percent) and diarrhea and distention following at a rate of 50.0 percent and 32.6 percent.[18] The mode of transmission isn't completely understood, although a few sources show evidence that contaminated water might be a source of infection.[19,20]

That being said, I've had a few guest experts on my podcast who don't believe that *Blastocystis hominis* is a problem in everyone. This includes Dr. Jason

Hawrelak and Dr. Nirala Jacobi, as they feel that in most cases *Blastocystis hominis* is commensal and doesn't cause harm. I can't say that I never treat *Blastocystis hominis* in my autoimmune thyroid patients, but it's very interesting how some practitioners will treat everyone with *Blastocystis hominis*, while others will leave it alone unless the person is experiencing gastrointestinal symptoms.

Entamoeba histolytica. *Entamoeba histolytica* is a protozoan that can live in the large intestine without causing damage, although sometimes it invades the colon wall, causing colitis, acute dysentery, or chronic diarrhea. The infection associated with this parasite is amebiasis, and it's responsible for an estimated one hundred thousand deaths annually, making it the second leading cause of death due to a protozoan parasite after *Plasmodium*.[21] In addition to causing gastrointestinal symptoms, there can also be extraintestinal manifestations which include amebic liver abscesses and other more rare manifestations such as pulmonary, cardiac, and brain involvement.[22]

How Do You Test for Gut Microbes?

There are different ways to test for microorganisms that inhabit the gut. Most of the time they are tested through the blood or the stool, although there are exceptions. For example, *H. pylori* can be tested through the blood, saliva, and stool, and through a urea breath test. Most doctors prefer stool and the urea breath test. Viruses can be tested for through the blood or stool, with the latter being more common when focusing on the gut. Parasites are also most commonly tested for through the stool.

It's important to understand that there is no perfect method of testing for gut microbes. I've seen *H. pylori* test negative on a stool antigen test and positive on a urea breath test, and vice versa. I've also seen both of these tests be negative and for *H. pylori* to show up on a DNA-based test such as the GI-MAP. It's also not uncommon for false negative readings when testing for parasites on a basic stool test. And while doing a comprehensive stool panel is more likely to pick up parasites, these tests are far from perfect.

So while in some cases I do like to test to determine if someone has *H. pylori*, parasites, or other gut microbes, you can't always rely on a negative result. This is especially true when it comes to testing for parasites through the stool. While at times you can try a different test and see if it gets picked up, there is a time and place for treating gut infections, even when the testing comes back negative. For example, if someone has a lot of gastrointestinal symptoms and it doesn't seem like it's related to a food sensitivity, yet a comprehensive stool panel, SIBO breath test, and/or other gut-related tests come back negative, it might still be worth following an antimicrobial treatment protocol (under the guidance of a healthcare practitioner).

How Do You Correct Gut Dysbiosis?

There are different ways to address potentially problematic gut microbes. One way is to simply "crowd them out" with beneficial microbes in the form of probiotic foods and supplements. Other times certain antimicrobial herbs can be beneficial. And of course there is a time and place for medication, including antibiotics, antivirals, and antifungals.

With my background, it shouldn't be a surprise that I try to take a natural approach whenever possible. But ultimately it's up to the patient. For example, if someone with Graves' disease tests positive for *H. pylori*, I prefer to use natural antimicrobial agents, although it's important to know that it usually takes longer to get rid of the bacteria this way. As a result, some people prefer to take antibiotics, even though there are negative consequences to taking them. In addition, with *H. pylori* most conventional medical doctors will recommend "triple therapy," which involves two antibiotics and a proton pump inhibitor.

If you do take antibiotics I would make sure to supplement with high-potency probiotics (at least 25–30 billion CFU). Just make sure you take them at least two hours away from the antibiotics so the antibiotics don't eradicate the beneficial microbes that are included in the probiotic.

What You Need to Know about Biofilm

A biofilm is a group of microorganisms (i.e., bacteria, yeast, etc.) which form a protective layer. Bacterial biofilms are resistant to antibiotics, disinfectant chemicals, phagocytosis, and other components of the innate and adaptive inflammatory defense system of the body.[23] *Candida albicans* can also form biofilms, which can make it resistant to certain antifungal medications such as fluconazole.[24] Since many people with thyroid and autoimmune thyroid conditions have these types of infections, it can be beneficial to understand how to disrupt these biofilms.

Many different microorganisms form biofilms, including *H. pylori*, *Yersinia enterocolitica*, *Borrelia burgdorferi*, *Klebsiella pneumoniae*, and *Candida albicans*. Some agents that can disrupt biofilm include N-acetylcysteine (NAC), proteolytic enzymes (when taken on an empty stomach), colloidal silver, lactoferrin, and bismuth.

2) REPLACE

This component involves replacing certain factors that play a role in digestion. I'm going to focus on digestive enzymes, betaine HCL, bile salts, and dietary fiber.

Digestive enzymes. These include enzymes to break down protein (proteases), carbohydrates (amylase), and fat (lipase).

What causes a deficiency of digestive enzymes? Some of the different factors that can cause a deficiency of digestive enzymes include damage to the microvilli, stress, nutrient deficiencies, and environmental toxicants.

Signs of a digestive enzyme deficiency: indigestion or a sense of fullness and bloating or flatulence two to four hours after eating a meal.

Plant vs. Animal Sources

Both plant and animal sources of digestive enzymes can be effective, although I usually recommend a non-vegetarian digestive enzyme to my patients that also includes betaine HCL and ox bile. For vegetarian sources, bromelain and papain are two of the more well-known plant-based enzymes, and digestive enzymes can also be derived from microbial sources, such as fungal organisms (e.g., *Aspergillus*). Pancreatin is an example of a digestive enzyme derived from an animal source (e.g., a porcine or bovine pancreas).

What You Need to Know about Hydrochloric Acid (HCL)

Many people have low gastric acid (stomach acid) and can benefit from taking betaine HCL with meals high in protein. Gastric acid consists mostly of hydrochloric acid, which is released from the parietal cells of the stomach. It plays a role in activating pepsinogen into the active enzyme pepsin, which in turn breaks down proteins. In addition, gastric acid has antimicrobial properties that can prevent the development of opportunistic bacteria and certain gut infections as well as SIBO.

What causes hypochlorhydria (low stomach acid)? Some of the different factors that can cause low stomach acid include nutrient deficiencies, hypothyroidism, and intestinal dysbiosis, including SIBO.

Signs of an HCL deficiency: sense of fullness during or after eating, bloating or belching immediately after eating, undigested food in the stool, one or more nutrient deficiencies (especially iron and vitamin B_{12}), and brittle fingernails. Just keep in mind that a mild HCL deficiency might not present with any symptoms.

Note: If taking betaine HCL, please make sure you do so with meals high in protein (at least 10 grams). You also want to start with a low dosage (i.e., one capsule with each meal), and if you experience heartburn or any other type of burning sensation, this is a sign that you are taking too much and should decrease the dosage. For example, if you were taking three capsules of betaine HCL with meals and were doing fine, but upon increasing the dosage to four capsules, you experienced burning, then you should decrease the dosage back to three capsules per meal and stick with this dosage.

One of the reasons why I usually recommend a digestive enzyme that includes betaine HCL is because it usually has lower amounts of betaine HCL when compared to a separate betaine HCL supplement. That means we can start with a lower dose, and then if absolutely necessary have the person take a separate betaine HCL supplement.

Foods That Promote the Production of Gastric Acid

Some foods that can increase gastric acid production include fermented vege-tables (e.g., sauerkraut, kimchi, and pickles), apple cider vinegar, and Swedish bitters. Since stress can reduce stomach acid levels, you might also want to consider doing some deep breathing for a few minutes before your meals.

Taking bitter herbs can also stimulate gastric acid production. Examples of bitter herbs include gentian, ginger, dandelion, and burdock. Whereas you would want to take betaine HCL with meals, if taking bitter herbs you would want to do so ten to fifteen minutes before meals.

Bile salts. Some people can also benefit from supplementing with bile salts, which are involved in fat emulsification. This is especially true for those who have had their gallbladders removed, as getting gallbladder surgery doesn't address the bile metabolism issues commonly associated with these conditions. Some other people can also benefit from taking bile salts, such as those who have problems emulsifying fats. Bile also plays an important role in estrogen metabolism, and, like gastric acid, also has antimicrobial properties. Ox bile can be a good source of purified bile salts.

I should add that a well-known influencer on YouTube mentions how you want to avoid supplementing with bile salts because they help with the conversion of T4 to T3, and he's concerned that taking bile salts can worsen hyperthyroidism. But there is no evidence to support this, and over the years I've had many people with hyperthyroidism supplement with bile salts in the form of ox bile and do fine. That being said, if you happen to supplement with bile salts and feel like it's exacerbating your hyperthyroidism then listen to your body and stop taking them.

Signs of bile insufficiency: the incomplete absorption of fats, which presents as steatorrhea (the excretion of abnormal quantities of fat with the feces); diarrhea is also common.

Foods that Promote Bile Production

Some of the foods that can help with the formation of bile include beets, ginger, radishes, and artichokes.

Dietary fiber. Although dietary fiber doesn't fall under the same category as digestive enzymes, betaine HCL, and bile salts, many people don't consume enough dietary fiber, which is important for many reasons. First, fiber helps to feed the good bacteria in your gut. Having sufficient dietary fiber is also important for having regular bowel movements, which is important for eliminating harmful chemicals from the body.

The Role of Butyrate

Eating a good amount of fiber can lead to higher butyrate levels. Butyrate is a short-chain fatty acid (SCFA) that is produced by the bacterial fermentation of fiber in the colon. Acetate and propionate are two other abundant SCFAs, although butyrate is the preferred energy source for epithelial cells located in the colon. SCFAs have a number of different functions, but one important function is to lower colonic pH, which can inhibit the growth of potential pathogens and at the same time promote the growth of beneficial bacteria, including bifidobacteria and lactobacilli.[25]

SCFAs also have anti-inflammatory effects and play a role in the regulation of immune system function. For example, evidence shows that butyrate can help increase regulatory T cells (Tregs) while decreasing Th17 cells.[26] T17 cells promote autoimmunity, while Tregs help to keep autoimmunity in check. As a result, if you have Graves' disease (or any other autoimmune condition), you want to do things to increase Tregs, while at the same time decreasing Th17 cells.

3) REINOCULATE

Although I commonly recommend probiotic supplements to my patients, it's important to understand that the bacteria in probiotic supplements don't permanently colonize the intestine themselves or modify the overall diversity of the intestinal microbiota.[27] However, studies have shown that taking probiotic supplements can significantly change the types of bacteria and, as a result, can have a significant capacity to remodel the microbiome.[27] In addition, our diet has a direct effect on our microbiome, which is why you want to eat plenty of prebiotic and probiotic sources of food.

While much research has been done involving the use of probiotic supplements, the approach we take now very likely won't be the approach we take in the future. When recommending probiotic supplements, some healthcare professionals recommend formulations with specific, well-researched probiotic strains, while other doctors don't pay as much attention to the specific strains included, but instead focus more on the diversity. In my practice I recommend probiotic supplements with well-researched probiotic strains, although this doesn't mean that I don't consider the diversity of the formulation.

Food sources of prebiotics and probiotics: While it can be beneficial to take a probiotic supplement, you should also eat food sources of probiotics, such as sauerkraut, pickles, kombucha, and even unsweetened coconut yogurt. Some examples of prebiotic foods include Jerusalem artichokes, asparagus, onions, chicory, bananas, and other fruit; even green tea is considered to be a source of prebiotics.[28,29] Prebiotic foods are important because they feed the good bacteria, such as bifidobacteria and lactobacilli, and they're good sources of short-chain fatty acids.

Which Strains of Probiotics Should You Take?

I can't say that I'm an expert on all of the different probiotic strains. However, when I recommend a probiotic supplement to my patients, I recommend probiotics that include well-researched strains, which greatly improve the chances of taking a supplement with therapeutic actions, because specific strains have specific functions. I will briefly mention the benefits of some of the strains I commonly recommend to my patients:

Lactobacillus acidophilus. This is probably the most well-known species, and it is resistant to gastric acid and bile salts, along with pepsin and pancreatin. The strains *Lactobacillus acidophilus* LA-5 and LA-14 have been shown to inhibit certain pathogens.[30,31]

Bifidobacterium lactis. This species produces large amounts of antimicrobial substances. It also modulates the immune system response to help against pathogens. The strains *Bifidobacterium lactis* BB-12 and HN019 are known for their antipathogenic and immune-enhancement effects.[32,33,34]

Lactobacillus casei. This probiotic also improves the health of the immune system, and can be effective against certain microbes such as *H. pylori* [35] and

Candida albicans.[36] Evidence indicates that the strain *Lactobacillus casei* CRL 431 (along with *Lactobacillus rhamnosus* CRL 1224) can be effective against *Aspergillus flavus*,[37] which is a fungus.

Lactobacillus plantarum. A few strains of *Lactobacillus plantarum* have proven to be beneficial. *Lactobacillus plantarum* 299v has been shown to provide effective symptom relief, particularly of abdominal pain and bloating, in patients with irritable bowel syndrome.[38,39] *Lactobacillus plantarum* Lp-115 also can benefit people with gastrointestinal disorders.[40]

Lactobacillus reuteri. In humans, *L. reuteri* is found in different body sites, including the gastrointestinal tract, urinary tract, skin, and breast milk.[41] Due to its antimicrobial activity, *L. reuteri* is able to inhibit the colonization of pathogenic microbes and remodel the commensal microbiota composition in the host. Some strains may reduce the production of pro-inflammatory cytokines while promoting regulatory T cell development and function.[41] *L. reuteri* DSM 17938 has been shown to shorten the duration of acute infectious diarrhea and improves abdominal pain in patients with colitis or inflammatory bowel disease.[42]

Lactobacillus rhamnosus. Numerous studies have shown the benefits of *Lactobacillus rhamnosus* GG in reducing the incidence of ear infections and upper respiratory infections in children[43] and antibiotic-associated diarrhea.[44] One study showed that *Lactobacillus rhamnosus* HN001 (along with *Bifidobacterium longum* BB536) can modulate the gut microbiota, which in turn can cause a significant reduction of potentially harmful bacteria and an increase of beneficial ones.[45] Another study I came across showed that taking *Lactobacillus rhamnosus* HN001 in early pregnancy may reduce the prevalence of gestational diabetes mellitus.[46]

Saccharomyces boulardii. *Saccharomyces boulardii* is a well-researched yeast-based probiotic with many different health benefits. It is well known for helping people who have a candida overgrowth.[47,48] It also can be useful in the maintenance treatment of Crohn's disease.[49] It can help to improve intestinal permeability[50] and help reduce inflammation and dysfunction of the gastrointestinal tract in intestinal mucositis.[51]

Other probiotic strains. Some other beneficial probiotic strains include *Bifidobacterium lactis* Bl-04, *Bifidobacterium longum* Bl-05, *Bifidobacterium bifidum* Bb-06, and *Lactobacillus casei* Lc-11.

What about Spore-Based Probiotics?

Two examples of spore-based probiotics include *Bacillus subtilis* and *Bacillus coagulans*. These are also known as *soil-based probiotics*. These bacterial spores offer the advantage of a higher survival rate during the acidic stomach passage and better stability during the processing and storage of the product.[52] One study involving a spore-based probiotic showed that it could help decrease proinflammatory cytokines and reduce the symptoms associated with a leaky gut.[53] Over the last few years, many healthcare professionals have started recommending spore-based probiotics to their patients with good results.

Should everyone take a probiotic, and if so, which one? I discuss probiotic supplements in the bonus chapter (which you can access in the resources at **savemythyroid.com/HHDNotes**), but I will say here that I usually recommend that my patients take a probiotic supplement with well-researched strains. As of writing this book, I can't say I have everyone specifically take a spore-based probiotic, although over the last few years I have had more people take it, and recently I started taking one as part of my supplement routine.

When choosing a probiotic supplement, keep in mind that you probably won't find one that includes all the strains I mentioned in this chapter, but you might want to consider taking a probiotic that has at least a few of them. I commonly recommend a probiotic supplement called SMT-Probio to my patients, which has a number of the different strains mentioned. If you want to check out all of the specific strains listed (eighteen in total) you can visit **www.ThyroSave.com.**

4) REPAIR

As you know, a leaky gut occurs when the intestinal barrier is compromised. Epithelial tight junctions form a selective permeable seal between the cells of the small intestine. In other words, these tight junctions of the small intestine allow some smaller molecules to pass through, but not other larger molecules. However, certain factors can disrupt these tight junctions, allowing larger proteins and other molecules to pass into the bloodstream, where they normally shouldn't be. Thus, the immune system sees them as being foreign and mounts an immune system response.

For example, the way gluten can cause a leaky gut is by causing a release of zonulin, a molecule that regulates the tight junctions of the small intestine, opening up the tight junctions between cells and allowing larger molecules to pass through into the bloodstream. Infections can also have a similar effect. Because of this, zonulin can be a marker of impaired gut barrier function.

As for how to repair the gut, a lot can be accomplished through diet. The different Hyperthyroid Healing Diets can help with gut healing by eliminating foods that can cause gut inflammation, along with an increase in permeability. In addition to avoiding foods that can have a negative effect on gut healing, certain foods can aid in healing the gut, which I'm about to discuss.

Foods That Can Support Gut Healing

Some of the foods that can help heal the gut include bone broth, fermented foods, and cabbage juice. I'd like to focus on bone broth, as many people are aware of the healing benefits of bone broth. Not only are more and more people drinking bone broth these days, but now people are adding bone broth protein powders to their smoothies.

I can't say that drinking bone broth is required to heal a leaky gut, but it can help because it has multiple gut healing agents, including collagen, glutamine, glycine, and proline. While making your own bone broth is probably the best option, I realize that this is time consuming, and I can't say that I regularly make bone broth. For those who don't have time to make their own bone broth, some companies, including Wise Choice Market and Kettle & Fire, sell premade organic beef bone broth from grass-fed cows.

Nutritional Supplements and Herbs That Can Help with Gut Healing

Some of the nutritional supplements and herbs that can benefit gut healing include L-glutamine, deglycyrrhizinated licorice, slippery elm, marshmallow root, aloe vera leaf, N-Acetylglucosamine, methylsulfonylmethane (MSM), zinc carnosine, and vitamin A. Remember that I have a bonus chapter where I discuss nutritional supplements and herbs that can support different areas of the body, including the gut. So for more information on these, including suggested doses, visit **savemythyroid.com/HHDNotes**.

5) REBALANCE

I'm not going to discuss this component in detail here, as I explain some of these factors in other chapters, mainly chapter 20. However, I do want to briefly discuss the parasympathetic nervous system, as this plays a big role in having optimal digestive health.

The parasympathetic nervous system is one of two branches of the autonomic nervous system, with the other branch being the sympathetic nervous system. The parasympathetic nervous system is also known as the "rest-and-digest system", and it consists of the vagus nerve, which, in turn, innervates most of the tissues involved in nutrient metabolism, including the stomach, pancreas, and liver.[54] Thus, activation of the parasympathetic nervous system will lead to activation of vagal efferent activity, which can influence how nutrients are absorbed and metabolized.[54] In other words, activation of the parasympathetic nervous system can increase the absorption of the nutrients you consume.

How do you activate the parasympathetic nervous system? One of the best ways is by practicing mind-body medicine, which I discussed in chapter 20. This includes meditation, yoga, and biofeedback. For example, evidence shows that yoga can directly stimulate the vagus nerve and enhance parasympathetic output.[55] In the same chapter, I also discuss how heart rate variability could help achieve a state of coherence, which is associated with a relative increase in parasympathetic activity.

Consider Incorporating Vagus Nerve Exercises

Chronic stress can have a negative effect on vagus nerve function. It's also important to mention that stress stimulates the sympathetic nervous system while inhibiting the parasympathetic nervous system. Stress causes a release of corticotrophin-releasing factor, and this can cause an increase in intestinal permeability (a leaky gut) and intestinal dysbiosis.[56] So hopefully you understand how chronic stress can lead to inflammation and affect the health of the gut.

One of the best ways to improve the health of the vagus nerve is to incorporate mind-body medicine. Further, Dr. Datis Kharrazian is the author of the amazing book *Why Isn't My Brain Working?*, and he wrote a blog post that discusses four vagus nerve exercises you can incorporate:

1. **Gargle (2 minutes of vigorous gargling).** Gargling with water a few times per day can activate the vagus nerve. Dr. Kharrazian recommends drinking several large glasses of water per day and gargling each sip until you finish the glass of water.

2. **Stimulate your gag reflex.** Dr. Kharrazian mentions that he has his patients purchase a box of tongue blades so they can stimulate their gag reflex throughout the day. You would just lay the tongue blade on the back of your tongue and push down to activate a gag reflex.

3. **Sing loudly in the shower.** Dr. Kharrazian recommends singing as loudly as you can when you are in the car or at home. I usually do this while taking a cold shower, which also can activate the vagus nerve!

4. **Coffee enemas.** Many people use coffee enemas as a form of detoxification, and I was surprised to learn that coffee enemas can help activate the vagus nerve.

Can You Focus on Multiple Components of the 5-R protocol Simultaneously?

You might wonder if you can address more than one component of the 5-R protocol simultaneously. For example, if someone has a gut infection, is it acceptable to take digestive enzymes and probiotics at the same time the infection is being eradicated, and perhaps even take some gut-healing agents? You can address multiple components simultaneously, and most healthcare professionals do so, including me. In fact, that's the purpose of my Gut Healing Bundle, as this includes a high-quality digestive enzyme, probiotic, and gut healing supplement, and you can learn more about this by visiting **www.GutHealingBundle.com.**

However, there also is nothing wrong with focusing on one *R* at a time. For example, it's perfectly fine to first focus on removing the factor that is causing the leaky gut. After all, you can't fully heal your gut until you address the first *R*, Remove. Then, once this has been accomplished, you can focus on the other components.

I will add that if you focus on the Remove component first, after you remove the factor that caused the leaky gut, you then might want to focus on the other components simultaneously. In other words, you might want to initially focus on removing the factor that caused the leaky gut, and then take measures to replace, reinoculate, repair, and rebalance the body.

Beyond the 5-R Protocol

I've heard some healthcare practitioners mention how incorporating the 5-R protocol isn't always sufficient when restoring the health of the gut microbiome. Some will say that you need to do other things first, such as support the liver and lymphatics. The truth is that when it comes to optimizing your gut health, most people will get great results following the 5-R protocol alone, but it is true that some people need to do other things to improve their health.

The biggest challenge for many is the first component of the 5-R protocol (Remove). Sometimes someone has to simply remove a food allergen (i.e., gluten) or take natural or prescription antimicrobials to eradicate gut microbes (i.e., *H. pylori*, parasites, SIBO). But it can be more complex than this at times. For example, someone might have a toxic mold problem resulting in small intestinal fungal overgrowth (SIFO), and while taking anti-fungal herbs in this situation might help to some extent, ultimately the source of the mold needs to be addressed.

Chapter 21 Highlights

- Having a healthy gut is important with any health condition, including hyperthyroidism.
- A leaky gut involves damage to the enterocytes (cells of the small intestine) and is part of the triad of autoimmunity.
- When it comes to having a healthy gut, you want to focus on the components of the 5-R protocol: (1) Remove, (2) Replace, (3) Reinoculate, (4) Repair, (5) Rebalance.
- The Remove component is perhaps the most important one of the 5-R protocol, as it involves removing anything that will disrupt the gut, including food allergens, infections, and even certain medications.
- It's important to understand that there is no perfect method of testing for gut microbes, and false negatives are possible.
- You also want to replace certain factors that play a role in digestion, including digestive enzymes, low stomach acid, and bile salts.
- SCFAs such as butyrate have anti-inflammatory effects and play a role in the regulation of immune system function.
- While it can be beneficial to take a probiotic supplement, you should also eat food sources of probiotics, such as sauerkraut, pickles, kombucha, and even unsweetened coconut yogurt.
- As for how to repair the gut, a lot can be accomplished through diet, although there is a time and place for nutritional supplements and herbs.
- Activation of the parasympathetic nervous system can increase the absorption of the nutrients you consume.
- When it comes to optimizing your gut health, most people will get great results following the 5-R protocol alone, although some people need to do other things to improve their health.

To access the book references and resources, visit
SaveMyThyroid.com/HHDNotes.

CHAPTER
22

Improve Sleep Quality and Duration

Many people with hyperthyroidism experience sleep issues. This shouldn't be surprising, as a lot of people with this condition have anxiety, which certainly can have a negative effect on sleep. Heart palpitations are also common, and they are frequently more noticeable during the night. (This definitely was the case with me when I dealt with Graves' disease.) There can also be other factors that can make falling and/or staying asleep challenging, which I will discuss in this chapter.

I'd like to start by discussing why it's important to get sufficient sleep. Yes, I'm sure you know that sleep is important so that we feel refreshed upon waking up. Sleep is important for the ability to think clearly and be alert, and getting proper sleep also enhances memory. Inadequate sleep can not only affect our cognition and memory but also decrease our stress handling abilities.

In fact, I came across a journal article that discussed a study where mood was observed following varying degrees of sleep deprivation.[1] The study found that people who were sleep-deprived responded to low stressors similar to how people without any sleep deprivation responded to high stressors. I already discussed the importance of stress management in chapter 20, and there is no question that getting quality sleep plays an important role in this.

Sleep and Immunity

Sleep is also important for optimal adrenal and immune health. One of the main reasons why many people have "compromised" adrenals is because they don't get enough sleep. And having a healthy immune system is dependent on the circadian rhythms and getting sufficient sleep. Not only does immune system activation alter sleep, but sleep in turn affects the innate and adaptive arm of our body's defense system.[2]

In chapter 21 I mentioned how autoimmunity is characterized by an increase in Th17 cells and a decrease in regulatory T cells (Tregs), and I came across a study that showed that chronic obstructive sleep apnea is also associated with an increase in Th17 cells and a decrease in Tregs.[3] I realize this is an extreme example, as not everyone who has sleep issues has obstructive sleep apnea, but I just wanted to demonstrate how certain sleep disorders can impact the immune system.

Sleep and Cardiovascular Health

A number of observational studies have demonstrated an association between insomnia and incident cardiovascular disease morbidity and mortality, including hypertension, coronary heart disease, and heart failure.[4] It's also important to mention that the increased risk isn't just associated with insomnia, but short sleep duration as well.

During my research I came across an interesting, albeit older journal article (from 1983), that looked at the mortality risk associated with different sleeping patterns.[5] This was assessed by use of the 1965 Human Population Laboratory survey of a random sample of 6,928 adults in Alameda County,

CA, and a subsequent nine-year mortality follow-up. The analysis indicated that mortality rates from ischemic heart disease, cancer, stroke, and all causes combined were lowest for individuals sleeping seven or eight hours per night. Men sleeping six hours or less or nine hours or more had 1.7 times the total age-adjusted death rate of men sleeping seven or eight hours per night.

How Much Sleep Should *You* Get?

Based on what I just mentioned, you probably don't want to average less than six hours of sleep per night. But I would aim for at least seven hours per night, and eight hours would be even better. And remember that this doesn't include the time it takes for you to fall asleep. For example, if you're aiming for eight hours of sleep but it takes you thirty minutes to fall asleep, then you'd want to be in bed for a total of eight and a half hours.

I should mention that some evidence shows that some people have genetic variations that allow them to do fine on a shorter night's sleep.[6] According to the research, the most well-known genes triggering shortening of sleep duration or sleep need, if mutated, are DEC2, NPSR1, mGluR1, and β1-AR genes.[6] So while many people do need to get seven to eight hours in order to avoid suffering from daytime sleepiness, this doesn't describe everyone.

The Dangers of Sleep Medication

Unfortunately, many people resort to sleep medication, and it's hard to blame someone who is only getting a few hours of sleep each night, or perhaps not getting any sleep at all. The problem is that people can become dependent on these medications, and the effectiveness of certain sleep medications can decrease over time. This may lead to the person taking a higher dose of the medication, or they might switch to a different medication altogether.

Are Nutritional Supplements and Herbs a Solution?

Although I do recommend supplements to some of my patients with sleep difficulties, there are a few things you need to keep in mind. First of all, taking supplements doesn't always help, and part of the reason for this is that not all supplements work the same way. For example, if someone is having difficulty falling asleep because they have low melatonin levels, then it makes sense that taking a melatonin supplement may help. But if a melatonin deficiency isn't the problem, then chances are taking melatonin won't have any impact.

We also need to consider the dosing of these supplements. Staying on the topic of melatonin, many people who take melatonin will start with 3 to 5 mg per day, and one of the main reasons for this is that many supplements have melatonin in this dosage. But for those who truly need melatonin, many times 1 mg or less is needed.

Finally, while supplements and herbs can be helpful at times, they shouldn't be seen as a long-term solution to the sleep issue. The goal should be to correct certain underlying imbalances so that eventually the person will be able to sleep without taking supplements. I realize that sometimes this is easier said than done, and I don't suggest that you abruptly stop taking any supplements that might be helping with sleep, as it very well might be a gradual process.

Can Cognitive Behavioral Therapy (CBT) Help?

Cognitive behavioral therapy (CBT) refers to a class of interventions that share the basic premise that mental disorders and psychological distress are maintained by cognitive factors.[7] The strongest support exists for CBT of anxiety disorders, somatoform disorders, bulimia, anger-control problems, and general stress.[8] But there is also evidence that it can help with some cases of insomnia. CBT for insomnia (CBTi) encompasses sleep hygiene, stimulus control, sleep restriction, cognitive therapy, and relaxation training.[9]

A meta-analysis looked to determine the efficacy of CBT on diary measures of overnight sleep in adults with chronic insomnia, and the authors concluded that CBT is an effective treatment for adults with chronic insomnia.[10] Another meta-analysis demonstrated that CBT produces clinically significant effects that last up to a year after therapy.[11] Another study showed that CBT is a safe and highly effective treatment for insomnia, but it is underutilized primarily because (1) there is a shortage of trained CBT practitioners, and (2) people with insomnia are much more likely to choose medication as a treatment.[12]

Focus on Lowering Your Thyroid Hormones

Although I'm about to discuss different things you can do to improve sleep quality and duration, briefly followed by supplements that may help with sleep, if you developed sleep issues around the time that you started experiencing your hyperthyroid symptoms, then lowering the thyroid hormones very well might be the solution. Initially this might be addressed by taking antithyroid medication such as methimazole, or natural antithyroid agents such as bugleweed or higher doses of L-carnitine. But of course the long-term goal should be to address the underlying cause of the hyperthyroid condition so that you won't have to rely on taking medication or supplements to keep your thyroid hormones in a healthy range.

12 Things to Improve Sleep Quality and Duration without Supplements

If lowering your thyroid hormones doesn't help with your sleep issues, then there most likely are one or more other factors that need to be addressed. While nutritional supplements and herbs can sometimes be helpful for sleep, I first wanted to discuss twelve things you can do to improve sleep quality and duration without relying on supplements. You won't necessarily have to incorporate all of these, but there is always the chance that multiple factors are preventing you from getting quality sleep.

1. **Balance your blood sugar.** This is one of the main reasons people wake up in the middle of the night and have difficulty falling back asleep. Incorporating the Hyperthyroid Healing Diet strategies should greatly help, although if you have a condition such as insulin resistance, then you might need to do more than change your diet. Refer back to chapter 14 where I discuss blood sugar imbalances in greater detail.

2. **Incorporate stress management daily.** Cortisol imbalances can cause problems with falling and/or staying asleep. While elevated cortisol is frequently the culprit, depressed cortisol levels can also be a factor. Even though stress management alone might not be the solution to everyone's sleep issues, in many cases it's an important piece of the puzzle. Refer back to chapter 20, where I discuss stress-management strategies in greater detail.

3. **Reduce inflammation in your body.** Studies show that sleep disturbance and long sleep duration, but not short sleep duration, are associated with increases in markers of systemic inflammation.[13] So if you have an elevated C-reactive protein (CRP), which is an inflammatory marker that can be measured in the blood, it can be related to your sleep issues. Just keep in mind that a negative CRP doesn't rule out inflammation.

4. **Decrease consumption of caffeine, alcohol, and/or nicotine.** If you drink coffee, alcohol, and/or consume nicotine, then any or all of these can interfere with sleep.

5. **Be active throughout the day.** While regular exercise is important, there are many people who exercise three to five days per week yet aren't too active in between exercise sessions. And when I say *active*, I mean that you want movement to be a part of your daily routine. I realize this can be challenging for someone who works a desk job, and if this is the case with you I would try to take frequent breaks. Perhaps you can take a walk during lunch, etc., and when you're not at work try not to be a couch potato!

6. **Avoid blue light an hour or two before going to bed.** Being exposed to blue light right before going to bed can interfere with sleep by having a negative effect on the circadian rhythm. Common sources of blue light include fluorescent and LED lights, smart phones, televisions, and computers. Ideally you should avoid blue light an hour or two before going to bed, which means saying no to being on your computer or smart phone, watching television, etc.

7. **Turn down the temperature before going to bed.** Try turning down the temperature to between sixty-five and sixty-eight degrees, as many people sleep better with a cooler temperature.

8. **Make sure your bedroom is completely dark.** You want higher melatonin levels when going to bed, and melatonin production is optimal when it's completely dark. If for any reason you can't make the room completely dark (i.e., with blackout curtains), then wear an eye mask when going to bed.

9. **Use an air purification system.** The research shows that air pollution concentration is negatively associated with sleep duration.[14] So having an air purifier in your bedroom might help with sleep duration by improving the air quality.

10. **Get a new mattress.** I wouldn't say that this is a priority, but as you know, most people spend at least one quarter to one third of their life in their bed, so I think purchasing a good-quality, non-toxic mattress is a great investment. If you recently purchased a mattress I'm not suggesting that you ditch your mattress for a new one, but the next time you're searching for a mattress, then perhaps you can consider a non-toxic one. If you want to know the mattress that I sleep on, I'll include the brand in the resources at **savemythyroid.com/HHDNotes**, along with a few other non-toxic mattresses you can consider.

11. **Reduce exposure to EMFs in your bedroom.** All electronic devices emit EMFs, and while this might not be the reason for your sleep issues, this is definitely one of the most overlooked causes. Ideally you should not have any electronics in your room, including but not limited to a television, DVR, computer, etc. The next best thing would be to unplug these devices when going to bed.

    Also, I would try not to be on electronic devices (i.e., cell phone, laptop) one to two hours before going to bed. I admit that sometimes I'm on electronic devices close to my bedtime, but one thing I almost always do before going to bed is unplug the Wi-Fi at night (or have my daughter do it). Finally, if you use your cell phone as an alarm clock, make sure it's at least six feet away from you during the night, and on airplane mode.

12. **Clear your mind.** A big reason why many people can't fall asleep and/ or why they wake up in the middle of the night and have a difficult time falling back asleep is that they are unable to clear their mind. My guess is that this happens to all of us at times in our lives, as there certainly have been times when I had a lot on mind and it affected my sleep. And it doesn't necessarily have to be negative thoughts, as for example, you might simply have a project for work that needs to get done sooner than later, and you don't know how in the world you're going to accomplish this. I find that expressing gratitude before going to bed can greatly help, and when other thoughts creep into your mind in the middle of the night try to think about those things you are grateful for.

Nutritional Supplements and Herbs That Can Support Sleep

As I mentioned earlier, you don't want to rely on supplements. And before you take supplements I would recommend incorporating the changes I mentioned earlier. That being said, if you need to take nutritional supplements or herbs, that's fine. Just make sure they are of good quality, and have the mindset that you're only going to take them on a temporary basis.

Some of the nutritional supplements and herbs that can support sleep include melatonin, magnesium, L-theanine, 5-HTP, GABA, valerian root, kava, and CBD oil. Remember that I have a bonus chapter where I discuss nutritional supplements and herbs that can support different areas of the body, including sleep. For more information on these, including suggested doses, visit **savemythyroid.com/HHDNotes.**

In summary, sleep issues are common in those with hyperthyroidism. While the elevated thyroid hormones themselves can be a factor, causing anxiety, palpitations, and other symptoms, there can also be other reasons why someone has a difficult time falling and/or staying asleep. While there is a time and place for sleep medication, most people who struggle with sleep can eventually improve both sleep quality and duration by addressing the underlying causes, and at times taking nutritional supplements or herbs on a temporary basis.

Chapter 22 Highlights

- Many people with hyperthyroidism experience sleep issues, which can relate to anxiety, heart palpitations, or other factors.
- Sleep is important for optimal adrenal and immune health.
- I would aim for at least seven hours of sleep each night, and eight hours would be even better.
- While there is a time and place for sleep medication, the problem is that many people become dependent on it.
- If you developed sleep issues around the time that you started experiencing your hyperthyroid symptoms, then lowering the thyroid hormones very well might be the solution.
- Some things you can do to improve sleep quality and duration include lowering thyroid hormones, balancing your blood sugar levels, incorporating stress management daily, reducing inflammation, being active throughout the day, avoiding blue light before going to bed, and making sure your bedroom is completely dark.
- Some supplements that may help with sleep include melatonin, magnesium, L-theanine, 5-HTP, GABA, valerian root, and CBD oil.

To access the book references and resources, visit
SaveMyThyroid.com/HHDNotes.

CHAPTER
23

Exercise and Hyperthyroidism

W

e all know how important it is to exercise. But it can be challenging to stay active when dealing with hyperthyroidism, especially when it's moderate to severe. Before I was diagnosed with hyperthyroidism I was a regular visitor to the gym, working out three to five times per week. After I was diagnosed with hyperthyroidism, it was bad enough that I had to make extreme changes to my diet, so the last thing I wanted to do was stop going to the gym.

And, no, I'm not going to tell you to stop exercising. That being said, for many people with hyperthyroidism, it's important not to exercise vigorously for a couple of reasons. First of all, many people with hyperthyroidism have an elevated resting heart rate, and it's not uncommon for people's resting heart rate to exceed 100 BPM when dealing with this condition. A second reason is because many people with hyperthyroidism (as well as other health conditions) have compromised adrenals, and ideally you want to optimize your adrenal health before you go all out.

Regular Exercise vs. Regular Movement

I'll talk more about what type of exercise I recommend shortly, but I first want to encourage everyone with hyperthyroidism to be active on a consistent basis. While it's great to block out sixty to ninety minutes a few days per week to exercise, it is just as important, if not more important, to incorporate regular movement on a daily basis. In other words, ideally you don't want to have periods where you're sitting for two to four hours consecutively.

Obviously this can be challenging when someone is working behind a desk all day. And what frequently happens is that the person who spends eight hours behind a desk comes home and does some more sitting. After a long day at work they may feel the need to relax on the couch watching television or sit at their desk at home while surfing the Internet. I'm not discouraging anyone from getting some rest and relaxation after working a long day, but if you work behind a desk, try to take frequent breaks, and perhaps even go for a walk during your lunch break.

If you work from home, it can be easier to incorporate regular movement. For example, at my home I have a treadmill desk, so I routinely walk at a slow pace on the treadmill while working on my computer. Another option is to invest in a standing desk. Both of these are better options than sitting throughout the day.

Should You Count Your Daily Steps?

These days it's common for people to use different devices to track how many steps they take in a day. Although my wife and older daughter do this, as of writing this book I can't say I do. But if you need this for motivation, then go for it! And it's not just for motivation, as I think it's great to set physical goals.

As for how many steps you should aim for in a day, the most common number people seem to aim for is 10,000. Some people will even have contests to see who can accomplish the most steps in a single day. Overall, I think this is a great way to make sure you're getting regular movement on a daily basis, but many people with hyperthyroidism need to be cautious about not overdoing it.

Once again, most people with hyperthyroidism can do some light walking. But everyone is different, and you need to listen to your body. You also need to remember that you might not be able to do what you were able to in the past . . . at least not at this point. For example, you might have been fine with 10,000 steps per day or more prior to being diagnosed with hyperthyroidism, but if this currently causes shortness of breath or other symptoms, then scale back to 5,000 or 7,500 steps per day for now.

I realize it's frustrating to not be able to do what you were once able to do with ease. But you'll eventually get back to where you were from an exercise standpoint. And if you weren't exercising prior to your hyperthyroidism diagnosis, I encourage you to start slow and not overexert yourself, and perhaps even hire a certified personal trainer for a few sessions.

Overtraining and Hyperthyroidism

I briefly mentioned earlier in this book that I overtrained prior to the development of my Graves' disease condition. When we think of stress, many people think of emotional stressors. But physical stressors can play a big role as well, and overtraining can put a great deal of stress on the body and affect the adrenals in a similar way as emotional stress. So while I'm sure that emotional stress played a role in my Graves' disease condition, I'm pretty confident that overtraining was also a contributing factor.

But it's not just the adrenals that overtraining affects. Overtraining causes an increase in oxidative stress, which can cause a lot of harm. I discuss oxidative stress in more detail in chapter 25. While a small amount of oxidative stress is fine, too much oxidative stress can cause mitochondrial dysfunction, decrease immune function, and even have a negative effect on cardiovascular health. So you want to try to do things to reduce the oxidative stress in your body.

One question you may have is whether or not I knew I was overtraining at the time, and the answer is no. Of course I knew I was exercising intensely, but overtraining didn't come to my mind at all. But when I look back, there is no doubt that this was the case. I bring this up because I'm sure there are some people reading this book who are currently overtraining as well and are not aware of it. Obviously this is subjective, as there is no test that can tell you if you are overtraining.

Signs That You're Overtraining

There can be a few signs and symptoms of overtraining. First of all, if right after the workout you're exhausted, then this is a pretty good sign. Obviously you're not going to have the same amount of energy that you had prior to working out, but you shouldn't feel the need to sit or lie down for a long period of time.

Other signs/symptoms include unusual muscle soreness, delays in recovering, prolonged general fatigue, and/or poor quality sleep. If you're a cycling woman, then it can also lead to irregular menstrual cycles, although hyperthyroidism itself can cause this as well.

3 Types of Exercises (And Which Ones You Should Do)

I just want to remind you that before starting any new exercise program it's wise to consult with a healthcare practitioner and get the proper clearance. I can't say that there are zero risks when exercising with hyperthyroidism, even when incorporating milder types. But this is why it's important to do things to safely manage the symptoms while addressing the underlying cause.

Let's go ahead and take a look at the three different types of exercises:

1. **Resistance training.** This is the most important type of exercise to help build muscle mass and increase bone density, both of which are negatively affected in hyperthyroidism. When I discuss resistance training, I'm not suggesting that you should do heavy weight lifting, and you don't even need to use weights at all if you don't want to, although this certainly is an option. Either way, you definitely don't want to overdo it.

It's important for me to remind you that you should do things to lower the thyroid hormones while doing weight-bearing exercises. And I'm guessing you'll also be doing things to address the cause of the hyperthyroidism, which is what this book is all about (along with my first book, *Natural Treatment Solutions for Hyperthyroidism and Graves' Disease*). In some cases when the hyperthyroidism is severe, it might be best to get the thyroid hormones under control before you start engaging in weight-bearing exercise.

What Type of Weight-Bearing Exercise Should You Do?

The purpose of this book isn't to give you an exercise routine to follow, and to be honest, this will vary depending on the person. Some people might choose to use weights, some might use resistance bands, and others will rely on their own body weight (i.e., pushups, lunges). If you haven't exercised in quite awhile, I would recommend starting slow, and you might even want to hire a personal trainer, even if it's just for a session or two. A big reason for this is to make sure you have the proper form so you don't injure yourself. It's not always easy to do this when viewing photos, or even when watching videos.

2. **Continuous aerobic exercise.** It's tough to be an avid runner or cyclist and then be told that you have to take a break from these activities. And while I'd love to say that those who are engaging in moderate or vigorous

aerobic exercise can keep this up without any risks, I'd be lying if I told you this. Of course everything comes down to risks vs. benefits, and you might argue that the risks of being sedentary are greater than the risks of exercising when dealing with hyperthyroidism. This may be true, but I'm not asking you to be sedentary. I'm just recommending that you slow down temporarily.

I know this is difficult for many people to do, as when I was diagnosed with hyperthyroidism I had been in an exercise routine for many years. Moderate to vigorous aerobic exercise was a big part of my exercise routine, so the last thing I wanted to do was slow down. But I did take this approach, and while it was frustrating, I'm glad I didn't push my body too hard while I was recovering.

So what type of continuous aerobic exercise should you do? Initially I would limit it to walking. And I'm not talking about taking a brisk walk, but just walking at a normal pace. I realize that some will be fine with this, but others can't imagine not going for their morning run. Once again, this is only temporary, and it won't be too long before you are able to get back into your old routine again.

You might wonder if it's okay to engage in other types of aerobic exercise, such as swimming. Swimming offers some wonderful health benefits, but I would still be cautious about doing anything that greatly increases your heart rate. That being said, if you're effectively managing your hyperthyroid symptoms, then you probably can engage in some swimming, but I just would make sure not to overdo it, and to listen to your body. Of course, always check with your doctor first before engaging in any type of exercise.

3. **High-intensity interval training.** There is no question that high-intensity interval training (HIIT) has numerous health benefits, and I recommend it for those who are in an optimal state of health. Unfortunately, this doesn't

describe most people reading this book. And when I say this, I realize that there are people with hyperthyroidism who have lived a healthy lifestyle and are absolutely shocked that they developed hyperthyroidism.

Even if this is true, you need to evaluate your current situation and understand that although you might be healthier than friends and family members who aren't dealing with hyperthyroidism, this is a time for healing. I'm not suggesting that everyone with hyperthyroidism is in a poor state of health. I'm just saying that at this time, your health is less than optimal, so if you enjoy HIIT I would take a break from it and understand that I encourage you to get back to doing this in the future. If anything, use this as a motivator to get your health back.

Decreased Muscle Mass and Hyperthyroidism

I mentioned earlier in this chapter how it's very common for people with hyperthyroidism to have a decrease in muscle mass. Not that you need any test to let you know that you're losing muscle mass, but the creatinine on a comprehensive metabolic panel is a marker that can be associated with decreased muscle mass. It's commonly low in those with hyperthyroidism. However, it's not a specific marker for muscle mass, and in fact, if it is elevated it can be an indication of chronic kidney disease (along with a low eGFR).

Anyway, while exercise can of course help to increase muscle mass, you also need to address the hyperthyroidism. If the thyroid hormone levels remain elevated, you probably won't see the muscle mass increase much, if at all, even if you are exercising regularly. So while I do recommend you do weight-bearing exercises to increase muscle mass, you also want to do everything you can to get those thyroid hormone levels within a healthy range. You might need to take antithyroid medication or an herb such as bugleweed on a temporary basis, and hopefully if you do this you'll also try to address the underlying cause.

I also need to remind you that in order to increase muscle mass, you need to eat sufficient protein. I discussed this in chapter 4, as ideally you want to eat at least 75 percent of your ideal body weight in protein. And remember that there is a difference between the bioavailability of animal vs. plant-based protein sources. I even came across a study that showed that plant protein is associated with a lower bone mineral density when compared to animal protein.[1] Since hyperthyroidism can have a negative effect on bone mineral density, this is a good reason to consider eating animal protein if you don't do so already, although I completely understand those who are a vegan or vegetarian due to ethical reasons.

Subclinical Hyperthyroidism and Exercise

If you have subclinical hyperthyroidism (low TSH with normal thyroid hormone levels) you might be wondering if you can engage in more vigorous exercise. If you have normal thyroid hormone levels, chances are you don't have an elevated resting heart rate. If you do then it might be related to something else. Either way, whether or not you can participate in more intense exercise really depends on the health of your adrenals.

What I would suggest is to first test your adrenals. I wouldn't rely on a blood test that just measures the morning serum cortisol, but instead I would recommend either doing an adrenal saliva test or a dried urine test such as the DUTCH, as both of these look at the circadian rhythm of cortisol, along with DHEA. If you have subclinical hyperthyroidism and your adrenals are in good shape, then perhaps you can exercise more vigorously. If not, you would want to work on improving your adrenal health first.

When Can You Start Your "Old" Exercise Routine?

So just to summarize, if you have elevated thyroid hormone levels along with tachycardia (resting heart rate >100 BPM), then you want to address this first before you can exercise more vigorously. But even if your thyroid hormone levels are within the optimal reference range, you want to make sure your adrenals aren't compromised. And if they are, you want to work on improving their health.

Quite frankly, even if your adrenals are in a good state of health, I would avoid vigorous aerobic exercise and high-intensity interval training until your thyroid hormone levels are within the optimal reference range without relying on antithyroid medication or natural antithyroid agents such as bugleweed. This doesn't mean you can't increase the intensity if your thyroid hormones are within the optimal reference range while taking medication or herbs. But ideally I wouldn't go all out until you're off antithyroid medication and/ or natural antithyroid agents and your adrenals are looking good on a saliva test or dried urine test.

Don't Have the Time to Lift?

For those who would like to incorporate some resistance training but don't have the time to do so, I came across a very interesting journal article entitled "No Time to Lift? Designing Time-Efficient Training Programs for Strength and Hypertrophy: A Narrative Review".[2]

The goal of the review was to determine how strength training can be carried out in a time-efficient manner. Essentially the authors concluded that weekly training volume is more important than training frequency, and they recommend performing a minimum of four weekly sets per muscle group, ideally using six to fifteen repetitions. In other words, you don't have to work out two to three days per week to benefit from exercise. In addition, they mention how stretching prior to resistance exercise is optional, and should only be prioritized if one of the goals is to increase flexibility.

In the journal article, the authors discussed a few studies that showed that you can achieve similar training effects by training once a week compared to a higher frequency (i.e., three days per week), as long as total weekly volume is equated. For example, they mentioned that a meta-analysis from 2018 compared strength gains from low training frequency (one day per week), medium training frequency (two days per week), and high training frequency (>three days per week) for each muscle group, and the authors reported only minimal greater increases in strength gains from higher frequencies. In addition, when training volume was matched (i.e., total number of repetitions), no significant effect of training frequency was observed for strength gains.

This isn't to suggest that there is no benefit to working out multiple times per week, as I still do this. But the main point I want to make is if you only have time to do resistance training once per week, you can still benefit from it. One more thing I'll mention that the authors brought up is *micro dosing*, where someone can work out multiple times per week but in very-short-duration sessions (i.e., fifteen minutes), as this can also be of benefit.

There is more to the journal article, so if this interests you then of course feel free to read it in its entirety. I just wanted to encourage you to do some resistance exercise, even if you don't have a lot of time. Whether you do a single 45-minute to one hour session per week, or three 15-minute sessions per week, you will gain some benefits, which is very important for those dealing with hyperthyroidism.

People with Hyperthyroidism Have a Lower VO_2 Max

One of the ways to determine how physically fit you are is by measuring your VO_2 max, which is the volume of oxygen that can be consumed while exercising at maximum capacity. The average sedentary male achieves a VO_2 max of about 35 to 40 mL/kg/min, and the average sedentary female scores approximately 27 to 30 mL/kg/min.[3] On the other hand, elite male runners have shown VO_2 maxes of up to 85 mL/kg/min, while elite female runners have scored up to 77 mL/kg/min.[3] One study I came across showed that VO_2

was lower in those with hyperthyroidism, although there was an appreciable improvement of exertion capacity after only thirty days.[4]

I wouldn't worry about measuring your VO_2 max at this time, as this usually is done by hooking up to a mask and heart rate monitor while running on a treadmill or riding a bike. The mask is connected to a device that measures the volume of oxygen you inhale and the amount of air you exhale. It can be challenging to check this on your own, and even if it is on the low side, this very well might be related to the hyperthyroidism, and not necessarily your level of fitness.

In summary, for those who were in the routine of exercising regularly prior to developing hyperthyroidism, it can be frustrating and discouraging to scale back. While you want to be cautious about engaging in high-intensity exercise, you still want to be somewhat active, and because many people with hyperthyroidism have a decrease in muscle mass and bone density, it's a good idea to do some resistance training. Once you have restored your health, you should be able to go back to your old exercise routine, although you want to make sure not to overtrain, as this puts a lot of stress on your body and in some cases can cause a relapse.

Chapter 23 Highlights

- It can be challenging to stay active when dealing with hyperthyroidism, especially when it's moderate to severe.
- That being said, I encourage everyone with hyperthyroidism to be active on a consistent basis.
- Overtraining can put a great deal of stress on the body, causing an increase in oxidative stress.
- Resistance training is the most important type of exercise to help build muscle mass and increase bone density, both of which are negatively affected in hyperthyroidism.
- Light walking is fine for most people with hyperthyroidism, and if you're effectively managing your hyperthyroid symptoms, then you probably can engage in some swimming.
- While exercise can help to increase muscle mass, you also need to address the hyperthyroidism.
- I would avoid vigorous aerobic exercise and high-intensity interval training until your thyroid hormone levels are within the optimal reference range without relying on antithyroid medication or natural antithyroid agents such as bugleweed.

To access the book references and resources, visit
SaveMyThyroid.com/HHDNotes.

CHAPTER
24

Reducing Your Toxic Burden

his is yet another chapter I could easily write an entire book on. It's no secret that we live in a toxic world, and there are basically two perspectives you can take. The first is to think that no matter what we do, there is no possible way to completely eliminate our exposure to these environmental toxicants, so what's the use of trying to reduce our toxic load? The second perspective is that while we can't completely eliminate our exposure, the lower the toxic load we have, the better.

It shouldn't surprise you that I choose the second perspective . . . even though I feel pretty good from a symptomatic standpoint. I say this because there are people who are highly sensitive to smoke, perfumes, fragrances, cleaning products, gasoline, etc. Of course, in this situation it makes perfect sense to do everything you can to reduce your exposure to these and other chemicals and environmental pollutants. But when someone doesn't feel any different when exposed to these toxicants, or when they do things to reduce their toxic load, then it can be more difficult to justify why such a person needs to reduce their toxic load.

When It Comes to Eliminating Toxins, Everyone Is Different

No two people are exactly the same when it comes to eliminating toxins. For example, two people can be exposed to the same toxic environment at home or at work, and one might be efficient at eliminating toxins from their body, while the other person might not be as efficient. As a result, the first person might feel perfectly fine, while the other person might experience a lot of symptoms.

One reason is related to certain genetic polymorphisms. I won't get into great detail about genetic polymorphisms in this book, but these are essentially common genetic variations. They can affect different areas of the body, including how we detoxify. For example, I have an MTHFR homozygous C677T polymorphism, which affects the phase 2 detoxification pathway known as *methylation*.

The bad news is that there is no way to reverse these and other genetic polymorphisms. But the good news is that you can still do things to support detoxification. While I don't require all of my patients to do a genetic panel as of writing this book, I will admit that this can come in handy when determining if someone needs additional nutritional support. For my MTHFR polymorphism, I take a methylation supplement that has certain nutrients to support this detoxification pathway.

Toxin vs. Toxicant

Although I and many other healthcare practitioners are guilty of using the word *toxin* when describing environmental chemicals, the correct term is really *toxicant*. Toxins are natural products. Examples include the ones found in poisonous mushrooms or snakes' venom. On the other hand, toxicants are man-made products that are introduced into the environment. So for example, pesticides are actually considered to be *environmental toxicants*, not *environmental toxins*.

In the past I exclusively used the term *environmental toxin* because I didn't know better. These days I still commonly use this term, but in many cases I should be using the word *toxicant*. In this book I use the terms interchangeably.

Can a Hyperthyroid Healing Diet Help Reduce Your Toxic Load?

There is no question that diet plays a key role in the detoxification process. In fact, although many people take nutritional supplements and herbs to support detoxification, you want to do as much as you can through the food you eat. The reason for this is that detoxification is a nutrient-dependent process. In other words, if you have one or more nutrient deficiencies, which is quite common, this will reduce your ability to biotransform and eliminate toxicants you're exposed to.

A Breakdown of Common Environmental Toxicants

There's no possible way I can discuss all of the different chemicals in a single chapter . . . not even the most common ones, so this isn't all-inclusive. However, the good news is that many of the detox strategies I'll discuss later in this chapter will help with most of the different types of environmental toxicants, not just the ones I mention in this chapter. Whenever I can, I will try to link the environmental toxicant to its effect on thyroid and/or immune system health, based on what I find in the research.

Heavy metals. Heavy metals are elements found in nature that accumulate in the environment, and we are usually exposed to them either through food we consume (i.e., seafood) or occupational exposure. They can contaminate the air and water and can be toxic even at very low concentrations. Some of the more concerning toxic metals include aluminum, arsenic, cadmium, lead, and mercury.

A few studies have shown evidence of a link between mercury exposure and thyroid autoimmunity, along with other autoimmune conditions.[1,2] Even though mercury can potentially trigger autoimmunity, the organ most affected by this heavy metal is the brain. Evidence indicates that mercury from dental amalgam fillings may contribute to the body burden of mercury in the brain.[3]

Although I didn't find any research that showed a link between aluminum exposure and hyperthyroidism, keep in mind that aluminum is a demonstrated neurotoxin and a strong immune stimulator.[4] This is why aluminum is commonly added to vaccines as an adjuvant.

A few studies have shown that cadmium exposure can cause thyroid dysfunction.[5,6] Just as mercury can potentially trigger autoimmunity, the same might be true of cadmium.[7] While lead might play a role in autoimmunity,[8] I wasn't able to find any correlation in the research between lead and hyperthyroidism, and the same is true with arsenic, as I couldn't find any evidence of a relationship between arsenic and hyperthyroidism.

Bisphenol A (BPA). Bisphenol A (BPA) is a chemical commonly found in plastic water bottles, but there are many other sources as well, including food packaging, dental materials, healthcare equipment, and thermal paper (i.e., receipts), as well as toys and articles for children and infants.[9] Due to its phenolic structure BPA has been shown to interact with estrogen receptors, and thus can play a role in the pathogenesis of numerous endocrine conditions, including male and female infertility, hormone dependent tumors (i.e., breast and prostate cancer), polycystic ovarian syndrome (PCOS), and other metabolic conditions.[9] This is why it is labeled as an *endocrine-disrupting chemical.*

Since 1997 there have been thousands of studies that have reported adverse effects in animals administered low doses of BPA.[10] BPA fits within the binding pockets of both estrogen receptor (ER)α and ERβ.[11] BPA is an antagonist of the thyroid hormone receptor, interfering with the normal binding of T3.[12,13]

There are numerous structural analogs to BPA, including bisphenol B (BPB), bisphenol E (BPE), bisphenol F (BPF), and bisphenol S (BPS).[14] Many people realize that there are risks associated with BPA, and as a result they use BPA-free products (i.e., BPA-free plastic water bottles). However, studies show that these structural analogs (BPB, BPE, BPF, etc.) have the same effects on the estrogen receptor and androgen receptor as BPA, and most of the alternatives are just as potent as BPA.[14]

There are a few studies showing an association between BPA and thyroid autoimmunity.[15,16] However, one of the studies showed a relationship between BPA and thyroid peroxidase (TPO) antibodies, but no relationship between BPA and TSH receptor antibodies,[16] which are the ones associated with Graves' disease. It's also worth mentioning that while the TSH receptor antibodies are associated with Graves' disease, many people with Graves' disease also have elevated TPO antibodies.

- **Formaldehyde.** Formaldehyde is a volatile organic compound (VOC) with numerous industrial and commercial uses as a solution, disinfectant, and preservative or to produce industrial resins used to manufacture adhesives and binders in wood, paper, and other products.[17] It is present in many household products, such as foam insulation, cleaning and personal care products, and pressed wood products such as particleboard and plywood, and as a result is a common indoor air pollutant found in virtually all homes and buildings.[17,18] Off-gassing of formaldehyde (and other VOCs) from new housing materials is also a big concern.[19]

- **Parabens.** Parabens have been widely used as preservatives in the cosmetic, food, and pharmaceutical industries for more than seventy years.[20] There is controversy over the safety of parabens, as while some sources claim that they are safe for use in cosmetics and pharmaceuticals within the recommended range of doses,[21] they are classified as endocrine-disrupting chemicals and may even play a role in obesity.[22,23] As a result, I definitely try to stay away from cosmetics (and foods) that contain parabens.

- **Polychlorinated biphenyls (PCBs).** PCBs are considered *persistent organic pollutants*, fat-soluble compounds that bioaccumulate in individuals and bio-magnify in the food chain.[24] PCBs were the first industrial compounds to experience a worldwide ban on production because of their potent toxicity.[24] Unfortunately, PCBs are still present in our food supply, and they can lead to reduced infection-fighting ability, increased rates of autoimmunity, cognitive and behavioral problems, and hypothyroidism.[24] A meta-analysis suggests that exposure to PCBs is also associated with an increased risk of cardiovascular-specific mortality in the general population.[25]

- **Flame retardants.** Polybrominated diphenyl ethers (PBDEs) also known as *flame retardants*, are commonly found in furniture such as couches and mattresses, as well as children's pajamas. Studies show that flame retardants can cause hormone disruption, thyroid cancer, and neurological toxicity.[26,27,28]

- **Volatile organic compounds (VOCs).** VOCs are solvents and include benzene and xylene. Identified emission sources include cigarette smoking, solvent-related emissions, renovations, household products, and pesticides.[29] Carpets act as a primary source of VOCs,[30] and they also commonly contain other environmental chemicals. Paint is also a potential source of VOCs, but the good news is that you can purchase zero-VOC paint.

  Tetrachloroethylene is also a VOC and is one of the common chemicals used in the dry cleaning industry. According to the Agency for Toxic Substances & Disease Registry, "Exposure to very high concentrations of tetrachloroethylene can cause dizziness, headaches, sleepiness, incoordination, confusion, nausea, unconsciousness, and even death".[31] As a result, if you dry clean your clothes you might want to consider going to an organic dry cleaners.

- **Per- and polyfluoroalkyl substances (PFAS).** In vivo, in vitro, and epidemiological evidence suggests that perfluoroalkyl substances (PFAS) may alter thyroid function in human health, with negative effects on maternal and fetal development outcomes.[32]

How to Optimize Detoxification

There are a few things you need to do to get the most out of your detoxification efforts. This is important even if you are relying mostly on food to support detoxification. First of all, you want to make sure you are having at least one daily bowel movement. Two or three would be even better.

Many people with hyperthyroidism have more frequent bowel movements due to the elevation in thyroid hormones, but of course the goal is to have regular bowel movements even if the hyperthyroidism is under control. If you experience constipation, please refer back to chapter 10 where I discuss Hyperthyroid Healing Diet troubleshooting.

In addition to having regular bowel movements on a daily basis, you want to drink plenty of fluids. In fact, doing this is necessary to avoid constipation, although there might be other things you need to do. There are many other benefits of keeping well hydrated by drinking plenty of fluids, and one of them is more frequent urination. While you might want to limit your fluid intake at night so you don't repeatedly wake up in the middle of the night to use the restroom, you do want to urinate every few hours to help with the elimination of toxins.

Water should be the main way you hydrate your body, and I recommend drinking at least half your weight of water in ounces. For example, if you weigh 150 pounds, then you should drink at least 75 ounces of water per day. Having pale yellow urine is a good indication that you're staying well hydrated. If you want to drink beverages other than water, please read chapter 9.

How Much Do You Sweat?

Another way to support detoxification is to make sure you do things to sweat. For many this isn't a problem. Some people actually sweat quite easily, even when engaging in mild activity. This is especially true for many people with hyperthyroidism, as it's common for people with this condition to experience excessive sweating.

On the other hand, some people have difficulty sweating, even when exercising vigorously or going into a sauna. This is referred to as *hypohidrosis* or *anhidrosis*. There can be numerous causes of anhidrosis, including certain medications that disrupt neural inputs from the anterior hypothalamus to the sweat gland,[33] but another potential cause is an imbalance in the autonomic nervous system. When this is the case, incorporating vagus nerve exercises might be beneficial (which I discussed in chapter 21), and even chiropractic care and acupuncture might be helpful in some cases. However, it's important to mention that many cases of anhidrosis are more complicated, and there can even be genetic factors.

You might be wondering whether or not you should incorporate sauna therapy to help you sweat. I will discuss this later in this chapter, as while I personally use an infrared sauna three times per week, many with hyperthyroidism will want to be cautious about using a sauna while trying to restore their health. And of course the same goes for vigorous exercise (in order to induce sweating), so initially you might need to focus on eliminating toxins through your bowel movements and urination.

Lymphatic Drainage 101

While I don't consider myself an expert when it comes to supporting the lymphatic system, the good news is that it's not too difficult to do this. But why should you support your lymphatic system? The lymphatic system is a component of the circulatory, immune, and metabolic systems, and it is composed of lymphatic fluid, lymphatic vessels, and lymphatic cells.[34] The spleen and thymus are lymphatic organs, and the lymphatics allow for the immune system to function properly as it carries antigens to lymph nodes, as well as carries immune cells such as macrophages to sites of infection to initiate the immune process.[34]

If you have experienced a lot of swelling/edema for quite awhile, then chances are you have a backed-up lymphatic system. While sometimes medical intervention is necessary, most of the time you can address this naturally. Just keep in mind that it can take a good amount of time to resolve this, although you should notice a gradual improvement over time.

So how can you "drain" your lymphatics? First of all, regular movement is a great way to support your lymphatic system. While you know from reading chapter 23 that you don't want to overexert yourself, this doesn't mean that you should be a couch potato. Even light walking can help, but so can light jumping (i.e., on a rebounder), stretching, practicing yoga, etc.

Staying well hydrated by drinking plenty of water is also very important. Dry brushing is another method of supporting the lymphatic system, and this involves the use of a soft, natural bristle brush on dry skin in order to manually activate the lymphatic system. I'll include a video on dry brushing you can check out in the resources, which you can access by visiting **savemythyroid.com/HHDNotes**. Homeopathic remedies can also be beneficial, and I'll include an example in the resources as well.

Understanding the 3 Phases of Detoxification

Phase 1. This phase is known as *biotransformation*, and it's where certain toxins are converted into intermediate metabolites which can actually be more harmful than the original compound. In fact, these intermediate metabolites can cause damage to the proteins, DNA, and RNA if they don't go through phase 2 detoxification.

Cytochrome P450 enzymes are produced by the liver, and are also found in the kidney, small intestine, lung, adrenals, and most other tissues. They are utilized in phase 1. There are fifty-eight different cytochromes, and different cytochromes play different roles in the metabolism of toxicants, which include medications. The cytochrome P450 enzyme can be inhibited or induced by certain drugs, as well as by certain nutrients. An inducing agent can increase the rate of another drug's metabolism, whereas an inhibiting agent can inhibit the drug's metabolism.

Phase 2. This is also known as the *conjugation process*, and in this phase the intermediate metabolites produced in phase 1 are combined with certain molecules and become less toxic and water soluble. While this might sound easy enough, it actually can be quite complex, as there are six different phase 2 pathways. This includes acetylation, glucuronidation, sulfur conjugation, methylation, glutathione, and amino acid conjugation. I'm not going to discuss these here, but just remember that having problems with any one of these pathways can affect phase 2 detoxification.

Phase 3. In this phase the water soluble molecules are excreted through the urine or bile. This is why drinking plenty of fluids and having regular bowel movements daily is essential for proper phase 3 detoxification.

How to Decrease Your Toxic Burden

Now I'd like to discuss some things you can and should do to reduce your toxic burden. After all, the lower the toxic burden you have, the better your overall health will be.

Avoidance of Toxicants. You of course want to do everything you can to minimize your exposure to environmental toxicants. You have the most control over this in your own home, where you can purchase organic food, drink purified water, use natural cleaners and cosmetics, get an air purifier, etc. On the other hand, once you step out of your house, you don't have much control over the environment.

Before I have an initial consultation with a patient, I have them complete a Toxin Exposure Questionnaire from the Institute for Functional Medicine. It helps me figure out if they are getting a lot of toxic exposure from the food they eat, their home, or their workplace; whether they use conventional cleaning chemicals and disinfectants; if they are getting toxin exposure from dental procedures (i.e., silver fillings), and if they are being exposed to electromagnetic radiation.

Food. As I mentioned earlier, eating whole, healthy foods is essential to support detoxification. And when trying to reduce your toxic burden it makes sense to try to eat as many organic foods as you can. If you can't eat all organic, at the very least prioritize vegetables, fruits, meat, and poultry.

Clean water. As I also mentioned earlier, you also need to drink plenty of water to eliminate toxicants from your body. And of course you want to try to drink purified water or a good-quality spring water. If you purchase any type of bottled water, you ideally want it to be glass (i.e., Mountain Valley Springs). While it's not a big deal if you drink out of a plastic water bottle and/or tap water on an occasional basis, you don't want to drink tap water or water out of plastic bottles on a consistent basis.

Air purifier. I wouldn't say this is a requirement for everyone, but a good-quality air purifier can help with air quality. This can be especially important to have if your home is located near a busy road (i.e., a highway). We have multiple air purifiers in our house and one in the office. To see what air purifiers I recommend, visit **SaveMyThyroid.com/HHDNotes**.

Sweating. This is another excellent way to excrete toxins and toxicants from the body, and I briefly mentioned earlier how important it is to sweat. You can sweat from exercising, or you can use a sauna. I use an infrared sauna three times per week to help reduce my toxic burden.

However, if you have unmanaged hyperthyroidism, you need to keep in mind that sauna will increase your heart rate, and if your resting heart rate is already high due to the hyperthyroidism, you don't want it to get even higher. In some cases you'll want to hold off on sauna therapy, although if your heart rate isn't elevated (i.e., because you're taking antithyroid agents) then doing sauna should be fine. To see what infrared sauna I recommend, visit **SaveMyThyroid.com/ HHDNotes**.

Support lymphatics. I briefly discussed this earlier, and I mentioned that jumping up and down is a great way to support the lymphatic system. You can do this using a rebounder, which essentially is a mini trampoline. Of course, you can also use a regular trampoline if you happen to have one. Or another option is to jump rope.

I also mentioned dry brushing, as this can help to support lymph flow, and I'll include a demonstration video of this in the resources. You also might want to check out an interview I did on my podcast with Kelly Kennedy, who is known as the Lymph Queen. Of particular interest is a device she has created to support the lymphatics called the *Flow Vibe*, which is an advanced bio sonic technology that supports lymphatic drainage of the neck, face, and other areas of the body. You can access the interview and learn more about the Flow Vibe, along with other ways to support your lymphatic system, by visiting **www.savemythyroid.com/123**.

Supporting Detoxification Through Nutritional Supplements and Herbs

Although you can do a great job of supporting your detoxification pathways through diet, taking certain nutritional supplements and herbs can also be beneficial. Some of the nutritional supplements and herbs which can support detoxification include milk thistle, NAC, alpha-lipoic acid, schisandra, acetylated or liposomal glutathione, trimethylglycine, and dandelion root. Remember that I have a bonus chapter where I discuss nutritional supplements and herbs that can support different areas of the body, including detoxification. For more information on these, including suggested doses, visit **savemythyroid.com/HHDNotes**.

Should Binding and/or Chelating Agents Be Used?

While it's important to support phase 1 and phase 2 detoxification, sometimes it can be beneficial to use certain binding and/or chelating agents. At times this can be beneficial for heavy metals. For example, if someone is trying to detoxify mercury (i.e., after getting their mercury amalgams removed), they might choose to eat cilantro and/or chlorella to bind to the mercury, and perhaps take NAC or alpha-lipoic acid. There are also prescription chelating agents such as dimercaptosuccinic acid (DMSA) and dimercaptopropane 1-sulfonate (DMPS). Ethylenediaminetetraacetic acid (EDTA) is another prescription chelator that is more commonly used for lead and cadmium. These prescription chelating agents can be taken orally or administered intravenously.

Getting back to some of the natural agents, silica can help bind to aluminum. Modified citrus pectin can help with the excretion of cadmium and lead. Zeolite and bentonite clay can not only bind to heavy metals, but to myco-toxins as well. The same is true with activated charcoal.

I need to let you know that there are risks of taking some of these agents ... especially prescription chelating agents. One concern is redistribution of the heavy metals in different areas of the body. For example, one case report involving a person who received intravenous EDTA showed that they exhibited increased tissue lead burden after treatment.[35] This is why it's important to have healthy glutathione levels when doing any type of chelation therapy.

Another concern is the loss of minerals. For example, one study showed that EDTA chelation not only causes the excretion of lead and cadmium, but zinc and calcium as well.[36] While taking a multimineral supplement might be a good idea when using such chelating agents, this is yet another reason why it's wise to work with a healthcare practitioner.

Other Detox Methods That Might Be Beneficial

- **Coffee enemas.** Unlike just about everything I've discussed so far to help with the elimination of environmental toxins from the body, I can't say that I personally do coffee enemas. And while some practitioners don't advocate coffee enemas due to the lack of published research, this doesn't mean that they can't be of benefit. For example, Gerson therapy is a well-known natural treatment regimen for cancer, and they aggressively use coffee enemas to help restore the health of people.

  It's important to understand that coffee enemas are not primarily used to empty the bowels, as they supposedly help support liver detoxification by increasing glutathione production. According to the brilliant Dr. Datis Kharrazian, coffee enemas can also help to stimulate the vagus nerve.

- **Colon hydrotherapy.** I'm sure some people reading this are wondering if colon hydrotherapy can effectively remove toxins, and the answer is yes. However, just as is the case with coffee enemas, there is controversy over the use of colon hydrotherapy. The late Dr. Walter Crinnion, author of the book *Clean, Green, and Lean*, was an expert on detoxification.

  He was also my instructor for a detoxification and biotransformation class I took while getting my master's in nutrition degree, and he told his students that if there was only one method he could use to remove toxins it would be colon hydrotherapy. However, some are concerned about whether colon hydrotherapy has a negative effect on the gut microbiome, and the research seems inconclusive.

- **Ionic foot baths.** I also don't have experience with ionic foot baths, but some practitioners swear by them. I wasn't able to find evidence proving that ionic foot baths can help with the elimination of toxicants from the body. Of course the lack of research doesn't confirm that it doesn't work, and I know other healthcare practitioners who get good results with their patients by recommending them. One of them is Dr. Wendy Myers, who discussed some of the benefits of ionic foot baths on the *Save My Thyroid* Podcast, and you can check out the interview by visiting **www.savemythyroid.com/131**.

The Impact of Electronic Pollution on Our Health

We are surrounded by electromagnetic fields, also known as EMFs. Every electronic device emits EMFs. This includes televisions, computers, refrigerators, cell phones, vacuum cleaners, and fluorescent lights. There is a great deal of controversy as to how EMFs affect the cells and tissues of the body.

EMFs might even have a negative effect on thyroid health. Studies in rats have found that exposure to both 50 Hz and 900 MHz EMFs decrease the production of thyroid hormone.[37] Cell phones emit about 900 MHz.

Of course not all studies translate to humans, although one study that looked at the correlation between cell phone use and thyroid health showed higher-than-normal TSH and lower thyroid hormone levels in those who used their cell phones more frequently.[38] The study concluded that there are possible harmful effects of mobile microwaves on the hypothalamic-pituitary-thyroid axis.

As for whether electromagnetic fields can be a factor in the development of Graves' disease, I did come across a journal article that looked at the relationship between electromagnetic fields and autoimmunity.[39] The authors mentioned how exposure to electromagnetic fields may induce a stress-like situation, which can be a factor in autoimmunity. While this is an interesting study, this doesn't confirm a direct relationship between EMFs and auto-immune conditions such as Graves' disease.

While there is no way to completely avoid your exposure to EMFs, I would try to do everything you can to minimize your exposure to them. Evidence suggests that EMFs can potentially cause infertility[40] and cancer,[41] although more research is needed. If you're interested in learning more about how to reduce electronic pollution, you might want to check out a two-part interview I did with EMF-expert Lloyd Burrell, by visiting **www.savemythyroid.com/73** and **www.savemythyroid.com/74.**

In summary, environmental toxicants can be a factor in the development of hyperthyroid conditions. While you can't completely eliminate your exposure to these toxicants, you can do a lot to reduce your toxic burden. In order to optimize your detoxification efforts, make sure you are having daily bowel movements, staying well hydrated, sweating, and doing some of the things I discussed to support your lymphatics. As for decreasing your toxic burden, trying your best to minimize your exposure to environmental toxicants is important by eating organic, drinking purified water, using natural cleaners and cosmetics, and doing some of the other things I discussed in this chapter. Also don't overlook the negative impact of electronic pollution on our health.

Chapter 24 Highlights

- No two people are exactly the same when it comes to eliminating toxins.
- Toxins are natural products, while toxicants are man-made products that are introduced into the environment.
- There is no question that diet plays a key role in the detoxification process, as it is a nutrient-dependent process.
- Some of the common environmental toxicants include heavy metals, BPA, formaldehyde, parabens, PCBs, flame retardants, VOCs, and PFAS.
- In order to optimize detoxification, make sure you're having regular bowel movements, drink plenty of water, do things to sweat, and support lymphatic drainage.
- Here are some things you can do to reduce your toxic burden: avoid toxicants as much as you can, eat whole, healthy, organic foods, drink clean water, get an air purifier, do things to make you sweat, support lymphatics.
- Some of the supplements that can support detoxification include milk thistle, NAC, alpha-lipoic acid, schisandra, acetylated or liposomal glutathione, trimethylglycine (TMG), and dandelion root.
- Sometimes it can be beneficial to use certain binding and/or chelating agents, especially when addressing heavy metals.
- Other detox methods that might be beneficial include coffee enemas, colon hydrotherapy, and ionic foot baths.
- We are surrounded by electromagnetic fields, which might have a negative effect on thyroid and immune health.

To access the book references and resources, visit
SaveMyThyroid.com/HHDNotes.

Correcting Nutrient Deficiencies and Optimizing Your Mitochondria

You probably have heard that mitochondria are the energy powerhouses of the cells. They are found in most cells in the body, and they rely on nutrients to convert into energy. They also need oxygen to convert the glucose from the food we eat into an energy-storing molecule called *adenosine triphosphate* (ATP).

This chapter will focus more on the importance of correcting nutrient deficiencies, although I feel it's important to mention that decreased oxygen consumption is common in those with hyperthyroidism.[1] This is yet another reason why it's important to do things to lower the thyroid hormones, whether it means taking antithyroid medication or natural agents such as bugleweed. Certain beta blockers such as propranolol that can decrease the peripheral conversion of free thyroxine (T4) to triiodothyronine (T3) can also decrease whole-body oxygen consumption significantly.[1]

What Is Oxidative Stress?

Chances are you've heard the term *free radical*. Free radicals are essentially unstable atoms that can damage cells. Examples of free radicals include hydrogen peroxide, superoxide anion, and peroxynitrite. It's normal to have free radicals, but you need to have sufficient antioxidants to prevent them from causing damage. In fact, free radicals can adversely alter lipids, proteins, and DNA and lead to a number of human diseases.[2]

Oxidative stress usually is caused by either an excess of free radicals and/or a decrease in antioxidants. Too much oxidative stress can cause damage to the cells, resulting in mitochondrial dysfunction. In order to reduce oxidative stress, you essentially want to do things to decrease free radicals and/or increase antioxidants.

There are numerous factors that can cause an increase in free radicals. This includes x-rays, ozone, cigarette smoking, air pollutants, and industrial chemicals.[3] Infections can also be a cause of free radicals, including viruses,[4,5] and perhaps even Lyme disease.[6] And it's also important to mention that hyperthyroidism can cause an increase in oxidative stress.

The way antioxidants can reduce oxidative stress is by donating an electron to a free radical, which in turn will neutralize it. Three of the main antioxidants derived from food include vitamin C, vitamin E, and beta-carotene. Two other antioxidants that are produced by the body but are also commonly given as supplements include CoQ10 and glutathione.

Next I'd like to discuss three steps you need to optimize the health of your mitochondria.

Step #1: Have Healthy Levels of Thyroid Hormone

Thyroid hormone affects virtually every organ system in the body. This includes the heart, gut, liver, adrenals, nervous system, etc. It's also important in supporting the brain, and therefore it can affect mood and cognition if someone doesn't have enough thyroid hormone . . . or too much thyroid hormone. The same is true with fertility, ovulation, and menstruation, as too little or too much thyroid hormone can have severe consequences.

Thyroid hormones play a very important role when it comes to optimal mitochondria health. First of all, they stimulate something called *mitochondriogenesis*, which is the formation of mitochondria. If you don't have enough thyroid hormone, you won't produce enough mitochondria. Of course people with hyperthyroidism don't have this problem, although those with hyperthyroidism will use up oxygen quicker, and if the hyperthyroidism is severe, this can result in an ATP deficiency.

Research also shows that hyperthyroidism can cause oxidative injury of the tissues. So essentially, hyperthyroidism can be a factor in mitochondrial dysfunction, which explains why some people with hyperthyroidism can experience fatigue (although there can be other reasons as well). The point here is that both low and high thyroid hormones can have negative consequences on the health of the mitochondria.

Step #2: Correct Nutrient Deficiencies

Everyone reading this book knows that it's not good to have nutrient deficiencies. While all nutrients are important, some of the more essential ones that relate to mitochondrial health include the B vitamins, vitamin C, vitamin E, selenium, zinc, coenzyme Q10, carnitine, lipoic acid, and taurine. B vitamins and lipoic acid are essential in the tricarboxylic acid cycle, while selenium, α-tocopherol, and coenzyme Q10 support the electron transfer system function.[7] Carnitine is essential for fatty acid beta-oxidation, while selenium is involved in mitochondrial biogenesis.[7]

Other important nutrients include iron, magnesium, and omega-3 fatty acids. I'm going to discuss some of the more important nutrients shortly, but I'll say here that before correcting nutrient deficiencies, you need to understand how nutrient deficiencies develop. One reason is that many people eat poorly. This is one of the main reasons I wrote this book, although I'm sure most people reading this already know that it's a good idea to eat whole, healthy foods, including many organic options. However, many people eat what they perceive as being healthy foods (i.e., grains), although in a lot of people they can cause problems.

Problems with digestion/absorption is another common cause of nutrient deficiencies. For example, you need sufficient stomach acid to break down minerals and protein. And having any problems with malabsorption due to SIBO, inflammatory bowel disease, or other causes can also lead to nutrient deficiencies.

Certain medications can also lead to specific nutrient deficiencies. For example, certain beta blockers can block the CoQ10-dependent enzymes.[8,9] Taking proton pump inhibitors (PPIs) can cause deficiencies in vitamin B_{12}, vitamin C, calcium, iron, and magnesium.[10] Oral contraceptives can cause deficiencies in folic acid; vitamins B_2, B_6, and B_{12}; vitamins C and E, and the minerals magnesium, selenium, and zinc.[11] Metformin can decrease vitamin B_{12} levels.[12, 13]

Focus on Nutrient Density

In 2023 I had the honor of interviewing Dr. Sarah Ballantyne on my podcast, and we had a chat about nutrient density. Dr. Sarah is the founder of the Autoimmune Protocol and the creator of the Nutrivore Score. The Nutrivore Score is a measure of the total nutrients per calorie in a food.

According to Dr. Sarah's research, a nutrient-dense powerhouse superfood is any food with a Nutrivore Score higher than 800. High nutrient-density foods have a Nutrivore Score between 400 and 8,000. Medium nutrient-density foods have a Nutrivore Score between 150 and 400. And, low nutrient-density empty-calorie foods have a Nutrivore score less than 150.

If this fascinates you as much as it does me, then you'll want to check out her website **www.Nutrivore.com**. Here you can learn about some of the foods with the highest Nutrivore Scores, and she also shares a lot of valuable information on her YouTube channel (Dr. Sarah Ballantyne). You might also want to check out her e-book, *Top 500 Nutrivore Foods*, which has the top five hundred most nutrient-dense foods according to their Nutrivore Score. And in May 2024 she is scheduled to release the book *Nutrivore: The Radical New Science for Getting the Nutrients You Need from the Food You Eat*. Plus don't forget to check out my interview with Dr. Sarah (**www.savemythyroid.com/83**).

Step #3: Address Other Factors That Can Reduce Oxidative Stress

In addition to balancing the thyroid hormones, you want to try to address any other factors that can cause oxidative stress. I briefly mentioned a few of these factors earlier, but I would especially focus on (1) reducing your toxic load, (2) addressing any underlying infections (i.e., Lyme disease, bartonella), and (3) increasing your antioxidants. I discussed how you reduce your toxic load in greater detail in chapter 24, so I won't discuss this here. Stealth infections such as viruses and Lyme disease can be challenging to treat, and many times the goal isn't eradication of the microorganism, but instead doing things to greatly improve your immune system health.

As for increasing your antioxidants, while you can take antioxidants in the form of nutritional supplements, I would try to do as much as you can through food. In fact, for those who are thinking about taking antioxidants in the form of supplements on a continuous basis to reduce oxidative stress, there is evidence that doing this might cause more harm than good.[14,15] This seems to be especially true with vitamin E and beta-carotene. This doesn't mean that there isn't a time and place for supplementing with antioxidants, and I commonly recommend vitamin C and glutathione supplements to my patients. But you want to rely more on whole, healthy foods.

The Impact of Antithyroid Medication on the Mitochondria

One of the concerns with antithyroid medication such as methimazole and PTU is the potential negative effects it can have on the liver. It's very common to see patients with elevated liver enzymes when taking antithyroid medication. This doesn't describe everyone of course, but it is one reason why some endocrinologists will pressure their patients to receive radioactive iodine or thyroid surgery (although many will do this even before they prescribe antithyroid medication).

Anyway, as for how antithyroid medication affects the liver, one mechanism might be by damaging the mitochondria of the hepatocytes, which are liver cells. One study showed that methimazole decreased liver mitochondrial ATP and glutathione; increased mitochondrial swelling, lipid peroxidation, and reactive oxygen species (ROS); and collapsed mitochondrial membrane potential when administered to mice.[16] However, I also need to mention that there was an in vitro (test tube) study that showed that methimazole not only caused no significant injury toward isolated liver mitochondria in vitro but also improved mitochondrial function and protected this organelle.[16]

Even though this is conflicting, there is no question that methimazole damages liver cells in a lot of people, so I definitely would rely more on the results of the study done on mice. I also need to mention another study that showed that taking taurine reduced the toxic effects of methimazole in isolated rat liver cells.[17] N-acetylcysteine (NAC) has hepatoprotective (liver-protecting) effects and therefore has been shown to be of benefit to those taking methimazole.[18]

Milk thistle also has been shown to have hepatoprotective effects. [19] I have a product called Hepatommune Supreme that includes both NAC and milk thistle, along with the herb schisandra, which also supports the liver.

Beta Blockers and Mitochondrial Health

Since it's common for people with hyperthyroidism to take beta blockers, it's also worth mentioning that certain beta blockers can decrease CoQ10 levels by inhibiting CoQ10-dependent enzymes. [20] I also found two case studies that showed that certain beta blockers aggravated the symptoms of mitochondrial disorders. [21,22] One of them involved propranolol, [21] which is commonly given to hyperthyroid patients since it also affects the conversion of T4 to T3. The other study involved metoprolol. [22]

I'm not trying to discourage people from taking beta blockers, as there definitely is a time and place to take them. But I just want to make you aware of some of the potential side effects. And if you do need to take a beta blocker, you might want to consider supplementing with 100 to 200 mg of CoQ10.

Common Nutrient Deficiencies That Affect Mitochondrial Health

Obviously all of the nutrients are important for optimal health, but I'm going to focus on some of the most important ones here.

Selenium. Although selenium has many roles in the body, the predominant biochemical action of this mineral in both animals and humans is to serve as an antioxidant via the selenium-dependent enzyme glutathione peroxidase and, thus, protect cellular membranes and organelles from oxidative damage. [23]

If someone is deficient in selenium, they will also be low in glutathione, and this is a concern because glutathione helps to protect the cells from the damaging effects of free radicals. While taking precursors such as N-acetylcysteine (NAC) can increase glutathione levels, you also need to have healthy selenium levels.

Although supplementing with selenium can be beneficial in some cases, you do want to be careful about supplementing with high doses of selenium supplements, as doing this can result in a selenium toxicity. A few years ago, 201 people were affected by an error in a liquid dietary supplement that contained two hundred times the labeled concentration of selenium.[24] Fortunately, only one person was hospitalized. The symptoms associated with selenium toxicity include diarrhea (78 percent), fatigue (75 percent), hair loss (72 percent), joint pain (70 percent), nail discoloration or brittleness (61 percent), and nausea.[24]

It's also worth mentioning that selenium can benefit the mitochondria. One study showed that selenium plays an important role in mitochondrial regeneration.[25] Another study demonstrated that selenium can preserve mitochondrial function and stimulate mitochondrial biogenesis.[26]

Zinc. Having a zinc deficiency is common due to inadequate intake, malabsorption, and impaired utilization, with inadequate dietary intake the primary cause.[27] A moderate to severe zinc deficiency can cause rough skin, poor appetite, mental lethargy, delayed wound healing, taste abnormalities, hypogonadism, oligospermia, and weight loss.[28]

Zinc deficiency impairs both the innate and the adaptive immune system and can be normalized by zinc supplementation.[29] Also, a few studies show that zinc can decrease Th17 cells, which promote autoimmunity.[30,31,32] In addition, zinc can increase Tregs, which suppress autoimmunity.[33] Finally, a zinc deficiency can make someone more susceptible to developing an infection,[34,35,36] which can trigger Graves' disease or subacute thyroiditis.

Zinc can also improve the health of the gut, which, of course, is important for a healthy immune system. One study showed that zinc substantially alters the gut microbiota and reduces the minimum amount of antibiotics needed to eradicate pathogens such as *Clostridium difficile*.[37] Zinc also plays a role in the function of the epithelial barrier, which seems to be due to modifications of the tight junctions.[38] If you recall, damage to these tight junctions is a factor in a leaky gut. Another study showed that zinc carnosine could help prevent an increase in intestinal permeability.[39]

Zinc can also benefit the health of the mitochondria in a few different ways. First of all, it can improve mitochondrial respiratory function.[40] Second, it prevents the generation of reactive oxygen species.[40]

Magnesium. Magnesium is a cofactor in hundreds of enzyme reactions. For example, magnesium plays a role in many ATP-generating reactions.[41] ATP is required for glucose utilization; the synthesis of fat, proteins, nucleic acids, and coenzymes; muscle contraction; methyl group transfer; and many other processes, and as a result, interference with magnesium metabolism also influences these functions.[41]

Magnesium can help to increase insulin sensitivity.[42,43] Also, evidence shows that chronic magnesium deficiency results in excessive production of oxygen-derived free radicals and low-grade inflammation.[44] One of the main reasons for this is that magnesium is a cofactor in the synthesis of glutathione. Thus, if someone has a moderate to severe magnesium deficiency, there is a good chance they have a glutathione deficiency as well, which will increase the chances of them having oxidative stress.

When I recommend magnesium supplements to my patients, I usually recommend magnesium glycinate/malate, or perhaps magnesium citrate if they are experiencing constipation. Other forms include magnesium oxide, magnesium taurate, magnesium lactate, magnesium threonate, and magnesium orotate. All of these can be beneficial, although I would try to avoid magnesium oxide unless it's part of a chelate that also includes a higher-quality form of magnesium, such as magnesium glycinate.

Iron. Iron is one of the most commonly deficient minerals seen in people. It's surprising that many medical doctors don't recommend an iron panel to all of their patients. It's even more surprising when someone is experiencing symptoms such extreme fatigue or hair loss, yet an iron panel isn't ordered.

It's important to understand that you can have an iron deficiency without having anemia, and you can have anemia without having an iron deficiency. To better understand this, let's discuss what happens when someone has anemia. Anemia results when the body doesn't produce enough red blood cells or hemoglobin.

Although many medical doctors don't perform an iron panel, most doctors routinely order a complete blood count to look at the red blood cells, hemoglobin, and hematocrit. When someone has anemia, one or more of these values are depressed. Hemoglobin is an iron-rich protein that gives blood its red color; thus, when iron is low, typically hemoglobin is low, along with the red blood cell count and hematocrit. But this isn't always the case. Thus, just because all three of these are normal doesn't mean you can't have an iron deficiency.

While a complete blood count is commonly recommended by primary care physicians when someone has a routine physical examination, in my opinion, an iron panel should also be ordered. If someone has a normal iron panel but has depressed red blood cells, hemoglobin, and/or hematocrit, then other potential causes of the anemia should be investigated, such as a vitamin B_{12} deficiency or even inflammation. However, if someone has an iron deficiency, regardless of whether or not they have anemia, the cause of the deficiency should be addressed.

What Are Common Causes of an Iron Deficiency?

Someone can become deficient in iron for one of three main reasons. One reason is due to blood loss, which is why some doctors will refer the patient with iron deficiency anemia to a gastroenterologist in order to rule out gastrointestinal bleeding. Not surprisingly, women who have a heavy menstrual flow are more likely to have an iron deficiency than women who have a lighter menstrual flow.

A second reason for an iron deficiency is iron malabsorption. This can be caused by a number of different factors, such as having an infection, inflammatory bowel disease, celiac disease, and, in some cases, small intestinal bacterial overgrowth. Even exposure to glyphosate can lead to the chelation of minerals such as iron, thus leading to an iron deficiency.[45] Glyphosate, the active ingredient in the herbicide Roundup, is discussed in chapter 26.

A third common reason for an iron deficiency relates to low dietary intake of iron. Iron is found in two different forms. Heme iron is found in foods such as meat, poultry, and fish. It is more absorbable than nonheme iron, which is found in plant-based foods.[46,47]

Thus, vegetarians and vegans are more likely to develop an iron deficiency than those who eat meat. It's also important to know that vitamin C and hydrochloric acid help to increase the absorption of iron; thus, having hypochlorhydria (low stomach acid) or low vitamin C levels can have a negative effect on iron absorption.

Iron Toxicity Concerns

If someone has a severe iron toxicity, they may experience vomiting, diarrhea, and abdominal pain initially, and liver failure can eventually develop. However, over the years, I have had a few patients with elevated iron markers in the blood who didn't experience such symptoms. Even in these cases, it's important to get the iron levels down, as too much iron can cause oxidative stress. This is why you never want to supplement with iron unless an iron deficiency has been confirmed. And then, even if taking an iron supplement is necessary, you want to address the cause of the deficiency.

While in this chapter I have discussed some of the benefits of the nutrients on the health of the mitochondria, there are concerns with too much iron when it comes to mitochondrial health. In fact, the research shows that iron overload can cause mitochondrial dysfunction, including damage to the mitochondrial DNA.[48,49] For this reason alone I think that everyone should consider getting a full iron panel done.

Vitamin A. Out of the four different fat-soluble vitamins (A, E, D, and K), vitamin A was the first fat-soluble vitamin to be discovered. Vitamin A has a number of important functions. It plays a very important role in immunity, which of course is important for anyone with an autoimmune thyroid condition such as Graves' disease. Vitamin A can help with the inflammatory and repair process. It helps greatly in preventing infections from developing, and an infection can potentially trigger autoimmunity.

Vitamin A is important when it comes to eye health. It can specifically help to decrease the incidence of cataracts.[50] Vitamin A also plays an important role in healthy skin.[51] Because of this, it can greatly help people who have acne. Vitamin A can also help prevent conditions such as cardiovascular disease.[52] In addition, it helps to maintain the epithelial tissues of the skin, gastrointestinal tract, respiratory tract, and genitourinary tract.[53]

Vitamin A also plays an important role in mitochondrial energy homeostasis.[54] Specifically, retinol is essential for the metabolic fitness of mitochondria,[55] as research shows that when cells were deprived of retinol, respiration and ATP synthesis decreased. Another study showed that vitamin A depletion causes oxidative stress and mitochondrial dysfunction.[55]

Vitamin D. Vitamin D is more of a prohormone than a nutrient, and you probably won't be getting most of your vitamin D from the food you eat. Vitamin D increases the intestinal absorption of calcium and phosphorus, which in turn promotes bone mineralization and remodeling. It is also involved in regulating serum calcium and phosphorus levels and plays a big role in immunity, which of course is important for those with autoimmune conditions such as Graves' disease.

I find that most people are deficient in vitamin D, and therefore need to work on getting more sun exposure, although many need to supplement with vitamin D_3. This describes me, as I definitely don't spend enough time in the sun, and therefore I take 5,000 IU/day of vitamin D_3 to maintain healthy levels (at least 50 ng/mL). It's also worth mentioning that for numerous reasons (i.e., genetics, air pollution), some people who get regular sun exposure will still need to supplement with vitamin D.

A few different studies also show that vitamin D can benefit mitochondrial health. One study showed that vitamin D supplementation improves mitochondrial function and reduces inflammation,[56] while another study showed that vitamin D modulates mitochondrial oxidative capacities in skeletal muscle.[57] And yet another study showed that the vitamin D receptor is necessary for mitochondrial function and cell health.[58]

Vitamin K. There are essentially three different forms of vitamin K. Vitamin K_1, also known as *phylloquinone*, is found in plant sources, especially leafy green vegetables. On the other hand, vitamin K_2, known as *menaquinones*, is found in mostly animal products, although there are other sources as well, such as natto, which is a fermented type of soy. Vitamin K_3, also known as *menadione*, is found in small amounts in certain foods, but essentially is considered to be a synthetic form of vitamin K.

Vitamin K_1 can be obtained through plants such as kale, spinach, beet greens, collards, broccoli, and Brussels sprouts. As I mentioned before, vitamin K_2 is mostly found in animal foods, such as eggs, cheese, butter, beef, and is also found in natto. There are two main types of vitamin K_2, which include menaquinone-4 (MK-4) and menaquinone-7 (MK-7).

MK-4 is what's mostly found in animal foods, while natto is a source of MK-7. Both of these can be excellent sources of vitamin K_2, although with regard to MK-4, the quality of the animal product is important, as eggs from pasture-raised chickens, and meat and dairy from grass-fed animals will contain higher levels of MK-4 than those from grain-fed animals.

While vitamin D is important for the absorption of calcium, vitamin K_2 is necessary to help "escort" calcium into the bones. If vitamin K_2 is low, then some of the calcium will end up in the soft tissues of the body, such as the arteries. The way vitamin K_2 works is by activating a protein called *osteocalcin*, which helps guide the calcium into the bones. Vitamin K_2 also activates another protein called *matrix Gla protein* (MGP), which is a potent inhibitor of arterial calcification,[59] as it helps to pull calcium out of the soft tissues. Protein-S is a vitamin-K dependent protein that can play a role in bone turnover and bone mass.[60]

As for how vitamin K_2 affects the mitochondria, I came across a study demonstrating that it regulates mitochondrial fission, mitochondrial fusion, mitophagy, and mitochondrial biogenesis, thereby alleviating mitochondrial dysfunction and maintaining mitochondrial homeostasis.[61]

Omega-3 fatty acids. It is important to have the proper ratio of omega-6 and omega-3 fatty acids. The optimal ratio of omega-6 to omega-3 fatty acids should be somewhere between 1:1 and 4:1, but most people eat somewhere in the range of 10:1 to 20:1. Since most people eat too many foods high in omega-6 fatty acids (i.e., vegetable, nut, and seed oils), it's not surprising that most people have a high ratio. Keep in mind that not all omega-6 fatty acids are bad for you. Gamma linolenic acid (GLA) is an omega-6 fatty acid, and numerous studies have shown this fatty acid to have anti-inflammatory effects.[62,63]

While having healthy omega-3 levels is important for everyone, regardless of the type of hyperthyroidism they have, it's arguably even more important for those with Graves' disease. Higher doses of EPA and DHA can help to reduce inflammation and downregulate proinflammatory cytokines.[64,65] Also, evidence indicates that they can help reduce Th17 cells,[66] which I've already mentioned are associated with autoimmunity.

Omega-3 fatty acids can also benefit the mitochondria in multiple ways. First of all, studies show that omega-3 fatty acids improve mitochondrial dysfunction in brain aging.[67] Omega-3 supplementation can also increase the capacity for the emission of mitochondrial reactive oxygen species and reorganize the composition of mitochondrial membranes.[68] It's also worth mentioning that fatty acid oxidation mainly occurs in the mitochondria. Fatty acid oxidation is what your body uses to break down fatty acids and use them for energy.

CoQ10. The primary biochemical action of CoQ10 is as a cofactor in the electron-transport chain, in the series of redox reactions that are involved in the synthesis of adenosine triphosphate (ATP). [69] As most cellular functions are dependent on an adequate supply of adenosine triphosphate (ATP), CoQ10 is essential for the health of virtually all human tissues and organs.[69] In addition to its well-established function as a component of the mitochondrial respiratory chain, CoQ10 also functions in the reduced form (ubiquinol) as an antioxidant.[70]

Ubiquinol protects membrane phospholipids and serum low-density lipoproteins from lipid peroxidation, as well as mitochondrial proteins and DNA from free radical–induced oxidative damage.[70] Some studies suggest that as people age, decreases in CoQ10 content may occur in mitochondria and that decreases of CoQ10 below the physiological levels can potentially affect mitochondrial respiratory function.[71]

Hyperthyroidism is especially linked with lower levels of CoQ10. A study looked at the circulating levels of CoQ10 in both hypothyroid and hyperthyroid conditions and found that these levels are higher in people with hypothyroidism.[72] This same study shows that the values of CoQ10 in hyperthyroid patients are among the *lowest* in different human diseases. Yet another study confirmed that serum CoQ10 levels in hyperthyroidism were significantly lower than that of euthyroid subjects, while in hypothyroidism, serum CoQ10 levels did not show any significant difference from that of euthyroid subjects.[73]

Other nutrients worth mentioning. The goal of this chapter wasn't to cover every single vitamin and mineral, but I do want to give a brief shout-out to some of the other important nutrients I didn't cover. Calcium has a lot of important functions, and while most people are aware of the benefits of calcium with regard to bone health, many are unfamiliar with the other roles this mineral plays in the body. Calcium plays a very important role in muscle contraction. I'm not just talking about the muscles in your arms, legs, and other extremities, but *all* of the muscles in your body, including your heart muscles. Proper nerve conduction also relies on adequate calcium levels.

I mentioned in chapter 3 how you don't need to rely on dairy as a source of calcium, as there are other good non-dairy sources, including arugula, cruciferous vegetables, and fish with bones.

Potassium is also an important mineral. Besides playing an important role in fluid and electrolyte balance, as well as neuronal transmission, potassium is necessary for the conversion of glucose into glycogen, as well as membrane polarization, muscle contraction, and hormone secretion. It also helps to regulate blood pressure.

Copper also has many different functions, as it also is involved in immunity, as well as the nervous system, reproductive system, and other bodily systems. And while you don't want a copper deficiency, you also don't want to have an excess of copper.

The B vitamins are also important for optimal health, and if you're dealing with a lot of stress, your body will tend to use up the B vitamins more quickly, and thus supplementation with a B complex might be a good idea.

In summary, having healthy mitochondria is important, and hyperthyroidism can be a factor in mitochondrial dysfunction. While balancing the thyroid hormones can benefit the health of the mitochondria, correcting nutrient deficiencies can also be extremely important. While it's important to eat whole, healthy foods that are nutrient dense, there is a time and place for supplementation when correcting nutrient deficiencies.

It's also worth mentioning that antithyroid medication and beta blockers can have a negative effect on the health of the mitochondria. This doesn't mean that if you're taking these that you should stop, as everything comes down to risks versus benefits.

Chapter 25 Highlights

- Mitochondria, the energy powerhouses of the cells, are found in most cells in the body, and they rely on nutrients to convert into energy.
- Three steps to optimize your mitochondria include (1) having healthy levels of thyroid hormones, (2) correcting nutrient deficiencies, and (3) addressing other factors that can increase oxidative stress.
- Thyroid hormones play a very important role when it comes to optimal mitochondria health.
- As for how antithyroid medication affects the liver, one mechanism might be by damaging the mitochondria of the liver cells.
- Since it's common for people with hyperthyroidism to take beta blockers, it's also worth mentioning that certain beta blockers can decrease CoQ10 levels.
- Common nutrient deficiencies that can affect mitochondrial health include selenium, zinc, magnesium, iron, vitamin A, vitamin D, vitamin K2, omega-3 fatty acids, and CoQ10.

To access the book references and resources, visit
SaveMyThyroid.com/HHDNotes.

CHAPTER
26

Bioengineered Foods and Glyphosate Dangers

hen I was growing up I remember a commercial related to a brand of margarine that supposedly tasted like butter. The actress in the commercial played Mother Nature, and the premise of the commercial is that she tastes the margarine and thinks it's butter, but when she finds out that it's margarine, she follows with the line, "It's not nice to fool Mother Nature!" You probably know how bad margarine is for your health, and while it's not the exact same situation with GMO foods, there is no question that we are trying to fool Mother Nature again.

There are numerous reasons why you should try to eat mostly organic food. There's the endocrine-disrupting pesticides sprayed on non-organic fruits and vegetables, the hormones and antibiotics given to conventional livestock, and countless other environmental toxicants we're exposed to in the food we eat. Of course organic food isn't perfect, but it still is a lot better than non-organic food. It's more nutrient dense and has fewer harsh chemicals, and these two reasons alone should be enough to convince you to eat mostly organic.

Genetically modified foods, also referred to as *bioengineered foods*, are yet another reason why you should eat mostly organic. While there is still controversy over the potential dangers of consuming bioengineered foods, why take the risk when it's easy enough to purchase food that isn't genetically modified? I realize that cost may be a big factor for some people, but in my opinion, the benefits of eating whole, healthy organic foods far outweigh the potential risks of eating bioengineered foods.

Which Foods Are Genetically Modified?

The following represents the main genetically modified foods as of 2023:[1]

- Alfalfa
- Apple (ArcticTM varieties)
- Canola
- Corn
- Cotton
- Eggplant (BARI Bt Begun varieties)
- Papaya (ringspot virus-resistant varieties)
- Pineapple (pink flesh varieties)
- Potato
- Salmon (AquAdvantage®)
- Soybean
- Squash (summer)
- Sugar beet

Why Does "Bioengineering" of Foods Take Place?

There are a few different reasons for the genetic modification of foods. One reason is to make crops that are resistant to herbicides, and they accomplish this by taking genes from one species and inserting them into another one. Some of these crops can also produce their own pesticides.

Another reason is because GMO crops make it easier for farmers to kill weeds, while at the same time allowing the GMO crops to be resistant to herbicides, including Roundup. And of course a final reason is to make more money. Once again, everything comes down to risks versus benefits, and while many people won't think twice about eating bioengineered foods, I would recommend doing everything you can to avoid them.

How Are We Exposed to GMOs?

There are two main ways we're exposed to GMOs:

1. **By eating the food directly.** If you eat anything that isn't organic or has the non-GMO label, there is a very good chance you are consuming genetically modified foods.

2. **By eating livestock that is fed GMO foods.** For example, if you eat non-organic poultry, there is a good chance it was fed GMO-corn or soy.

What's the Concern with GMOs?

There are a few concerns with genetically modified foods. One concern is that the body may not process these foods the same way as non-GMO foods. The reason for this is that when you genetically modify foods, you are changing their DNA. This potentially can cause the immune system to see the proteins in these foods as being foreign, which in turn can cause an immune system response.

Then there is a concern with the Bt toxin. *Bacillus thuringiensis* is a gram positive bacterium used as a microbial insecticide. The genes of these bacteria have been incorporated into several major crops, making them resistant to insects. Essentially, the crops' DNA has been altered to produce what's called the *Bacillus thuringiensis* (Bt) toxin, which breaks open the stomachs of insects, thereby killing them. Although we were initially told that only insects would be negatively affected by the Bt toxin, some are concerned about it potentially harming some of the cells of the human digestive system, perhaps contributing to an increase in intestinal permeability (leaky gut), which is part of the triad of autoimmunity I discussed in an earlier chapter.

What You Need to Know about Glyphosate

You may have heard of glyphosate, which is the active ingredient in the herbicide Roundup. How does glyphosate relate to GMOs? Well, it is used primarily on genetically modified crops, and in my opinion (as well as the opinion of many others) it is a big factor in the increased prevalence of chronic health conditions, including autoimmune conditions such as Graves' disease. If you are eating processed or refined foods, then there is an excellent chance you are consuming glyphosate. This is especially true if these foods are not organic.

Monsanto is a corporation that was the leading producer for Roundup and genetically engineered seeds until Bayer successfully acquired the company in 2018. As for Roundup, the reason why many farmers use it is because it kills everything with the exception of the genetically engineered crop. So why is this a problem? Well, these crops contain high levels of glyphosate, which as I already mentioned can be a factor in the increase of chronic health conditions.

You might wonder why glyphosate is used on these crops if they can potentially cause chronic health problems. Not surprisingly, the main reason has to do with making a very large profit. It's unfortunate that some businesses will do whatever it takes to make a lot of money, even if it means risking the health of millions, if not billions of people.

More Toxic When Combined with Other Chemicals?

Most research studies that test for the toxicity of different chemicals test these chemicals in isolation. The problem with this approach is that most herbicides and pesticides, as well as other chemicals (i.e., household cleaners) include multiple compounds, which, when combined, make the product even more toxic.

Most of these pesticide and herbicide formulations contain adjuvants to enhance the herbicidal action of the formulation. For example, Roundup contains not only glyphosate but also ethoxylated adjuvants, and this combination makes the formulation even more toxic.[2] So while glyphosate alone can cause health issues, the combination of glyphosate with these adjuvants makes it even more toxic.

The Glyphosate-Hyperthyroidism Connection

I think it's safe to say that most cases of hyperthyroidism aren't directly caused by consuming glyphosate. However, I do think that our increased exposure to environmental chemicals overall is a big reason why more and more people are developing thyroid and autoimmune thyroid conditions. And while we can't blame glyphosate alone, it is one of the major environmental toxins most people are exposed to on a consistent basis.

I think it's safe to say that if glyphosate didn't exist, there would still be many cases of hyperthyroidism due to the other chemicals we're exposed to in the food we eat, the water we drink, and the air we breathe, not to mention the increased levels of chronic stress just about everyone deals with. But while we can't blame glyphosate for all of our health issues, I do think it is a major culprit.

This is especially true since it's been shown that glyphosate causes intestinal dysbiosis.[3] This is a factor with autoimmune conditions such as Graves' disease. It also can affect estrogen metabolism,[4] which is one of the main causes of toxic multinodular goiter, and it even can play a role in the development of other hyperthyroid conditions. For example, subacute thyroiditis is usually viral induced, but since most of the immune system cells are located in the gut, being exposed to glyphosate can compromise the immune system, making someone more susceptible to a viral infection.

Should You Test for Glyphosate?

I can't say I have all of my patients test for glyphosate, as I usually just assume that everyone has some levels of glyphosate in their body. In fact, I've had some patients do a urinary glyphosate test, and I'm pretty sure I have seen some levels of glyphosate in everyone who has tested. In some cases it's within the acceptable limits, while in other cases it's well above the lab reference range. I must admit that I did test my glyphosate levels as well (I used Mosaic Diagnostics), and while it was within the lab reference range, I still wanted to do things to decrease the levels, which I did (confirmed later through retesting).

You can also test your water for glyphosate, although I have not done this as of writing this book. But truth to be told, we probably should all be testing our water for glyphosate. And if you filter your water like I do, it might be a good idea to test the filtered water to make sure it's doing the job!

Gluten vs. Glyphosate

While it's very common for natural healthcare practitioners to recommend that their patients avoid gluten, there is some debate as to whether the problem is actually with glyphosate. One of the main reasons is because many crops are sprayed with glyphosate right before they are harvested, including wheat and other grains. This very well may explain why some people do fine when eating foods with gluten in a different country, or a healthier type of wheat (i.e., einkorn, sourdough).

If you have celiac disease, it's important to avoid *all* types of gluten on a permanent basis. While there can be an argument that some people are reacting to glyphosate and not gluten, with celiac disease, the person will have an autoimmune response to gluten. Although some earlier studies suggest that it might be okay for people with celiac disease to eat sourdough bread, later studies have shown that this isn't the case.[5]

Is Changing Your Diet Enough?

Although nothing you do will completely eliminate your exposure to glyphosate, eating mostly organic foods and drinking certain types of purified water (i.e., reverse osmosis) will decrease your exposure. And in this day and age that's probably the best we can do, as I don't know any way to completely eliminate glyphosate exposure. This is especially true if you don't eat at home 100 percent of the time.

What Can You Do to Minimize Your Exposure?

As I just mentioned, the best thing you can do to minimize your exposure to glyphosate is eat whole, healthy, organic foods, as well as drink purified water where the glyphosate is filtered out, such as reverse osmosis.[6] Once again, if you're concerned about the minerals being removed, you can always add minerals to your water. If you use a different water filter, make sure you do your own research to make sure that it filters out glyphosate. If you eat packaged foods, I also would make sure they're organic, and you can also look out for brands that have a "glyphosate-free" seal on the label, such as One Degree Organic Foods, Chosen Foods, and Heavenly Organics.

Can You Detoxify Glyphosate from Your Body?

Dr. Stephanie Seneff is a senior research scientist who is a well-known expert on glyphosate, as she has written journal articles on glyphosate and has been interviewed on many podcasts and other platforms on this topic. She mentions a paper that shows how the application of charcoal, sauerkraut juice, and humic acids can result in a significant reduction of glyphosate.[7] Glycine might also be beneficial.

Although I haven't seen any research showing that sweating can help with the elimination of glyphosate, after I initially did a urinary test for glyphosate, I started using my infrared sauna more consistently, and the levels decreased on my follow-up test. Now, as I mentioned earlier, they weren't too high to begin with, as they were actually within the lab reference range, but I still wanted to see if I could get the levels lower.

Also, there might have been other factors that resulted in the decreased levels of glyphosate. But sweating can of course help with the excretion of many other environmental toxicants, so it's something to consider. Just keep in mind that not everyone with hyperthyroidism should use an infrared sauna, which I discussed in chapter 24.

Concerns with GMO 2.0

I had the honor of interviewing GMO expert Jeffrey Smith on my podcast, which you can check out by visiting **www.savemythyroid.com/119**. Jeffrey briefly discussed concerns with gene editing, and you can learn more about it by watching a six-minute animated film at **www.responsibletechnology.org** called "Seven Reasons Why Gene Editing Is Dangerous and Unpredictable." What's even more scary is that according to Jeffrey Smith, anyone can create a gene-edited food.

A big concern with gene editing is genetically engineered microbes and the impact this can have on our health, including our gut microbiome. There is concern about these genetically engineered microbes making their way to the gastrointestinal tract, resulting in a state of dysbiosis, and playing a role in the development and/or exacerbation of autoimmune conditions such as Graves' disease. Once again, you can hear Jeffrey Smith chat about this during our conversation.

In summary, if you weren't aware of the potential risks associated with genetically modified foods before reading this chapter, I hope you are well aware at this point and will take action to minimize your exposure to them. Eating mostly organic foods is a great place to start. As for glyphosate, even if you eat 100 percent organic, you probably won't be able to avoid this completely, but you can still minimize your exposure to it, and you should always do things to support detoxification.

Chapter 26 Highlights

- Genetically modified foods, also referred to as bioengineered foods, are yet another reason why you should eat mostly organic.
- The following represent the main genetically modified foods since 2023: alfalfa, canola, corn, papaya, pineapple, potato, soybean, squash, and sugar beets.
- The two main ways we're exposed to GMOS is (1) by eating the food directly and (2) by eating livestock that is fed GMOs.
- One concern is that the body may not process these foods the same way as non-GMO foods.
- Glyphosate is the active ingredient in the herbicide Roundup, and it is used primarily on genetically modified crops.
- Roundup contains not only glyphosate but also ethoxylated adjuvants, and this combination makes the formulation even more toxic.
- Glyphosate causes intestinal dysbiosis, which is a factor with auto-immune conditions such as Graves' disease.
- Although nothing you do will completely eliminate your exposure to glyphosate, eating mostly organic foods and drinking purified water will decrease your exposure.
- A big concern with gene editing is genetically engineered microbes and the impact this can have on our health, including our gut microbiome.

To access the book references and resources, visit
SaveMyThyroid.com/HHDNotes.

CHAPTER
27

Tests to Consider

'm not going to go into great detail with all of the different tests you can get, as that's beyond the scope of this book. However, I do want to go over the more important blood tests I recommend, as well as briefly discuss some additional tests I recommend to my hyperthyroid patients.

Blood Tests I Commonly Recommend:

I'm going to focus on ten of the more common blood tests I recommend to patients. But before doing this, I want to mention that there is a difference between lab reference ranges and optimal ranges. If something is on the high or low side, this can be a cause for concern. And unfortunately, most medical doctors will dismiss anything that's within the lab reference range, regardless of whether or not the values are on the high or low side.

Test #1: Thyroid panel with antibodies. A basic thyroid panel includes the TSH, free T3, and free T4. Some practitioners will recommend the total T4 and/or total T3, but I prefer looking at the free thyroid hormones. Of course, you can also test for both the free and total thyroid hormones, but in most cases I find that if the free thyroid hormones are elevated, the total thyroid hormones will also be elevated. And even if one or both of the free thyroid hormones were high while the total thyroid hormones were normal, you would still want to take action to lower the free thyroid hormones.

As far as testing for the thyroid antibodies, the antibody associated with Graves' disease is the thyroid stimulating immunoglobulin (TSI), which is a type of TSH receptor antibody (TRAB). Some practitioners will recommend the TRAB alone. The problem with only testing the TRAB is that the TSI is not the only type of TRAB. That being said, if someone has hyperthyroidism and a positive TRAB, that pretty much is diagnostic of hyperthyroidism. I do need to add that I have seen situations where the TRAB was within the lab range and the TSI was elevated, so if the TRAB is negative in someone with hyperthyroidism I wouldn't rely on it alone.

Then there are thyroid peroxidase (TPO) antibodies. These are common in both Graves' disease and Hashimoto's. They are a little more closely associated with Hashimoto's, but the majority of people with Graves' test positive for these.

There are also anti-thyroglobulin antibodies. These are more specific to Hashimoto's, although there are people who have all three of these antibodies. In other words, some people have elevated TSI, TPO, and anti-thyroglobulin antibodies.

There is also a marker called *reverse T3*. I used to test this on everybody, but I no longer do so with my hyperthyroid patients. And the reason for this is that reverse T3 is elevated in most people with hyperthyroidism. There are exceptions, but this is a very common finding.

An elevated reverse T3 won't change my treatment recommendations when working with hyperthyroid patients. On the other hand, if someone has hypothyroidism, then it's a pretty good idea to test the reverse T3.

th
el
w

T
(l
li

v
I
v
F

(
l
l
i
l
i

Another marker I don't test for on a regular basis but will bring up here is thyroid binding globulin. This is a carrier protein thyroid hormones bind to. There are situations where I test for this, but most of the time, I do not.

How frequently do you want to test these thyroid-related markers? It depends on the person. I usually want to see a thyroid panel, not including the antibodies, at least every two months. If it's every four to six weeks, that's fine. If someone absolutely can't do it every two months and they have to stretch it to three months, then of course we'll make it work.

While it would be great for you to test the thyroid antibodies every time you do a thyroid panel, if you're paying out of pocket and money is tight, it's fine to test them every other time you do a thyroid panel. For example, if you get the thyroid panel every two months, you can do antibodies every four months. Just keep in mind that if you have Graves' disease, it's just as important, if not more important, to see the thyroid antibodies decrease as it is to see the thyroid hormones decrease. The reason for this is that if the thyroid antibodies decrease and eventually normalize, the thyroid hormones should eventually normalize, too, although the reverse isn't true.

Test #2: Complete blood count (CBC) with differential. I recommend a CBC with differential to just about all of my patients. The main purpose of this test is to see if there are any disorders related to the red and white blood cells. This test seems very basic, but it can provide a lot of useful information. If someone has anemia, polycythemia, a possible infection, clotting disorders, or nutrient deficiencies, then this test can be of value.

Some common findings on a CBC with differential include a low white blood cell count, as well as low neutrophils or high lymphocytes. Neutrophils and lymphocytes are types of white blood cells. It's important to mention that if you just get a regular CBC done without the differential, it won't look at the neutrophils, lymphocytes, eosinophils, basophils, and monocytes. That's why

you want to get the differential. Some medical doctors will just recommend a basic CBC. But once again, I do recommend the CBC with differential to all of my patients.

Then there is the mean corpuscular volume (MCV). Seeing this marker elevated, or even on the high side of the reference range, can indicate certain nutrient deficiencies, such as vitamin B_{12}. A high red cell distribution width (RDW) can indicate an iron deficiency. A low red blood cell count (RBC) along with a low hemoglobin and/or hematocrit can indicate anemia.

Test #3: Comprehensive metabolic panel (CMP). This is another test I recommend to just about all of my patients. The main purpose of this test is to see if there are any disorders related to the liver or kidneys, or if there are electrolyte imbalances. It also tests for glucose and some markers related to protein. Some common findings include a high fasting glucose, low serum potassium, and low sodium.

Sometimes people will have low calcium, but more frequently I see higher calcium levels, which could sometimes indicate hyperparathyroidism. That being said, it's important to mention that a high serum calcium is very common with hyperthyroidism too. This doesn't mean you want to dismiss it and not keep an eye on it if it's elevated, as in some cases a person could have both hyperthyroidism and hyperparathyroidism. It's also common to see a high bilirubin on this panel, and this commonly is related to a genetic condition called Gilbert's syndrome, although sometimes this can also be directly related to the hyperthyroidism.

Elevated liver enzymes are also common to see on a CMP in those with hyperthyroidism. These include aspartate transaminase (AST) and alanine transaminase (ALT), with ALT more commonly elevated. Elevated liver enzymes are especially common in those who take antithyroid medication. Elevated alkaline phosphatase is also common in those with hyperthyroidism, and while this can be an indication that there is a liver problem, the reason it usually is elevated in hyperthyroidism is due to the bone turnover. So while you will want to monitor this, in most cases this will decrease and normalize over time.

Test #4: Lipid panel. This looks at total cholesterol, high density lipoprotein (HDL), low-density lipoprotein (LDL), triglycerides, and very-low-density lipoprotein (VLDL).

With hyperthyroidism it's very common to see a low total cholesterol and/or LDL. On the other hand, if someone has lower thyroid hormone levels (i.e., when taking antithyroid medication), then cholesterol may be high. A lot of people taking antithyroid medication will also have low HDL levels.

Getting back to total cholesterol, I usually like to see it above 150 mmol/L. Most medical doctors are concerned if it gets above 200; when this happens I don't get too concerned unless if it is significantly above 200. If cholesterol is elevated, you might want to do an advanced lipid panel to look at LDL particle size, although decreased thyroid hormone levels as a result of taking antithyroid medication can also cause a high total cholesterol and LDL.

When cholesterol is below 150, if it's related to hyperthyroidism, then frequently, when we correct the hyperthyroidism, the cholesterol levels will increase. I won't panic over low cholesterol related to hyperthyroidism, but it's something I don't want to see on a long-term basis because cholesterol is so important. Even though many doctors get concerned when cholesterol is too high, cholesterol is the precursor for estrogen, progesterone, testosterone, cortisol, and other hormones, so it's very important to have healthy levels of cholesterol.

It's very common to see higher levels of triglycerides. Sometimes it's within the lab reference range, so it might be 120–130 mg/dl, but ideally you want it less than 100 mg/dl, and less than 75 mg/dl is even better. With most labs, below

150 is normal according to their range, but just a reminder that "normal" isn't the same as "optimal". Also, you want to do a lipid panel while fasting. If you don't fast, then the triglycerides might be over 150, which wouldn't be a surprise if you weren't fasting.

The triglyceride-to-HDL ratio is one of the better predictors of heart disease.[1] Ideally you want this ratio to be below 2, and there is especially a concern when it is 2 or higher.

Test #5: Iron panel. This includes serum iron, ferritin, iron saturation, and TIBC (total iron-binding capacity). One reason I recommend an iron panel to most patients is because many people have an iron deficiency. And you can't always rely on a single marker to determine this. Ferritin is related to the iron stores, and many labs will consider anything over 10 ng/mL to be normal, or sometimes over 15 ng/mL. However, you want ferritin to be at least 40–45, some sources will say between 70 and 90 is ideal. This is a good example of why you need to pay attention to the optimal reference ranges.

However, it's important to point out that someone can have an iron deficiency even if ferritin is normal or elevated. Ferritin is also known as an *acute phase reactant*, which means that it can increase in response to inflammation. I would also pay close attention to the serum iron levels and iron saturation, as if one or both of these are low or on the low side, then this usually indicates an iron deficiency, even if ferritin is looking good.

Another reason you want to consider doing an iron panel is that some people have an iron overload. It could be genetic, or perhaps you're taking too high of a dose of iron supplementation. Even hyperthyroidism itself can sometimes cause the serum iron and iron saturation to increase.

Once again, if ferritin is elevated but the serum iron and iron saturation look okay, then it's probably related to inflammation. On the other hand, if the serum iron and/or iron saturation are both high, then you might be looking at an iron overload situation. That's why you want to look at a full iron panel.

That being said, some practitioners will test ferritin by itself. Others will just test for serum iron on its own. If this is the case with you, then you might need to ask your doctor if they can test the other markers, or you might have to pay out of pocket to have them tested.

Test #6: 25-OH vitamin D. Vitamin D is commonly deficient in a lot of people in general, not just those with hyperthyroidism. Vitamin D is known for its importance when it comes to bone health but also plays a very important role in immune system health. So while it's important for everyone to have healthy vitamin D levels, it is even more important in those with autoimmune conditions, including Graves' disease.

There are a few different ways to test for vitamin D in the blood. You specifically want to test for 25-hydroxy vitamin D (also known as 25-OH vitamin D). Another option that labs have is 1-25- dihydroxyvitamin D, but when I was getting my master's in nutrition degree, I was taught that this is not a reliable indicator of vitamin D status. The reason for this is that 1,25-dihydroxyvitamin D is regulated by parathyroid hormone, and when someone has a vitamin D deficiency, it results in a compensatory increase in the parathyroid hormone levels. This in turn will increase 1,25-dihydroxyvitamin D, so 1,25-dihydroxyvitamin D is usually normal or elevated, even in the presence of a vitamin D deficiency.

However, there is some controversy over this, as a number of years ago I attended a health conference taught by Dr. Ben Lynch, author of the excellent book *Dirty Genes*, and he was a proponent of testing the 1,25-dihydroxyvitamin D marker instead of 25-OH vitamin D. Then in 2023 I had thyroid physiology expert Dr. Eric Balcavage on my podcast, and he also recommended to test for 1,25-dihydroxyvitamin D. Even though I and most other healthcare practitioners recommend focusing on 25-OH vitamin D, Dr. Balcavage feels that most people are overdosing on vitamin D_3

So for many years I and other practitioners have recommended having a 25-OH vitamin D level between 50-80 ng/mL, and as of writing this book that still is the case. For years I have also personally taken 5,000 IU of vitamin D_3 per day (with vitamin K_2) to maintain "healthy" vitamin D levels. One of the concerns with vitamin D is that if you take too much it can cause hypercalcemia (elevated blood calcium levels), but you can easily monitor this by doing a comprehensive metabolic panel.

It's very interesting, and while as of writing this book I still recommend to test for 25-OH vitamin D, this very well might change in the future. The current research I've come across still doesn't favor testing 1,25-dihydroxyvitamin D over 25-hydroxyvitamin D, and I haven't seen any harmful effects with a vitamin D level between 50-80 ng/mL.

That being said, I mentioned earlier that vitamin D can increase serum calcium, and if it becomes elevated this can be a concern. The challenge is that hyperthyroidism itself can also cause elevated serum calcium levels in some cases, and so if you have hyperthyroidism and have elevated serum calcium levels then you might want to test for parathyroid hormone (PTH), which normally should be low if serum calcium gets too high. If PTH is low then this probably relates to hyperthyroidism or taking too much vitamin D3, but if PTH is normal or high, then it very well might indicate primary hyperparathyroidism. This is caused by an adenoma, which is a benign tumor.

Test #7: Blood sugar markers. While many medical doctors rely on a fasting glucose, which is part of a CMP, I recommend testing hemoglobin A1C and fasting insulin. Hemoglobin A1C gives an average of the blood glucose levels over a period of two to four months. Although testing the fasting glucose and hemoglobin A1C can be valuable to determine if someone has blood sugar imbalances, doing a fasting insulin can provide a lot of value as well. In fact, some functional medicine practitioners don't pay much attention to the hemoglobin A1C or the fasting glucose.

For hemoglobin A1C, most labs consider a value less than 5.7 percent as being normal, but many healthcare practitioners consider 5.0 percent or lower to be optimal. That being said, I can't say that I get too concerned if someone's hemoglobin A1C is a tad higher, such as 5.2 or even 5.3 percent. As for fasting insulin, I like to see it no higher than 7 μIU/mL, but many consider less than 5 to be optimal.

Test #8: High sensitivity C reactive protein (hs-CRP). This is a marker related to inflammation in the body. It relates specifically to what's called *interleukin 6* (IL6). Because it's related to a specific inflammatory cytokine, a normal CRP does not rule out inflammation in the body.

On the other hand, if you have an elevated CRP, you definitely want to pay attention to this. There could be many causes of CRP being elevated. Two common causes of an elevated CRP are inflammatory foods and infections. Not getting enough sleep can also be a factor. Of course there are many people who don't get enough sleep and their CRP looks fine. Just another example demonstrating that everyone is different.

Another marker related to inflammation is the erythrocyte sedimentation rate, also known as ESR. That's something you could also test for. Some practitioners will recommend both the CRP and the ESR.

Test #9: Homocysteine. Homocysteine is a sulfur amino acid, and its metabolism requires folate, vitamin B_6, and vitamin B_{12}. A high homocysteine can indicate problems with something called *methylation*, which is part of the phase 2 detoxification process. Methylation involves conjugating phase 1 intermediates with methyl groups. Three of the more important nutrients required to help support methylation include folate, vitamin B_{12}, and vitamin B_6. These are the main cofactors of S-Adenosyl-l-methionine (SAMe), which is the main methyl donor.

A number of years ago I had elevated homocysteine. However, it wasn't detected until a few years after I was in remission from Graves' disease, so I can't say it played a role when I was working on getting into remission. In addition to relating to methylation, elevated homocysteine levels have been associated with conditions such as increased total and cardiovascular mortality, increased incidence of stroke, increased incidence of dementia and Alzheimer's disease, increased incidence of bone fracture, and a higher prevalence of chronic heart failure.[2]

Test #10: Gamma-glutamyl transferase (GGT). GGT plays a role in glutathione homeostasis. High levels are correlated with glutathione depletion in the liver. Just as a reminder, glutathione is a master antioxidant that neutralizes and scavenges free radicals, detoxifies harmful compounds from the body, promotes cellular repair, and is used in DNA synthesis and repair. Glutathione is made and recycled mainly in the liver, but it is found in every cell in the body.

An elevated GGT can sometimes be an indication of liver disease, although most of the time this isn't the case. Elevated values can also indicate obstructive jaundice, cholangitis, and cholecystitis. If the GGT is greater than 100 IU/L, then I definitely would pay closer attention to this. I'd say from an optimal perspective you want this below 30, and below 20 is even better.

Other blood tests. There are also other blood tests I recommend, including RBC magnesium, vitamin B$_{12}$, viruses (i.e., Epstein-Barr), and a fatty acid profile, just to name a few. In some cases testing the sex hormones can be beneficial, including progesterone, estrogen (estradiol, estrone, estriol), and free and total testosterone. So while the ten blood tests I listed in this chapter are ones I recommend to just about all of my patients, at times I will recommend additional markers.

Specialty Tests I Recommend

I'm about to discuss some of the "specialty" tests I recommend to my patients. Keep in mind that I don't recommend all of these to every single person I work with. And once again, I'm not going to get into too much detail with regard to each test.

Adrenal testing. As I discussed in chapter 20, there are a few different ways to test for the health of the adrenals, but I'm going to focus on saliva and dried urine testing. For many years, I have conducted saliva testing on my patients, and I also used saliva testing when I was dealing with Graves' disease. One of the main advantages of saliva testing is that it allows the patient to collect a few different samples throughout the day.

The reason this is important is that cortisol follows a circadian rhythm, as it should be at the highest level upon waking up and at the lowest level when you are ready to go to bed. This is one of the main advantages of saliva testing for cortisol over blood testing. Another advantage is that it is non-invasive, and you can do it from the comfort of your home.

You might wonder if saliva testing is as accurate as blood testing when it comes to evaluating the adrenals. Numerous studies show that using saliva testing to measure the cortisol levels is either just as good or even better than blood testing.[3,4,5] While most medical doctors in general don't utilize saliva testing in their practice, many medical doctors who practice functional medicine understand the benefits of saliva testing. When I order a saliva test for a patient, I not only want to look at cortisol levels throughout the day, but I also like to test for the DHEA, 17-OH progesterone, and secretory IgA in order to get a full picture of their adrenal health.

Companies I have used for saliva testing: Diagnos-Techs Adrenal Stress Index, Genova Diagnostics Adrenocortex Stress Profile, ZRT Laboratory Adrenal Stress Profile

Although I still recommend saliva testing to a lot of my patients, over the last few years I've also had a lot of patients use dried urine testing. I specifically recommend the DUTCH test, which stands for Dried Urine Test for Comprehensive Hormones. This test looks at the circadian rhythm of cortisol by measuring the free cortisol and cortisone levels throughout the day. In addition, it looks at the cortisol metabolites, along with DHEA-S.

The cortisol metabolites evaluated include a-Tetrahydrocortisol, b-Tetrahydrocortisol, and b-Tetrahydrocortisone. It's very common for one or more of these metabolites to be elevated in those with hyperthyroidism. This should make sense, as in hyperthyroidism there is an increase in cortisol clearance due to the increased metabolism.

It's worth mentioning that many conventional labs offer a twenty-four-hour urine free cortisol test, but this is not the same as dried urine testing. Keep in mind that the twenty-four-hour urine free cortisol test doesn't look at the circadian rhythm of cortisol. This confuses some people, as they think it does look at the circadian rhythm since it requires collecting urine samples over a twenty-four-hour period. However, you are collecting all of the urine samples in a single plastic container, and because of this, it's impossible to evaluate the circadian rhythm.

Companies I have used for urinary adrenal testing: Precision Analytical DUTCH Test

Sex hormones. Most healthcare professionals test the sex hormones (i.e., estrogen, progesterone, testosterone) through the blood, and I recommend blood testing at times for the sex hormones as well. This is especially true for men and postmenopausal women, as in these people a one-sample test is sufficient. Although a cycling hormone test is a great option for cycling women, another option is to do a one-sample blood test in the early second half of the cycle, usually between days nineteen through twenty-one, although this may vary depending on the average length of the woman's menstrual cycle.

It's also important to understand that blood testing for the sex hormones usually involves measuring the "total" hormone, unless you specify the free form. For example, regarding blood testing for testosterone, many healthcare professionals recommend testing for both the total and free testosterone. Total testosterone involves testing for mostly the bound form of the hormone, while free testosterone involves only looking at the free hormone.

Although some labs do offer tests for free estradiol and free progesterone, the "total" estradiol and progesterone are usually ordered. When testing for sex hormones in the blood, it can be beneficial to test for the pituitary hormones, which include follicle stimulating hormone (FSH) and luteinizing hormone (LH).

I mentioned dried urine testing for adrenals earlier, and this also is an option for testing the sex hormones. The main benefit of dried urine testing for the sex hormones is the ability to measure the hormone metabolites. Estradiol and estrone both lead to the formation of estrogen metabolites, which include 2-hydroxyestrone (2-OH-E1), 4-hydroxyestrone (4-OH-E1), and 16α-hydroxyestrone (16α-OH-E1). These metabolites have different biological activity, as the 2-OH metabolite has weak estrogenic activity, and thus is labeled as being the "good" estrogen.

In contrast, the 4-OH and 16α-OH metabolites have a greater amount of estrogenic activity. Evidence shows that those with higher amounts of 4-OH and 16α-OH metabolites have an increased risk of developing certain types of cancers.[6] What are the benefits of testing the metabolites? Well, if someone has a greater ratio of the "bad" metabolites to the "good" metabolites, then they can take measures to increase the 2-OH metabolites by eating cruciferous vegetables regularly or in some cases taking a sulforaphane or diindolyl-methane (DIM) supplement.

In addition to these metabolites, some companies test for other hormone metabolites. This includes a-pregnanediol, b-pregnanediol, 5a-androstanediol,

5b-androstanediol, and 2-methoxy-estrone. Looking at these can also have some benefits. For example, you can compare the ratio between 2-methoxy-E1 and 2-OH-E1 to get an idea of methylation activity.

Companies I have used for urinary testing of the sex hormones: Precision Analytical DUTCH Test, ZRT Urine Metabolites Profile, Meridian Valley

Gastrointestinal health testing. A comprehensive stool panel is one of the best, and perhaps *the* best test, for determining the health of the digestive system. This is why many natural healthcare professionals recommend this test to their autoimmune patients, as you can't have a healthy immune system without having a healthy gut. I don't recommend a comprehensive stool panel to all of my patients with hyperthyroidism, although over the years I have recommended a good number of comprehensive stool tests.

A comprehensive stool panel tests for commensal, opportunistic, and potentially pathogenic bacteria, along with yeast and parasites, and many companies also test for markers of digestion and absorption (i.e., pancreatic elastase and fecal fat), gut inflammation (i.e., calprotectin), short-chain fatty acids (i.e., n-butyrate), and beta-glucuronidase.

You might wonder what the difference is between a comprehensive stool panel you would obtain at a specialty lab and a stool panel from a conventional lab such as LabCorp or Quest Diagnostics. The stool panels ordered through local labs usually don't evaluate for the presence of as many microbes as comprehensive stool panels. Thus, a negative finding doesn't always rule out a gut infection.

In addition, many doctors will recommend a stool culture, which relies a lot more on the skill of the lab technician when compared to DNA/PCR technology. This also results in more false negatives when compared to DNA-based testing. However, some of the specialty labs also do culture testing.

While DNA/PCR technology is great, there are limitations. First of all, when it comes to testing for parasites, it can't test for as many parasites as microscopic O&P. In addition, there have been healthcare professionals who have submitted different stool samples from the same patient to two different labs at the same time, only to have one panel come back positive and the other negative. At times, the DNA/PCR testing has come back negative, whereas other diagnostic methods such as a stool culture or a trichome stain has resulted in positive findings. That being said, if given the choice, I'd go with DNA/PCR technology, but you need to keep in mind that false negatives are possible regardless of the method used.

Companies I have used for stool testing: Genova Diagnostics GI Effects, Doctor's Data Comprehensive stool panel, Diagnostic Solutions GI-MAP, US BioTek Microbiome Profile

I also want to briefly mention organic acids testing. This isn't primarily a gastrointestinal test, although it does look at markers of yeast and bacterial overgrowth, which relate to the health of the gut. The organic acids test from Mosaic Diagnostics (formally Great Plains Laboratory) also tests for several Clostridia bacteria markers that are associated with gastrointestinal diseases and neuropsychiatric disorders.

How about leaky gut testing? The classic method of determining whether someone has an increase in intestinal permeability (leaky gut) is through the lactulose-mannitol test, which is a urine test that involves swallowing a solution of lactulose and mannitol. Lactulose is a larger sugar molecule, and if someone has a healthy gut, this molecule shouldn't be absorbed. Therefore, if someone does this test and has large amounts of lactulose in the urine, then this usually confirms that the person has a leaky gut.

How accurate is the lactulose-mannitol test? A study in 2008 concluded that the lactulose-mannitol ratio had the highest diagnostic value to assess intestinal permeability.[7] Another study looked to determine the value of the lactulose-mannitol test in detecting intestinal permeability in those people with celiac disease.[8] The study showed that the sensitivity of the test was 87 percent in the screening situation and 81 percent in the clinical situation. So it definitely isn't a perfect test, and while the evidence is strong that everyone with Graves' disease (and other autoimmune conditions) has a leaky gut, I've seen this test negative in some patients who had elevated thyroid autoantibodies.

Some newer testing methods have been developed in recent years. The company Cyrex Labs has a test called the Intestinal Antigenic Permeability Screen (the Array #2), which is a blood test that measures the immune system response to an increase in intestinal permeability. It specifically tests for the presence of antibodies against actomyosin, occludin/zonulin, and lipopolysaccharides.

Before briefly discussing these markers, I want to mention that intestinal permeability can occur through two pathways. With the paracellular pathway, the antigen (e.g., food particle, infection) is transported between the cells of the small intestine, while with the transcellular pathway, the antigen goes through the body of the cell.

Actomyosin helps to regulate intestinal barrier function, and when there is damage to the cells of the small intestine via the transcellular pathway, this results in antibodies to actomyosin. This is very common in those who have celiac disease. Occludin and zonulin are considered to be tight junction proteins, as occludin helps to hold together the tight junctions, and zonulin helps to regulate the permeability of the small intestine. If someone has antibodies to occludin or zonulin, then this indicates that the tight junctions between the cells of the small intestine have been compromised.

Lipopolysaccharides (LPS) are large molecules found in gram-negative bacteria, and if they are absorbed, they elicit a strong immune response. These lipopolysaccharides, in turn, can cause an increase in intestinal permeability.[9,10] However, they apparently don't always cause a leaky gut, as I've seen patients who have had antibodies to LPS but not to actomyosin or occludin/zonulin.

Zonulin plays a role in regulating intestinal barrier function, and it is a marker that can be added to some comprehensive stool panels. If elevated it is indicative of an increase in intestinal permeability. The problem is that false negatives are possible, so if you test for this marker and it's negative, it doesn't rule out a leaky gut.

Companies I have used for measuring intestinal permeability: Cyrex Labs Intestinal Antigenic Permeability Screen (Array #2), Genova Diagnostics Lactulose-Mannitol Test, Zonulin from Diagnostic Solutions and US BioTek

Environmental toxins. While I think hair and urine testing for heavy metals can provide some value, there obviously isn't a single test that looks at all the environmental toxins. I feel this is an important message to convey, as someone might get a test for heavy metals that looks good, but there are a few things they need to keep in mind. First of all, false negatives are possible on these tests, and perhaps even false positives.

For example, if someone just does a single hair or urine test for heavy metals and everything looks good, this doesn't mean that there aren't any heavy metals embedded in the tissues. This is why some practitioners use provoked testing with these tests, especially urinary testing for heavy metals. With pre- and post-provocation testing, the patient collects a baseline urine sample, then takes some type of oral chelating agent, such as dimercaptosuccinic acid (DMSA), dimercaptopropanesulfonate (DMPS), or ethylenediaminetetraacetic acid (EDTA), followed by a second urine collection. The purpose of the chelating agent is to mobilize heavy metals from the tissues, which will greatly increase the chances of one or more heavy metals being elevated on the second urine test.

Provoked urine testing is somewhat controversial. First, while most people seem to do fine when taking an oral chelating agent, adverse effects are possible. While in some cases this might be due to a detoxification reaction, in other cases it's due to an immune system reaction to the chelating agent.

In addition, there is some concern that mobilized heavy metals from the tissues might be redeposited in other areas of the body.[11] I briefly mentioned this in chapter 24. For example, if someone has a compromised blood-brain barrier, then it's possible that these metals will be redeposited in the tissues of the brain, which can lead to neuroinflammation.

However, this can be minimized by making sure that you have healthy glutathione levels. Thus, for anyone who takes an oral chelating agent or receives chelation therapy, it probably is wise to take measures to increase glutathione levels, which I discuss in chapter 24.

Another limitation of heavy metal testing is that there are many other environmental toxicants that can cause problems. So regardless of whether or not someone has one or more heavy metals show up on such a test, there will be other environmental toxicants in the tissues that of course won't show up on this test. And while there are tests available that look at different chemicals, such as the GPL-TOX from Mosaic Diagnostics, there is no single test that looks at all of the environmental toxicants.

One more limitation of many tests for environmental toxicants is that they look at the levels of specific chemicals. While this can be useful, it's very possible for someone to have an immune system response to an environmental toxicant, even if the actual levels are low. This is one advantage of the Cyrex Labs Chemical Immune Reactivity Screen (the Array #11).

Unlike most tests that measure the levels of certain chemicals, the Array #11 is a blood test that measures the immune system response to some of the more common environmental toxicants. This can be a very valuable test, as you can have low levels of heavy metals on one of the other tests I discussed yet have an immune system response to one or more of these. What happens is that certain chemicals can bind to our tissues, and the immune system will not just attack the chemical, but our own tissues as well. This is one mechanism of how an environmental toxicant can be a trigger for an autoimmune condition such as Graves' disease.

For example, someone can have most of their mouth filled with mercury amalgams yet not have an immune system response to the mercury. This doesn't mean that there aren't negative health consequences associated with the mercury exposure, but in this situation it means that the mercury probably isn't an autoimmune trigger. However, someone with only one or two mercury amalgams can have an immune system response to the mercury.

This is dependent on whether or not the person has what's referred to as *chemical tolerance*. If the person has a loss of chemical tolerance, also referred to as *toxicant-induced loss of tolerance* (TILT), then their immune system is likely to react to the mercury and other chemicals. Thus, while one can make a valid argument that having ten mercury amalgams is worse than having two mercury amalgams, if the person with ten mercury amalgams has chemical tolerance, while the person with two mercury amalgams has a loss of chemical tolerance, then the person with only two silver fillings is much more likely to develop an immune system reaction.

It's also important to mention that the Array #11 doesn't just test for mercury. It tests for antibodies to other heavy metals, as well as antibodies to other common environmental toxicants, including bisphenol A (BPA), aflatoxins, formaldehyde, isocyanate, benzene, parabens, and tetrachloroethylene. Because this test measures antibodies, there is always a possibility of a false negative result; thus, before doing this test, it probably is a good idea to get your serum immunoglobulin G, M, and A levels tested.

Based on what I've said here, should you consider doing the Array #11 instead of testing that measures the levels of heavy metals and/or other environmental toxicants? Perhaps, but you also need to keep in mind that the Array #11 has limitations as well. Just as is the case with all other tests for environmental toxicants, the Array #11 only looks at some of the more common chemicals that are likely to provoke an immune response. But there can be countless others that can cause problems that aren't measured, which is why I don't do this test on all of my patients.

Nutrient deficiencies. I use blood testing to measure some of the nutrients. First, I usually recommend a complete iron panel and vitamin B_{12}. RBC magnesium can also provide some value. However, there are limitations when it comes to testing nutrients through the blood, although this is the case with other methods as well. Although vitamin D is more of a prohormone than a vitamin, I still need to remind you that I recommend for all of my patients to test for 25-OH vitamin D.

There are also companies that focus on micronutrient testing, which involves evaluating all of the vitamins, minerals, and antioxidants. One of the more well-known labs tests the micronutrients through the white blood cells, specifically the lymphocytes. These lymphocytes are supposed to represent a history of an individual's nutrient status and the intracellular deficiencies.

I like the hair tissue mineral analysis (HTMA) test, although I'd never rely on this test for evaluating all of the minerals. However, this test isn't just evaluating mineral deficiencies, but it also looks for excess mineral levels (i.e., copper) and certain patterns. Thus, interpreting this test on the surface might seem easy, but it can be very challenging.

While the HTMA evaluates the heavy metals, it also isn't perfect in this regard. Just as is the case with urine testing, hair testing won't reveal all of the heavy metals because most people have toxic metals stored in their tissues. This is the reasoning behind provoked urine testing, although this also isn't perfect, and as I mentioned earlier, it comes with certain risks. The truth is that there is no perfect test that will give us all of the answers regarding detecting mineral imbalances and heavy metal toxicities. Nevertheless, HTMA can provide some valuable information at a very reasonable cost.

I should also mention organic acids testing will look at metabolites related to some of the nutrients, including a few of the B vitamins (vitamins B_{12}, B_6, B_5, B_2, and biotin), as well as CoQ10. But this test does so much more than look at some of the nutrient deficiencies, as it looks at yeast and bacteria, oxalates, some of the neurotransmitters, mitochondrial markers, and indicators of detoxification.

Should You Do Iodine Testing?

A few different methods of iodine testing exist. Unfortunately, no consensus about which is the most accurate method has been established. Blood testing doesn't seem to be too accurate, as it doesn't test for the levels of iodine in the tissues. Urine testing seems to be the most accurate, although there are limitations with this type of testing as well. In addition, different types of urine tests can make testing for iodine confusing.

You can do a one-sample iodine spot test, a twenty-four-hour urinary iodine test, and a twenty-four-hour urinary iodine loading test. Although I like the iodine loading test, as this is the test I used when I was diagnosed with Graves' disease, the dilemma is that this test involves taking a 50 mg tablet of potassium iodide before collecting the urine samples. While many people do fine when taking this high dose of potassium iodide, there is always a risk of someone having a negative reaction.

A safer option would be to do an iodine spot test, or a twenty-four-hour urinary iodine test. If you choose to do an iodine spot test, I would also recommend testing the bromide levels, as when these levels are elevated, this almost always indicates an iodine deficiency, even in the presence of normal iodine levels. As for what lab to use for iodine testing, a number of different labs conduct urinary iodine testing, although I usually use Hakala Labs (**www.hakalalabs.com**).

Elevated serum thyroglobulin levels can also be an indication of an iodine deficiency.[12,13] Keep in mind that I'm discussing testing for thyroglobulin and not thyroglobulin antibodies. Some healthcare professionals aren't familiar with the thyroglobulin marker on a blood test, and they commonly order the thyroglobulin antibodies instead; thus, you want to specify when requesting to get this measured.

It's also important to realize that elevated thyroglobulin levels can be an indication for thyroid cancer.[14,15] Keep in mind that I have worked with many patients who had elevated thyroglobulin values, and I don't recall a single person having thyroid cancer; nevertheless, it's something to be aware of. I should also mention that I did an interview with Dr. Angela Mazza, who is an integrative endocrinologist, and she said that having a larger thyroid can result in elevated thyroglobulin levels, and she usually doesn't get concerned if it's elevated unless if someone has a history of thyroid cancer and has received a thyroidectomy.

Food sensitivity testing. I discussed this in chapter 12, as over the years I haven't been a big fan of food sensitivity testing, although I did do some IgG testing on some patients. More recently I have started recommending mediator release testing (MRT) to some patients, in combination with an elimination diet (i.e., Level 3 Hyperthyroid Healing Diet). However, I can't say that all of my patients do the MRT, as while it can be very valuable, it's also quite expensive, and therefore many people rely on the elimination diet.

Conservative vs. Comprehensive Testing

Of course there are other tests besides the ones I listed here, but the point is that while food is very important, many people need to dig deeper to find their triggers. As for how much testing you should do, this does vary from person to person. When it comes to testing, I'm more on the conservative side, but I almost always give additional options to patients. For example, I commonly recommend adrenal testing, an HTMA, and blood testing to my patients, but on the follow-up email I send to all of my new patients I may also list a comprehensive stool panel as an optional test. Then again, if I think a stool panel or any other test is truly necessary then I will recommend it and not list it as optional (although ultimately it is still up to the patient).

The truth is that it's not always easy to know what tests someone needs. Getting back to the comprehensive stool panel, if someone is presenting with certain digestive symptoms, then it probably makes sense to do this test, or perhaps a SIBO breath test (or in some cases both of these). However, you can't always go by symptoms, so it's possible that the person might have a gut infection (i.e., *H. pylori*) even though they aren't experiencing any symptoms.

In summary, while improving one's diet can lead to dramatic changes in your health, because there are usually other underlying imbalances, you might want to consider doing certain tests. In addition to doing a thyroid panel with antibodies, other blood tests can be valuable, including a CBC with differential, comprehensive metabolic panel, lipid panel, iron panel, and vitamin D test. Many times specialty tests can also provide some valuable information, including adrenal, gastrointestinal health, organic acids, and nutrient deficiency tests, along with others. And while I tend to be on the conservative side when it comes to testing, there definitely is a time and place for more comprehensive testing.

Chapter 27 Highlights

- Ten blood tests I commonly recommend are (1) thyroid panel with antibodies, (2) CBC with differential, (3) comprehensive metabolic panel, (4) lipid panel, (5) iron panel, (6) 25-OH vitamin D, (7) blood sugar markers, (8) hs-CRP, (9) homocysteine, and (10) GGT.
- Other blood tests include RBC magnesium, vitamin B_{12}, viruses, a fatty acid profile, and the sex hormones.
- With regard to adrenal testing, the two main tests I recommend are saliva testing and dried urine testing.
- The main benefit of dried urine testing for the sex hormones is the ability to measure the hormone metabolites.
- A comprehensive stool panel tests for commensal, opportunistic, and potentially pathogenic bacteria, along with yeast and parasites, and many companies will also test for markers of digestion and absorption, gut inflammation, short-chain fatty acids, and beta-glucuronidase.
- There isn't a single test that measures all environmental toxins, although I like hair and urine testing, and there are other interesting tests, including the Array #11 from Cyrex Labs.
- I use both blood testing and hair mineral analysis testing to evaluate the minerals.
- As for how much testing you should do, it varies from person to person.

To access the book references and resources, visit
SaveMyThyroid.com/HHDNotes.

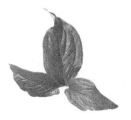

Hyperthyroid Healing Diet Wrap-up

CHAPTER
28

What to Eat, What to Avoid Summary

Just to warn you, this chapter is repetitive, as pretty much everything in this chapter you can find in the three Hyperthyroid Healing Diet chapters in section 2. I just want to make it easy for you, and while the reason why I wrote a chapter on each of the diets is so you will understand the reasoning behind why you should eat and avoid certain foods, I realize that some people don't want to understand this. In the case that you're one of those people who just want to know what to eat and what to avoid, without the additional information, this chapter is for you.

If you want even greater detail, you can access the yes/no lists that relate to each diet by visiting the resources page at **savemythyroid.com/HHDNotes**.

What You *Can* Eat on a Level 3 Hyperthyroid Healing Diet	What You *Can't* Eat on a Level 3 Hyperthyroid Healing Diet
• Meat (beef, lamb, pork, etc.) • Poultry (chicken, turkey, duck, etc.) • Organ meats • Fish and other seafood low in mercury and not too high in iodine (i.e., wild salmon, sardines) • Vegetables (excluding the nightshades) • Fruit (preferably lower in sugar such as wild blueberries, strawberries, and cranberries) • Mushrooms • Cassava, green bananas, green mangos, green plantains, jicama, parsnips, rutabaga, sweet potatoes, taro, tiger nuts, turnips, and yucca • Coconut products (unsweetened coconut yogurt, coconut milk, coconut kefir, etc.) • Ghee • Spices (excluding nightshade-based spices such as cayenne, chili powder, and paprika) • Honey and pure maple syrup (in moderation) • Certain flours in moderation (coconut flour, tapioca flour, cassava flour) • Green tea in moderation (due to the caffeine), herbal teas • Bone broth • Kombucha • Collagen powder • Hydrolyzed beef powder	• Eggs • Nuts and seeds • Nightshades • Legumes and lentils • Gluten • Grains (even gluten-free) • Dairy • Soy • Dark chocolate • Sea vegetables • Seafood very high in iodine (i.e., cod, lobster, and oysters) • Alcohol • Coffee • Bread • Sugary beverages • Artificial ingredients • Unhealthy oils (corn, cottonseed, peanut, safflower, soy, sunflower) • Partially hydrogenated oil • Monosodium glutamate

What You *Can* Eat on a Level 2 Hyperthyroid Healing Diet	What You *Can't* Eat on a Level 2 Hyperthyroid Healing Diet
• Meat (beef, lamb, pork, etc.) • Poultry (chicken, turkey, duck, etc.) • Organ meats • Fish and other seafood low in mercury and not too high in iodine (i.e., wild salmon, sardines) • Vegetables (excluding the nightshades) • Fruit (preferably lower in sugar such as wild blueberries, strawberries, and cranberries) • Mushrooms • Cassava, green bananas, green mangos, green plantains, jicama, parsnips, rutabaga, sweet potatoes, taro, tiger nuts, turnips, and yucca • Eggs • Nuts and seeds that aren't high in lectins and oxalates (pistachios, macadamia nuts, sprouted pumpkin seeds, sprouted sunflower seeds) • Coconut products (unsweetened coconut yogurt, coconut milk, coconut kefir, etc.) • Ghee • Spices (excluding nightshade-based spices such as cayenne, chili powder, and paprika) • Honey and pure maple syrup (in moderation) • Certain flours (coconut flour, tapioca flour, cassava flour) • Green tea in moderation (due to the caffeine), herbal teas • Bone broth • Kombucha • Collagen powder • Hydrolyzed beef powder • Dark chocolate in moderation	• Nightshades • Legumes and lentils • Gluten • Grains (even gluten-free) • Dairy • Soy • Sea vegetables • Seafood very high in iodine (i.e., cod, lobster, and oysters) • Alcohol • Coffee • Bread • Sugary beverages • Artificial ingredients • Unhealthy oils (corn, cottonseed, peanut, safflower, soy, sunflower) • Partially hydrogenated oil • Monosodium glutamate

What You *Can* Eat on a Level 1 Hyperthyroid Healing Diet	What You *Can't* Eat on a Level 1 Hyperthyroid Healing Diet
• Meat (beef, lamb, pork, etc.) • Poultry (chicken, turkey, duck, etc.) • Organ meats • Fish and other seafood low in mercury and not too high in iodine (i.e., wild salmon, sardines) • Vegetables (excluding the nightshades) • Fruit (preferably lower in sugar such as wild blueberries, strawberries, and cranberries) • Mushrooms • Cassava, green bananas, green mangos, green plantains, jicama, parsnips, rutabaga, sweet potatoes, taro, tiger nuts, turnips, and yucca • Eggs • Nuts and seeds that aren't high in lectins and oxalates (pistachios, macadamia nuts, sprouted pumpkin seeds, sprouted sunflower seeds) • Coconut products (unsweetened coconut yogurt, coconut milk, coconut kefir, etc.) • Ghee • Spices (excluding nightshade-based spices such as cayenne, chili powder, and paprika) • Honey and pure maple syrup (in moderation) • Certain flours (coconut flour, tapioca flour, cassava flour) • Green tea in moderation (due to the caffeine), herbal teas • Bone broth • Kombucha • Collagen powder • Hydrolyzed beef powder • Dark chocolate in moderation • Up to three servings per week of pressure-cooked lentils, legumes, white basmati rice, millet, sorghum	• Nightshades • Gluten • Dairy • Soy • Sea vegetables • Seafood very high in iodine (i.e., cod, lobster, and oysters) • Alcohol • Coffee • Bread • Sugary beverages • Artificial ingredients • Unhealthy oils (corn, cottonseed, peanut, safflower, soy, sunflower) • Partially hydrogenated oil • Monosodium glutamate

To access the book references and resources, visit
SaveMyThyroid.com/HHDNotes.

CHAPTER
29

Will Eating (Insert Food) Prevent You from Healing?

This was one of the last chapters I decided to add, as while I of course want people to restore their health, I also don't want them to be afraid of food. So for example, those who are familiar with the AIP Diet probably weren't surprised to see that eggs are excluded as part of a Level 3 Hyperthyroid Healing Diet. On the other hand, someone who isn't familiar with the AIP Diet might have been shocked to see that I recommend avoiding eggs.

The truth is that everyone is different, so when asking the question, "Will eating (insert food) prevent me from healing?" for many of these foods the real answer is I don't know. For this reason I probably shouldn't have included this chapter, but I decided to do so anyway.

Will Eating Eggs Prevent You from Healing?

Eggs are a nutrient-dense food, and while they of course can be eaten with any meal, many people eat eggs for breakfast. If someone doesn't have an egg allergy, then eating eggs probably won't prevent them from restoring their health. As I mentioned in chapter 5, another reason why eggs are excluded from an AIP/Level 3 Hyperthyroid Healing Diet is because the compounds in egg whites can have a negative effect on gut healing. Theoretically this can prevent someone from healing even in the absence of an egg allergy, but I think in most people this isn't the case, which is why if you like eating eggs, they should be one of the first foods reintroduced.

Will Eating Nightshades Prevent You from Healing?

Just as is the case with eggs, nightshade foods such as tomatoes, eggplant, and peppers have some nice health benefits. While many people tolerate nightshades and would restore their health even if they continued eating them, I have seen a lot more people not do well with nightshades when compared with some other foods, including eggs. So I do think that initially it's a good idea to take a break from them, and then you can reintroduce them in the future and see how you do.

Will Eating Gluten Prevent You from Healing?

Most natural healthcare practitioners recommend that their autoimmune patients avoid gluten, and in chapter 3 I discussed five reasons why I strongly suggest avoiding gluten. Does this mean it's impossible to restore your health if you eat some gluten, even in small amounts? It really depends on the person, as some people might be able to get away with small and occasional exposures to gluten, but why take the chance when there really is no health benefit of eating gluten? In addition, I already discussed that it can increase permeability of the gut, which is a factor in autoimmune conditions such as Graves' disease, so I would completely avoid it while healing.

But what if you have a non-autoimmune hyperthyroid condition? Since gluten can be inflammatory, I would still recommend for those with non-autoimmune hyperthyroid conditions to at least take a break from gluten while healing. Once again, there is no health benefit from eating gluten, and you can always choose to reintroduce it and see how you respond after you restore your health.

Will Eating Gluten-Free Grains Prevent You from Healing?

You might already be convinced that you should strictly avoid gluten in your diet, but is it okay if you eat some gluten-free grains? A few servings of certain grains are allowed on a Level 1 Hyperthyroid Healing Diet (discussed in chapter 7), and this wouldn't be the case if grains were a problem with everyone. But they tend to be harsher on the gut, and from a nutrient perspective they're not required, so while eating some gluten-free grains might not prevent you from healing, there is also the chance that they might affect your progress.

Will Eating Legumes Prevent You from Healing?

Similar to grains, a few servings of legumes each week are allowed on a Level 1 Hyperthyroid Healing Diet. If you are a strict vegan, you almost definitely need to eat some legumes as a source of protein. And if you properly prepare them (i.e., soaking, pressure-cooking) this will greatly decrease the amount of lectins, which is the main reason why legumes are excluded from both a Level 2 and Level 3 Hyperthyroid Healing Diet.

There is an argument for properly prepared legumes to be included in all three diets, and perhaps they will be in future editions of this book, but until I see more people restore their health while eating legumes, I'm going to err on the side of caution. It's a bit of a catch-22 situation, as the only way to know if eating properly prepared legumes will greatly affect the progress of my patient population is by allowing them to eat them, and the same argument can be made for gluten-free grains. On the other hand, you would think that Dr. Gundry wouldn't allow properly prepared legumes if he didn't have success with his patients, although I'm not sure what percentage of his patient base has an autoimmune condition.

Will Eating Soy Prevent You from Healing?

Soybeans are a type of legume, and I just discussed how many people with thyroid and autoimmune thyroid conditions will probably do fine eating properly prepared legumes. So how about organic fermented soy? Well, let's start out with non-fermented sources first, such as organic soy milk. Because it's organic, you don't have to worry about the GMOs, so what's the problem with this and other non-GMO sources of soy?

The main problem is that soy is a common allergen, so while there absolutely are some people who can tolerate soy, we can say the same with other allergenic foods. And because of this you have the choice to eat soy or any other allergen (i.e., dairy, corn) and see how you progress, and then eliminate them later if your health doesn't improve. But many natural healthcare practitioners, including me, recommend that their patients avoid the common allergens while restoring their health.

Getting back to organic fermented soy, the main reason this isn't allowed with any of the three diets is that soy is a common allergen. But if someone is pretty certain they don't have a soy allergy, then just as is the case with other legumes, they probably would do okay eating some organic fermented soy. I think that even with properly prepared legumes, including soy, there is always a concern that it still might interfere with healing of the gut, which is the main reason I'm hesitant to include properly prepared legumes (including organic fermented soy) as part of a Level 3 or Level 2 Diet.

Will Eating Dairy Prevent You from Healing?

Like gluten, dairy is another common allergen many natural healthcare practitioners recommend that their patients avoid. When it comes to giving up dairy, I think I get more resistance from people when compared to giving up gluten. And I understand, as unlike gluten, there are some good health benefits to dairy, and it's very tasty. I can't say with certainty that eating dairy will prevent you from healing, especially healthier forms such as raw dairy, but many people have a dairy sensitivity and don't know it.

Keep in mind that this is different than a lactose intolerance, which is an enzymatic deficiency in the enzyme lactase. If you have a lactose intolerance and eat some dairy, you might experience some symptoms, but it shouldn't prevent you from healing. On the other hand, if you have a dairy sensitivity then this can result in inflammation and very well might prevent you from receiving optimal results.

Will Eating High-Oxalate Foods Prevent You from Healing?

Only recently have I become more aware of the negative impact of high-oxalate foods, as in 2016 I did my first organic acids test and realized that I had high urinary oxalates, and as a result I eliminated spinach from my smoothies. But up until that point I can't say that I had people avoid high-oxalate foods, and even currently I can't say I focus on this a lot.

For example, although I commonly recommend that people avoid spinach since there are other lower oxalate alternatives (i.e., arugula, collard greens, red and green leaf lettuce), I still give the green light to sweet potatoes. Ultimately, it's up to you. I included the chapter on oxalates for greater awareness, and I do think it's a good idea to avoid the higher-oxalate foods where there are good substitutes (nuts are another example). I can't say that eating high-oxalate foods will prevent most people with hyperthyroidism from healing, since I didn't pay too much attention to oxalates for years yet still had most patients receive excellent results.

Will Eating Moldy Foods Prevent You from Healing?

Similar to high-oxalate foods, I can't say that I have told my patients to avoid moldy foods over the years. However, many of the patients I've worked with are avoiding the most common moldy foods. For example, if someone follows a Level 3 Hyperthyroid Healing Diet, then they will be avoiding grains (especially corn), nuts, seeds, and coffee, all of which can be contaminated with mold. There is a chance they might eat some moldy fruit however, and if someone is mold sensitive, this might be enough to prevent them from healing.

The more foods you eat that have the potential to be contaminated with mold, the greater the chance you have of hitting a roadblock in your recovery, but I wouldn't stress out too much about this. I included the chapter on mold in food (chapter 17) to bring greater awareness.

Will Eating Unhealthy Oils Prevent You from Healing?

Just as a reminder, the oils that are allowed on all three diets include coconut oil, olive oil, avocado oil, and palm oil (depending on the source). One of the main problems with some of the unhealthy oils is that they are very high in omega-6 fatty acids, so if, for example, you consume organic canola oil on a regular basis, the oil itself won't necessarily cause inflammation, but it can throw off the omega-3/omega-6 fatty acid ratio, which can potentially be inflammatory. If you eat non-organic canola oil, there is the concern with GMOs, which I discussed in detail in chapter 26.

Will Eating Sugar Prevent You from Healing?

I've always had a sweet tooth, so I can understand how difficult it can be to avoid sweets. Without question, eating refined sugars, especially on a regular basis, can prevent you from healing. This isn't only due to the inflammatory effects of sugar, but also because sugar feeds yeast such as *Candida albicans*. This in turn can cause a candida overgrowth, which can have a negative effect on gut healing. Eating a lot of refined sugars can also cause blood sugar imbalances, including insulin resistance, which can have a negative effect on your recovery. So I would try your best to avoid the refined sugars.

But how about natural sources of sugar, such as honey and maple syrup? Or eating fruit? As for the honey and maple syrup, having small amounts of these won't prevent someone with hyperthyroidism from healing. And the same is true with eating a few servings of fruit per day.

Will Eating Dark Chocolate Prevent You from Healing?

You might have noticed that dark chocolate is excluded from a Level 3 Hyperthyroid Healing Diet but is allowed on a Level 2 or Level 1 Diet. But will eating a small square or two of dark chocolate really prevent someone from healing if they are avoiding everything else? Chances are it won't, and there is a good argument for including a small amount of dark chocolate on a Level 3 Hyperthyroid Healing Diet. I just exclude it for the same reasons it's excluded from an AIP Diet, and I discussed this in chapter 6.

Will Eating Nuts and Seeds Prevent You from Healing?

When I was dealing with Graves' disease, I was eating nuts and hit a roadblock in my recovery. Perhaps if I properly prepared the nuts and/or only ate the nuts allowed on a Level 2 or Level 1 Hyperthyroid Healing Diet I would have progressed without a problem. Either way, nuts make an excellent snack food, and many people can restore their health while eating nuts. That being said, if you choose to eat them and your health doesn't improve in a timely manner, then you might choose to take a break from them.

Will Drinking Coffee Prevent You from Healing?

Many people find giving up coffee more difficult than giving up gluten and dairy. If you have compromised adrenals, which is quite common, then drinking coffee might prevent you from restoring your adrenal health, which in turn can prevent you from healing. This may also depend on how many cups of coffee you drink on a daily basis, along with whether you're a slow or fast metabolizer of caffeine, which can be determined through genetic testing. If someone with compromised adrenals drinks multiple cups of coffee per day and/or is a slow metabolizer of caffeine, then drinking coffee might negatively affect their progress.

Will Drinking Alcohol Prevent You from Healing?

Since alcohol can increase the permeability of the gut, it shouldn't be surprising that if you drink alcohol regularly, then it can prevent you from restoring your health. But how about having an occasional beer, or a glass of red wine every now and then? As for beer, if it's gluten-free, then perhaps having an occasional beer is okay, although it also depends on what other ingredients are included.

How about a glass of organic red wine every now and then? Just as is the case with every food discussed in this chapter, it really does depend on the person, and without question some people will be able to get away with drinking an alcoholic beverage on an occasional basis. There certainly are worse things you can drink than a glass of wine.

To access the book references and resources, visit
SaveMyThyroid.com/HHDNotes.

CHAPTER
30

Common Food-Related Questions

W hile I'm hoping most of your questions were answered within the first 29 chapters of this book, I realize that there might be some additional questions. The purpose of this chapter is to answer some potential "leftover" questions you may have. Obviously there will be some questions people have that aren't answered in this book, and while I can't say that I have the answer to every single question related to hyperthyroidism and diet, if you have unanswered questions, I would definitely be on the lookout for some of the live thyroid-related events I host online a few times per year, where I answer a lot of questions.

Just make sure you're on my email list, which you can get on by visiting **savemythyroid.com/HHDNotes**. And for those who are on Facebook, you might want to join my free Hyperthyroid Healing community by visiting **SaveMyThyroid.com/community**, as once or twice a month I do Facebook lives where I answer questions.

What Are My Thoughts on the Dirty Dozen and Clean Fifteen Lists?

The Dirty Dozen and Clean Fifteen lists are from the Environmental Working Group (**ewg.org**). The Dirty Dozen list includes the fruits and vegetables with the greatest amount of pesticides, while the Clean Fifteen list includes the fruits and vegetables with the least amount of pesticides. These lists are updated each year, and I do think they are valuable if you are unable to purchase organic produce. For example, strawberries have always been high on the Dirty Dozen list, so if you're unable to purchase organic strawberries, then it's probably best to avoid them.

On the other hand, avocados are usually high on the Clean Fifteen list. And so while it would be great to purchase organic avocados if possible, these are one of the safer foods to eat non-organic. My approach is to try to purchase all fruit and vegetables organic, but if I'm out and about and organic isn't an option, then I'll try to stick with the Clean Fifteen list. For example, if I'm at a restaurant, I have no problem eating steamed broccoli if it's not organic, but I'll try my best to avoid non-organic strawberries and kale.

Which Diet Should Be Followed For Thyroid Eye Disease?

Most people with thyroid eye disease (TED) have Graves' disease. Thyroid eye disease also involves the immune system, as the immune system attacks the tissues of the eyes, and can lead to signs and symptoms such as eye pain, swelling, bulging, and double vision. Since TED is also related to auto-immunity I would recommend a Level 3 Hyperthyroid Healing Diet, although if someone finds this to be too restrictive they can always start with a Level 1 or Level 2 Hyperthyroid Healing Diet.

What Should I Eat For Breakfast If Following a Level 3 Diet?

A lot people enjoy eating eggs for breakfast, but of course eggs are excluded from a Level 3 Hyperthyroid Healing Diet. Many following a Level 3 diet choose to eat leftovers they had for dinner as their breakfast. Some might choose to have a healthier chicken or turkey sausage with some vegetables, while others will prefer a smoothie with added protein powder.

How Can I Get Sufficient Protein For Breakfast?

This is almost a continuation of the previous question, as whatever you have for breakfast, you want to make sure to eat a sufficient amount of protein. I find that many people get enough protein for lunch and dinner, but don't get enough protein with breakfast. If you follow a Level 1 or Level 2 Diet then you can eat eggs, but even if this is the case it still might not be enough protein. For example, I frequently will eat two or three eggs for breakfast, but when doing this I will also have another source of protein, such as a smoothie with protein powder.

Without question it is easier to get sufficient protein with your meals if you eat meat. But as I just mentioned, I frequently eat eggs and a smoothie for breakfast, and so I can't say that I usually eat dinner for breakfast, or have chicken or turkey sausage. Everyone is different, and so you might prefer eating meat with all three meals in order to get sufficient protein, especially if you're following a Level 3 Diet. But even in this situation you might choose to rely on a smoothie with protein powder for breakfast. If this is the case just make sure you add a sufficient amount of protein to your smoothie, and it of course should be a healthier protein powder.

If you're a vegan then getting enough protein with any meal can be more challenging. That's why a Level 1 Diet allows legumes, and you might also need to rely on supplemental forms of protein powder, such as one that includes organic pea protein. If you're a vegetarian and eat eggs then this makes it easier to get protein, although in some cases it can still be challenging.

Is Eating a Small Amount of Gluten and Dairy Okay?

I discussed this in the previous chapter, at least with regard to gluten, but I'll expand on this here. The truth is that everyone is different, and there are people who might be able to get away with eating small amounts of gluten and dairy on an occasional basis. Heck, there might be people who are able to eat gluten and dairy on a daily basis and still restore their health. But without question a lot of people are sensitive to gluten and dairy, and both can be inflammatory and in many cases prevent someone with hyperthyroidism from healing. With regard to dairy, I'm not suggesting that it is inflammatory in everyone, and in fact many people can reintroduce dairy in the future.

Gluten is a different story, as while I can't say that I've been 100 percent gluten-free since being in remission from Graves' disease, there really are no health benefits of eating gluten, and for the most part I do try to avoid it. This is especially true when I'm at home, but even when I go out, I usually try to avoid gluten. The key is preparing in advance, as if you're in a situation where there are no good gluten-free options and you're hungry, then you'll probably end up eating gluten.

However, cross-contamination can be an issue, and I can't say that if I'm eating out that I go out of my way to make sure there isn't the possibility of cross-contamination. But it's still something to consider, as for some people this can make a difference in their recovery. And just a reminder that you can't always go by symptoms, as while some people experience symptoms when consuming even small amounts of gluten, others don't feel bad when eating larger amounts. However, this doesn't always mean that smaller amounts won't be problematic, especially when it comes to the health of your gut.

Can I Eventually Reintroduce Gluten and Dairy?

Ultimately this is up to you, but if you choose to reintroduce gluten and/or dairy, in most cases I would recommend waiting until after you have restored your health. In the book I admitted that I reintroduced gluten and dairy after getting into remission, and thankfully it hasn't caused a relapse thus far. However, everyone is different, and I'll also say that I don't eat gluten and dairy regularly. In fact, I really do try to avoid gluten, although whenever I have a cauliflower crust pizza, I don't use vegan cheese. On the other hand, if I have ice cream, I have no problem eating coconut ice cream, and the same goes with yogurt, as I actually prefer coconut yogurt over dairy-based yogurt.

Where Do You Recommend Buying Fruits and Vegetables?

Ideally, you want to purchase your produce from a local farmer's market, and the reason for this is that local produce is more nutrient dense. The reason for this is that fruits and vegetables begin to lose their nutrients shortly after being picked, so the longer vegetables go uneaten after being picked, the less nutrient dense they will be. That being said, you may be able to find some locally grown produce at a grocery store, and this doesn't mean that you won't get any benefits if you purchase fruits and vegetables that weren't grown locally. Either way you want to try to purchase organic produce.

Can I Take Fish Oils If I Don't Like Eating Fish?

In the book I discuss how you should limit your consumption of seafood due to numerous factors. However, I'm definitely not advising that people completely avoid fish, as everything comes down to risks versus benefits, and I think you should try to get at least some omega-3 fatty acids from the food you eat. That being said, if you don't eat fish, then not only can you take fish oil supplements, but you really do need to take them in order to prevent being deficient in them.

If you'd like, you can also do an omega-3 index and see if it's at least 8 percent. Omegaquant is a company that provides this, and you can learn more by visiting **www.omegaquant.com**. Not only did I take fish oils while I was dealing with Graves' disease, but I currently take them on a daily basis to maintain healthy omega-3 levels.

Is Juicing Allowed on Any of the Hyperthyroid Healing Diets?

Without question juicing has some wonderful health benefits, but the main reason I recommend taking a break from juicing while trying to restore your health is that it removes the fiber, and therefore has a very high insulin index. That being said, if someone is very insulin sensitive (i.e., has a lower hemoglobin A1C and fasting insulin), then they might be able to get away with juicing. On the other hand, smoothies retain the fiber, which is why I prefer smoothies over juicing.

Can I Eat Gluten-Free Oats?

Out of all of the different grains, I probably get asked about oatmeal the most. In other words, many people ask if they can eat oatmeal. One problem with oatmeal is that it's commonly contaminated with gluten, although someone can get around this by eating certified gluten-free oatmeal. However, the main reason to avoid oats is the same reason why I and many other healthcare practitioners recommend avoiding other grains when trying to heal: they tend to be harsher on the gut. So while it certainly is possible to heal if eating certified gluten-free oats, and one can even argue that they should be allowed on a Level 1 Hyperthyroid Healing Diet, just to play it safe I recommend avoiding oats while healing.

Is It Okay to Consume Raw Dairy?

I discussed this in chapter 3, as while many people who react to homogenized/pasteurized dairy do fine with raw dairy, this isn't the case with everyone. Some people will still react to the casein in raw dairy, so while restoring your health I recommend taking a break from it.

If I Avoid Dairy, Where Will I Get My Calcium?

I also discussed this in chapter 3, as while dairy is a good source of calcium, there are other non-dairy foods high in calcium, including kale, Chinese cabbage, collard greens, broccoli, blackstrap molasses, and fish with the bones in them (i.e., sardines).

Can I Gradually Incorporate One of These Diets?

While some people choose to strictly follow one of the Hyperthyroid Healing Diets right away, everyone is different, and it's perfectly fine to make changes to your diet slowly. Some people will start by simply avoiding gluten, while others will initially focus on adding more vegetables. Sure, there are people who will immediately cut out all food allergens and strictly follow one of the diets mentioned in this book, and if this describes you, that's awesome. But if you prefer to make gradual changes, that's perfectly fine.

Can I Use a Vegetable Powder Instead of Eating Vegetables?

I can relate to those who absolutely don't like vegetables, as I used to be one of those people. A big reason for this is that I simply wasn't exposed to them when I was younger. At the time I'm sure I thought it was great that I didn't have to eat vegetables, but it honestly took years to get to the point where I not only was eating them on a regular basis but also was enjoying them. Don't get me wrong, as if everything were equal from a health perspective, I would always choose eating pizza over eating steamed broccoli, but of course this isn't the case.

There is no question that vegetable powders and other "veggie supplements" aren't a substitute for eating vegetables. This isn't just my opinion, as Consumer Labs showed that you don't get nearly the amount of nutrients by consuming fruits and vegetables in the form of supplements.[1] That being said, when I have smoothies, I do add some extra protein in the form of protein powder, and one of the protein powders I like is an organic pea protein with added greens. I don't look at this as a substitute for adding vegetables to my smoothie, as I still usually add five to seven different vegetables to my daily smoothie, along with eating vegetables separately during the day.

Is Eating a Lot of Animal Protein Harmful?

I think that eating a lot of unhealthy animal protein can be problematic, but if you stick with organic and pasture-raised meat and poultry, then not only is this not harmful, but it can have immense health benefits as well. Keep in mind that I'm not suggesting that you follow a carnivore diet, although I realize that some people with certain health conditions have received great benefits from following such a diet. But if you read section 2, then you realize that while I think animal protein is by far the best source of protein, I also recommend eating a lot of plant-based foods.

That being said, there is some controversy if someone has the APOE4 gene, which can increase the risk of developing dementia.[2] Approximately 25 percent of people carry one copy of APOE4, and 2 to 3 percent carry two copies.[2] If someone has two copies of the APOE4 gene, which can be determined through testing, then they might see some of the lipid markers increase (i.e., total cholesterol and LDL), and when this is the case, they might want to limit their consumption of animal protein, as well as other sources of saturated fat, including MCT oil, coconut oil, and coconut milk.

Should I Work with a Dietician or Nutritionist?

It certainly isn't a bad idea to work with someone who can help support you while following one of the Hyperthyroid Healing Diets. Of course this doesn't describe everyone, as some people will do perfectly fine on their own. On the other hand, some people like to be held accountable, and it can also be helpful to be able to ask questions, get recipe suggestions, etc.

As for whether you should see a dietician or nutritionist for support, it really depends. Just keep in mind that many dieticians and nutritionists wouldn't agree with the advice given in this book. Even with the explanations given and the research provided, many would still question the elimination of dairy, nightshades, grains, legumes, and other foods. Once again, I'm not suggesting to eliminate these on a permanent basis, but some would question eliminating these foods at all.

As part of my Hyperthyroid Health Restoration and Optimal Health Program, I do have nutritional health coaches to help guide people with the diet. This doesn't mean that you can't receive support elsewhere, as you can definitely work with someone who is familiar with Paleo principles, or even an AIP-certified health coach. However, you might want to give them this book to read so they are familiar with the variations.

Why Are Mushrooms Allowed? Aren't They Immune Stimulating?

Mushrooms have some wonderful health benefits, and most people with Graves' disease tolerate them well. If you enjoy eating mushrooms, I say go for it! That being said, everyone is different, so just as is the case with any food, if you don't feel well when eating mushrooms, then don't eat them. And I can't say that I have noticed mushrooms exacerbating the autoimmune component for those who have Graves' disease.

What Should I Do If I Stray from the Diet?

While I can't say there won't be any negative consequences if you stray from the diet, if this happens, all you can do is try your very best to get back on track. After all, you're human, so while I'm not giving you permission to cheat every now and then while restoring your health, if this happens, then get back on track.

Do I Need to Take a Probiotic Supplement If I Eat Fermented Foods Daily?

I usually recommend doing both, and there are a few reasons for this. First of all, most people don't eat enough fermented foods on a regular basis. If you eat multiple servings of fermented foods per day, then perhaps you don't need to take a probiotic supplement. That being said, if you take a probiotic supplement with a good number of strains (i.e., at least ten), chances are some of these will be different than what you're getting from fermented foods. And the more diversity you have, the better.

Do You Have Any Advice for Picky Eaters?

I was a picky eater growing up, and while I eat a greater variety of food these days, I still would consider myself to be picky. If I had to follow any of the Hyperthyroid Healing Diets two or three decades ago, I would have found it extremely difficult to do so. And since I didn't eat vegetables as a teenager or young adult, if I had to follow any of these diets way back then, I would most likely have failed, although I'll admit that a lot of this would be related to the lack of support.

If you are a picky eater, I recommend gradually introducing new foods, and it really does help when someone else is there to support you. For example, when I was in chiropractic school, not only did I not eat vegetables the first couple of years, but I never ate fish. And while I spoke about some of the risks associated with fish in this book, it's still an excellent source of omega-3 fatty acids, and I think it's fine to eat fish two to three times per week, as long as it's not too high in iodine, and also isn't a large fish that is more likely to be high in mercury and other environmental toxins.

Anyway, I had no idea how to prepare fish at the time, or which fish wouldn't have a strong "fishy" taste. But thankfully one of my best friends in chiropractic school (and still one of my best friends to this very day) and his wife showed me how to prepare fish and encouraged me to eat some. I can't say that I loved it, but I ate it because I knew I had to start eating better. The same thing applied to vegetables, as I didn't start eating them because I wanted to, but because I knew they had some amazing health benefits.

If you're a picky eater, I'm not saying that you absolutely have to eat foods you don't like and/or never thought you would eat, but I will also say not to rule anything out. In other words, you might think you won't eat a certain food, but eventually end up eating it. And to be honest, there are foods I still haven't tried eating, such as organ meats. I just can't get myself to eat organ meats, which to some people is silly since I have no problems eating animal flesh in other forms. The same goes for some other foods, such as lobster, as I never ate it and never plan to, and I'm cool with that.

Do I Have to Drink Bone Broth to Heal My Gut?

You definitely don't need to drink bone broth to heal your gut. The reason I can say this with confidence is that when I dealt with Graves' disease back in 2008/2009, I didn't drink any bone broth. Back then bone broth wasn't as popular, but over the last five to ten years not only do you see more and more different brands being sold, but there are even bone broth protein powders available! In chapter 8 I discussed why bone broth can help support the gut, so if you're willing to drink some, it can definitely help, but if you prefer not to drink bone broth, that's okay too.

Is It Okay to Eat a Lot of Leafy Green Vegetables If I'm Taking Blood-Thinning Medication?

If you are taking a blood thinner such as Coumadin, this doesn't mean that you need to completely avoid leafy green vegetables. Because Coumadin interferes with the way your body uses vitamin K_1, which is involved in clotting, some feel that they should avoid all food sources of vitamin K_1, including leafy green vegetables. While there may be a concern with eating large amounts of leafy green vegetables while on certain blood thinners, this doesn't mean that it's harmful to eat one or two cups per day. That being said, I would talk with your doctor about increasing your intake and simply request to have your blood tested more frequently and see if the dosage needs to be adjusted. It's also worth mentioning that the blood thinner Eliquis doesn't seem to interact with vitamin K_1.

Which Foods Can Help Increase Bone Density?

Just remember that while eating a healthy diet is important for healthy bones, the elevation in thyroid hormone needs to be addressed as well. In the book, I mentioned that eating sufficient protein is important from a bone density standpoint, so make sure to eat at least 75 percent of your ideal body weight in protein. For example, if your ideal weight is 120 pounds, you would want to eat at least 90 grams of protein per day.

And while you might not need to take a calcium supplement, you do need to eat foods rich in calcium, and I discussed some of these in chapter 3, as I mentioned vegetarian sources of calcium (kale, Chinese cabbage, collard greens, broccoli). I also mentioned fish with the bones, such as sardines, being an excellent source of calcium. Also make sure you have healthy vitamin D and vitamin K_2 levels, as vitamin K_2 is necessary to guide the calcium into the bones.

Is There a Special Diet to Follow for a Candida Overgrowth?

Some might wonder why I included chapters on mold in food and SIBO, but not one that focused on yeast overgrowth. Like mold, candida is a fungus, and it can be difficult to eradicate. If you follow a Level 2 or Level 3 Hyperthyroid Healing Diet, this should help with a candida/yeast overgrowth by limiting the amount of carbohydrates and sugars. Remember that having candida and other yeast in your body is normal, but an overgrowth can occur when your immune system is compromised, and this book should help you optimize your immune system health. That being said, there is a time and place for herbal or prescription antifungals.

Can I Eat Fermented Foods If Dealing with a Candida Overgrowth?

There is controversy when it comes to yeast overgrowth and fermented foods. Because some fermented foods include yeast (i.e., kombucha), some health-care practitioners recommend that those with a yeast overgrowth avoid all fermented foods. There are a few problems with this. First, not all fermented foods include yeast. Second, the healthy yeast in fermented foods won't necessarily worsen an existing yeast overgrowth. At least that's what I have found in my patient population over the years. That being said, everyone is different, and if you have a yeast overgrowth and feel better taking a break from eating fermented foods then that's perfectly fine.

Can't Iodine-Rich Foods Help to Lower Thyroid Hormones?

While I recommend avoiding very-high-iodine foods in this book, some reading this may wonder if eating high-iodine foods can actually benefit those with hyperthyroidism. After all, in some cases high-dose iodine can lower thyroid hormones. The problem is that this isn't the case with everyone, as while some people would tolerate higher-iodine foods such as seaweed, kelp, and shellfish without a problem, for others it can exacerbate their hyperthy-roidism and/or the autoimmune component for those with Graves' disease. Just remember that I personally had a good experience with high-dose iodine supplements many years ago, so I'm not anti-iodine, but I'm just very cautious because too much iodine can prevent some people from healing, and in some cases can even worsen their condition.

What Do You Think About the Eat Right For Your Blood Type Diet?

Eat Right 4 Your Type is a very popular book, and I found it very interesting when I read it many years ago. While there are some people who to this day still swear by this diet, there really isn't any research behind it. That being said, I think it's a fascinating concept that you should follow a specific diet based on your specific blood type, and if you choose to follow the recommended diet based on your blood type and notice an improvement in your symptoms and/or blood tests then perhaps you should continue to follow it!

Can Gut Microbiome Testing Determine Which Foods I Should And Shouldn't Eat?

Certain companies such as Viome will use a stool sample to determine which foods you should eat and which foods you should avoid. In other words, the specific foods you can and can't eat are based on your gut microbiome findings. Viome uses artificial intelligence to determine this, and it really is an interesting concept. However, there is a lot of room for improvement with this technology, and as of writing this book I wouldn't rely on this testing to determine what diet you should follow.

That does it for the questions in this chapter, but once again, if there are questions you still have that weren't answered, definitely be on the lookout for some of the live thyroid-related events I host online a few times per year, where I answer a lot of questions. I also should add that I commonly have a "Your Thyroid Questions Answers" podcast episode, where I answer actual questions submitted by people with hyperthyroidism (and Hashimoto's). In order to ask a question and have me respond on the podcast, make sure you get on my email list, which you can do by visiting the resources page.

**To access the book references and resources, visit
SaveMyThyroid.com/HHDNotes.**

References, Recipes and Bonus Chapters

Please make sure you check out the resources where you can access the book references, Hyperthyroid Healing Diet Recipes, along with a couple of bonus chapters, one related to nutritional supplements, and the other one related to iodine. Throughout this book I also mentioned other topics, along with product recommendations that you can also find in the resources.

To access the book references and resources, visit
SaveMyThyroid.com/HHDNotes.

Thank you for reading my book!

I really appreciate all of your feedback and
I love hearing what you have to say.

I need your input to make the next version of this book
and my future books better.

Please take two minutes now to leave a helpful review on
Amazon letting me know what you thought of the book.

You can do so by visiting **savemythyroid.com/HHDreview**

Also, I'd love to read your review, and so after you leave it
please let me know by sending an email to
info@naturalendocrinesolutions.com

Want to work with my team and I?

If you have hyperthyroidism and want to do everything you can to save your thyroid, then there are a few factors that can prevent someone from restoring their health:

1. Overlooking the fundamentals
2. Lack of full commitment
3. Lack of accountability
4. Not working with a practitioner who has experience with hyperthyroidism

By reading this book you should have a good grasp of the foundations when it comes to using diet and lifestyle to restore your health, although you can also check out my Foundations of Overcoming Hyperthyroidism Online Course at **www.savemythyroid.com/foundations**. Of course only you can make the commitment to do what is necessary to save your thyroid, but if you want more guidance and accountability and would like to learn what it's like to work with my team and I visit **www.workwithdreric.com**.

About The Author

Dr. Eric Osansky is a licensed chiropractor with a masters degree in nutrition, and is also an Institute for Functional Medicine Certified Practitioner (IFMCP). Dr. Eric was diagnosed with Graves' disease in 2008, and restored his health through natural treatment methods. Dr. Osansky graduated summa cum laude from Life Chiropractic College in March of 1999, and like most other chiropractors he initially focused on musculoskeletal conditions, and did so for 7 1/2 years. But after restoring his health he began to exclusively see people with thyroid and autoimmune thyroid conditions, and approximately 85% of his patient base consists of those with hyperthyroidism.

In addition to his extensive background in nutrition and functional medicine he has obtained hundreds of hours of post-graduate training in neuroendocrinology, immunology, biotransformation and detoxification, and phytotherapy. He has also received a certificate of practical herbal therapy from the Australian College of Phytotherapy.

While Dr. Osansky feels that most people with hyperthyroidism should give natural treatment methods a try, he does realize that there is a time and place for conventional medical treatment such as antithyroid medication, and even thyroid surgery in certain situations. And while he of course wants to help everyone with hyperthyroidism, Dr. Osansky won't hesitate to refer someone out if he feels as if they are not a good candidate for a natural treatment approach.

As of writing this book Dr. Osansky does accept a limited number of new patients each month for people with thyroid and autoimmune thyroid conditions looking to restore their health naturally. Those who are interested in working with Dr. Eric should visit **workwithdreric.com**.

Dr. Osansky lives in Matthews, NC, with his wife Cindy, and his two teenage daughters, Marissa and Jaylee.

Index

Made in the USA
Monee, IL
30 May 2024

59103090R00243